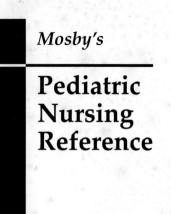

Mosby's

Pediatric
Nursing
Reference

Mosby's

Pediatric Nursing Reference

Third Edition

Cecily Lynn Betz, PhD, RN
Associate Director
UCLA University Affiliated Program
UCLA Neuropsychiatric Institute
Los Angeles, California

Linda A. Sowden, MN, RN
Nursing Department Director
All Children's Hospital
St. Petersburg, Florida

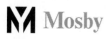 Mosby

St. Louis Baltimore Boston
Carlsbad Chicago Naples New York Philadelphia Portland
London Madrid Mexico City Singapore Sydney Tokyo Toronto Wiesbaden

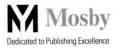

Mosby

Dedicated to Publishing Excellence

A Times Mirror
Company

Publisher: Nancy L. Coon
Senior Editor: Sally Schrefer
Associate Developmental Editor: Michele D. Hayden
Editorial Assistant: Lisa P. Newton
Project Manager: Mark Spann
Production Editor: Julie Eddy
Designer: Judi Lang
Production and Editing: Carlisle Publishers Services
Manufacturing Supervisor: Tony McAllister

A NOTE TO THE READER:
The author and publisher have made every attempt to check dosages and nursing content for accuracy. Because the science of pharmacology is continually advancing, our knowledge base continues to expand. Therefore we recommend that the reader always check product information for changes in dosage or administration before administering any medication. This is particularly important with new or rarely used drugs.

Printed in the United States of America
Composition by Carlisle Communications, Ltd.
Printing/Binding by R. R. Donnelley & Sons Company

Mosby–Year Book, Inc.
11830 Westline Industrial Drive
St. Louis, Missouri 63146

International Standard Book Number 0-8151-0599-1
96 97 98 99 00 / 9 8 7 6 5 4 3 2 1

Contributors

Vicky Armstrong, MSN, RNC
Clinical Nurse Specialist
Perinatal Outreach Program
Children's Hospital
Columbus, Ohio

Susan Givens Bell, BSN, RNC
Nursing Education Specialist
Neonatal Unit
All Children's Hospital
St. Petersburg, Florida

Debora Nash Cahill, MS, RN
Instructor
California State University–Dominguez Hills
Division of Nursing
Carson, California

Joan Calandra, MN, RN, CS
Psychiatric Clinical Nurse Specialist
Kaiser Permanente Medical Center
Department of Psychiatry/Medical Social Services
San Pedro, California

Sandra J. Czerwinski, MS, RN, CCRN
Director, Nursing Education
All Children's Hospital
St. Petersburg, Florida

Kelly Depue, MS, RN
Clinical Nurse Specialist
Children's Hospital
Columbus, Ohio

Sharon DiSano, BA, RN, CCTC
Heart/Renal Transplant Coordinator
All Children's Hospital
St. Petersburg, Florida

Peg Fitzgerald, MS, RN, FNP
Assistant Professor
Simmons College, Graduate School of Health Sciences
Andover, Maryland

Bonnie F. Gahn, MSN, MA, RNC
Director
Pediatric Nursing Services
Ross Products Division
Abbott Laboratories
Columbus, Ohio

Valerie Hammel, MSN, RN
Clinical Nurse Specialist
Department of Pediatrics
Kaiser Permanente Medical Center
Fontana, California

Judith Harr, MS, RN
Instructor
University of San Francisco
San Francisco, California

Michele S. Holecek, MSN, RN, CCRN
Clinical Nurse Specialist
Pediatric Intensive Care Unit
Children's Hospital of Orange Country
Orange, California

Jody A. Holland, MN, RN
Pediatric Clinical Specialist
Doernbecher Children's Hospital
Portland, Oregon

Mary Mikolajcik Kaminski, MS, RN, NNP
Coordinator, Neonatal Nurse Practitioner Program
Children's Hospital
Columbus, Ohio

Erin L. Keels, BSN, RN, NNP, C
Neonatal Nurse Practitioner
Children's Hospital
Columbus, Ohio

Sally Kimpel, MN, RN
Clinical Nurse Specialist
Kaiser Permanente Medical Center
San Diego, California

Norma L. Liburd, MN, RN, C
Clinical Nurse Specialist
All Children's Hospital
St. Petersburg, Florida

Karen Mathias, MSN, RN
Clinical Nurse Specialist
Emergency Services
Children's Health Care—Minneapolis
Minneapolis, Minnesota

Corinne McCarthy, MSN, RN, CPN
Pediatric Outreach Coordinator
Children's Hospital
San Diego, California

Kay Stump, MS, RN
Pediatric/Adolescent Clinical Nurse Specialist
Sarasota Memorial Hospital
Sarasota, Florida

Ellen P. Tappero, MN, RNC, NNP
Neonatal Nurse Practitioner
Lutheran Medical Center
Wheat Ridge, Colorado

Teresa Frances Vaughn-Davies, MSN, RN
Nursing Instructor
Los Angeles County Medical Center
School of Nursing
Los Angeles, California

Ronda M. Wood, MN, RNC
Nursing Instructor
Long Beach City College
Department of Nursing
Long Beach, California

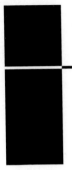

Reviewers

Carol L. Avent, MSN, RN, PNP
Professor
California State University—Fresno
School of Nursing
Fresno, California

Patricia A. Castaldi, MSN, RN
Assistant Dean
Elizabeth General Medical Center
School of Nursing
Elizabeth, New Jersey

Joyce Grant-Scott, MSN, RN
Nursing Educator
Jefferson Regional Medical Center
School of Nursing
Pine Bluff, Arkansas

Melissa Lickteig, MSN, RN
Instructor
Jefferson Regional Medical Center
School of Nursing
Pine Bluff, Arkansas

Nancy O'Donnell, MSN, RN
Associate Professor
J. Sargeant Reynolds Community College
Richmond, Virginia

Lisa Philichi, MN, RN, CCRN
Clinical Assistant Professor
Pacific Lutheran University
School of Nursing
Tacoma, Washington

Barbara Redding, EdD, RN
Associate Professor
University of South Florida
Department of Nursing
Tampa, Florida

Mary Reuland, MS, RN
Assistant Professor
College of St. Catherine—Minneapolis Campus
Department of Nursing
Minneapolis, Minnesota

Kathleen Paone Unger, MN, MSEd, RN
Assistant Professor
Cedar Crest College
Department of Nursing
Allentown, Pennsylvania

Preface

Mosby's Pediatric Nursing Reference is designed to serve nurses and nursing students who care for children and their families. Its small size and concise format were purposefully created for the nurse who wants an easily accessible reference. This book is divided into two parts. Part One contains information about frequently encountered medical and surgical conditions in the pediatric population. Part Two presents diagnostic procedures and tests. For the user's convenience, the chapters in each part are listed in alphabetical order. In the appendixes, the nurse will find valuable information about growth and development, immunizations, laboratory values, and guidelines for taking blood pressure measurement and conducting complete nursing assessments for each body system. Appendixes on pain in children, psychosocial interventions, home care, and height and weight growth curves are new to this edition.

The organization of the care-planning guidelines reflects our philosophical orientation—a family-centered approach. The needs of the child and family are addressed from a biopsychosocial perspective. The care-planning guidelines reflect a holistic approach to the child's and the family's short-term and long-term needs.

It is our hope that this compact yet powerful tool will prove a useful resource in the delivery of high-quality bedside care for children and the associated care required by their families.

Cecily Lynn Betz
Linda A. Sowden

A Note on Pediatric Drug Dosages

Because children vary widely in weight, age, body surface area, and their ability to absorb, metabolize, and excrete medications, extreme caution should be used when determining the proper dosage for a particular patient. Although the physician is responsible for writing the order correctly, the nurse is responsible for administering medications, always being careful to determine whether the dosage is correct. The nurse is urged to use the body surface method for calculating dosages (see Appendix G, *West Nomogram*).

The authors of this reference have endeavored to provide pediatric dosages consistent with safe practice. The nurse is advised, however, to rely on her or his own calculations, experience, judgment, and authoritative pharmacologic sources when administering drugs to specific patients.

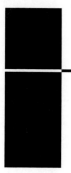

Contents

PART ONE
Pediatric Medical and Surgical Conditions

1   Anorexia Nervosa 2
2   Aplastic Anemia 9
3   Apparent Life-Threatening Event 15
4   Appendicitis and Appendectomy 20
5   Asthma 25
6   Attention Deficit/Hyperactivity Disorder 29
7   Bronchiolitis 36
8   Bronchopulmonary Dysplasia 41
9   Bulimia Nervosa 47
10 Burns 52
11 Cellulitis 62
12 Child Abuse and Neglect 67
13 Cleft Lip, Cleft Palate, and Repair 73
14 Coarctation of the Aorta and Coarctectomy 80
15 Congenital Dislocation of the Hip 87
16 Congestive Heart Failure 93
17 Croup 98
18 Cystic Fibrosis 103
19 Cytomegaloviral Infection 110
20 Diabetes Mellitus: Insulin-Dependent
    (Type I) 115
21 Disseminated Intravascular Coagulation 125
22 Drowning and Near-Drowning 130

23 Epiglottitis 138
24 Foreign Body Aspiration 143
25 Fractures 148
26 Gastroenteritis 155
27 Gastroesophageal Reflux 164
28 Glomerulonephritis 168
29 Hemolytic-Uremic Syndrome 173
30 Hemophilia 180
31 Hepatitis 186
32 Hernia (Inguinal) and Hernia Repair 194
33 Hirschsprung's Disease and Surgical Repair 198
34 Hodgkin's Disease 205
35 HIV and AIDS 212
36 Hydrocephalus and Surgical Repair 225
37 Hypertension 231
38 Hypertrophic Pyloric Stenosis 236
39 Idiopathic Thrombocytopenic Purpura 241
40 Imperforate Anus 247
41 Inflammatory Bowel Disease 254
42 Iron Deficiency Anemia 265
43 Juvenile Rheumatoid Arthritis 270
44 Kawasaki Disease 281
45 Lead Poisoning 289
46 Leukemia, Childhood 299
47 Meningitis 317
48 Mental Retardation 323
49 Muscular Dystrophy 329
50 Nephrotic Syndrome 334
51 Neuroblastoma 341
52 Nonaccidental Trauma 347
53 Non-Hodgkin's Lymphoma 351
54 Osteogenic Sarcoma and Amputation 358
55 Osteomyelitis 365
56 Otitis Media 370
57 Patent Ductus Arteriosus 375
58 Pneumonia 383
59 Poisoning 390
60 Renal Failure: Acute 393
61 Renal Failure: Chronic 401
62 Renal Transplant 409
63 Respiratory Distress Syndrome 414

64 Respiratory Syncytial Virus 420
65 Reye's Syndrome 423
66 Rheumatic Fever: Acute 430
67 Scoliosis 436
68 Seizure Disorders 443
69 Short Bowel Syndrome 451
70 Sickle Cell Anemia 460
71 Spina Bifida 467
72 Sudden Infant Death Syndrome 474
73 Tetralogy of Fallot 480
74 Urinary Tract Infections 492
75 Ventricular Septal Defect and Repair 496
76 Wilms' Tumor 503

PART TWO
Pediatric Diagnostic Tests and Procedures

General Nursing Action 510
77 Cardiac Catheterization 512
78 Computed Tomography 516
79 Electrocardiography 518
80 Endoscopy 520
81 Intracranial Pressure Monitoring 522
82 Intravenous Pyelogram 524
83 Magnetic Resonance Imaging 526
84 Peritoneal Dialysis 528

APPENDIXES

A Nursing Assessments 532
B Growth and Development 538
C Immunizations 563
D Taking Blood Pressure and Age-Appropriate Cuff Size 568
E Laboratory Values 570
F Abbreviations 578
G West Nomogram 585
H Height and Weight Growth Curves 587
I Pain in Children 596
J Psychosocial Interventions 610
K Home Care 614

PART ONE

Pediatric Medical and Surgical Conditions

1

Anorexia Nervosa

PATHOPHYSIOLOGY

Anorexia nervosa is an eating disorder characterized by refusal to maintain body weight that is within the minimal range of normal. The affected individual has a distorted body image, perceiving self as globally overweight or obsessing about shape and size of particular body parts (see the box on p. 3).

There are two subtypes of anorexia nervosa. One form is the restricting type, wherein the individual severely restricts food intake and compulsively exercises. The binge eating and purging type is marked by restricted dietary intake coupled with intermittent episodes of binge eating, followed by purging through self-induced vomiting or use of ipecac, laxatives, diuretics, or enemas. The excess use of appetite suppressants or diet pills is seen in both types.

Purging behaviors and semistarvation may induce electrolyte imbalance and cardiac problems that may ultimately lead to death. When normal eating is reestablished and laxatives stopped, the individual may develop peripheral edema.

A variety of psychologic factors are associated with the development of behaviors characteristic of anorexia nervosa. Low self-esteem often plays a significant role. Weight loss is viewed as an achievement, and self-esteem becomes dependent on body size and weight. There is also a relationship between eating disorders and mood disorders. In some cases,

Diagnostic Criteria for Anorexia Nervosa

A. Refusal to maintain body weight at or above a minimally normal weight for age and height (e.g., weight loss leading to maintenance of body weight less than 85% of that expected; or failure to make expected weight gain during period of growth, leading to body weight less than 85% of that expected).

B. Intense fear of gaining weight or becoming fat, even though underweight.

C. Disturbance in the way in which one's body weight or shape is experienced, undue influence of body weight or shape on self-evaluation, or denial of the seriousness of the current low body weight.

D. In postmenarcheal females, amenorrhea, that is, the absence of at least three consecutive menstrual cycles. (A woman is considered to have amenorrhea if her periods occur only following hormone, e.g., estrogen, administration.)

Specify type:

Restricting type: during the current episode of anorexia nervosa, the person has not regularly engaged in binge eating or purging behavior (i.e., self-induced vomiting or the misuse of laxatives, diuretics, or enemas)

Binge eating and purging type: during the current episode of anorexia nervosa, the person has regularly engaged in binge eating or purging behavior (i.e., self-induced vomiting or the misuse of laxatives, diuretics, or enemas)

Modified from American Psychiatric Association: *Diagnostic and statistical manual of mental disorders,* Washington, DC, 1994, The Association, pp. 544-545.

major depression may result from nutritional deprivation. Individuals with anorexia nervosa may lack spontaneity in social situations and may be emotionally restrained.

Family dynamics may play a role in development of symptoms. Parents may be controlling and overly protective. Eating behaviors may emerge in an unconscious attempt to gain control over the environment. Also contributing to this eating disorder is a societal ideal slimness that the adolescent strives to emulate. In some cases, diminished weight and loss of secondary sexual characteristics may be related to difficulty in accepting maturation into adulthood.

INCIDENCE

1. Cardiac complications occur in 87% of affected youth.
2. Renal complications occur in approximately 70% of affected youth.
3. Approximately 5% of anorexics are male.
4. Anorexia nervosa affects 1% of white female individuals between 16 and 24 years.
5. Peak age of onset is between 14 and 18 years.
6. Mortality rates range between 2% and 8%.
7. Incidence rates are increased in higher socioeconomic groups.
8. Five percent of children affected are under 12 years of age.

CLINICAL MANIFESTATIONS

1. Sudden, unexplained weight loss
2. Emaciated appearance, loss of subcutaneous fat
3. Changes in eating habits, unusual eating times
4. Excessive exercise and physical activity
5. Amenorrhea
6. Dry, scaly skin
7. Lanugo on extremities, back, and face
8. Yellowish discoloration of skin
9. Sleep disturbances
10. Chronic constipation or diarrhea, abdominal pain, bloating
11. Esophageal erosion
12. Depressed mood
13. Excessive focus on high achievement (becomes distressed when performance is not above average)

14. Excessive focus on food, eating, and body appearance
15. Erosion of tooth enamel and dentin on lingual surfaces (late effects)

COMPLICATIONS

1. Cardiac: bradycardia, tachycardia, arrhythmias, hypotension, cardiac failure
2. Gastrointestinal: esophagitis, peptic ulcer disease, hepatomegaly
3. Renal: serum urea and electrolyte abnormalities (hypokalemia, hyponatremia, hypochloremia, hypochloremic metabolic alkalosis), pitting edema
4. Hematologic: mild anemia and leukopenia (common) and thrombocytopenia (occurs rarely)
5. Skeletal: osteoporosis, pathologic fractures
6. Endocrine: reduced fertility, elevated cortisol and growth hormone levels, elevated gluconeogenesis
7. Metabolic: decreased basal metabolic rate, impaired temperature regulation, sleep disturbances

LABORATORY AND DIAGNOSTIC TESTS

1. Electrocardiogram (ECG)—may demonstrate bradycardia
2. Erect and supine blood pressure—to assess for hypotension
3. Serum urea, electrolytes, creatinine (in severe cases, monitor every 3 months)—may show low blood urea nitrogen (BUN) level due to dehydration and inadequate protein intake; metabolic alkalosis and hypokalemia due to vomiting
4. Urinalysis, urine creatinine clearance (in severe cases, monitor annually)—pH may be elevated; ketones may be present
5. Complete blood count (CBC), platelet count (in severe cases, monitor every 3 months)—usually normal; normochromic, normocytic anemia may be present
6. Serum glucose (in severe cases, monitor every 3 months)
7. Liver function (in severe cases, monitor every 3 months)
8. Thyroid-stimulating hormone (TSH), cortisol levels (in severe cases, monitor semiannually)

9. Bone density (in severe cases, monitor annually)—demonstrates osteopenia
10. Body composition (in severe cases, monitor annually using calipers, or water immersion)
11. Presence of hypercarotenemia—due to vegetarian diets or decreased metabolism

MEDICAL MANAGEMENT

Treatment is provided on an outpatient basis unless severe medical problems emerge. An interdisciplinary approach is needed to ensure optimal outcomes. Outpatient treatment includes medical monitoring, dietary planning to restore nutritional state, and long-term psychotherapy to work through underlying issues. Psychopharmacologic treatment may be initiated to treat symptoms of depression, anxiety, and obsessive-compulsive behaviors. Hospitalization is indicated if the adolescent weighs less than 20% of ideal body weight or is unable to adhere to the treatment program on an outpatient basis, or when neurologic deficits, hypokalemia, and cardiac arrhythmias exist.

The following medications may be used:

1. Antidepressants—the selective serotinin reuptake inhibitors (SSRI) are also used, particularly if compulsive exercising is a component of the illness (imipramine, desipramine, fluoxetine, sertraline, paroxetine)
2. Estrogen replacement for ammenorrhea

NURSING ASSESSMENT

1. Assess psychologic status with psychologic inventories: Eating Attitudes Test (EAT), EAT-26, Eating Disorders Inventory (EDI), Beck Depression Inventory.
2. Assess height and weight through use of growth charts (weight measurements taken after patient has undressed and voided).
3. Assess pattern of elimination.
4. Assess exercise pattern for type, amount, and frequency.
5. Assess for signs of depression.

NURSING DIAGNOSES

- Altered nutrition: less than body requirements
- Self-concept disturbance

- High risk for fluid volume deficit
- Activity intolerance
- Ineffective individual coping

NURSING INTERVENTIONS

1. Include family in forming dietary supplementation plan.
2. Provide information about adequate nutritional intake and the impact inadequate intake has on energy level and psychologic well-being.
3. Initiate specific plan of exercise as reinforcer for positive behavioral outcomes.
4. Establish trusting relationship that promotes disclosure of feelings and emotions.
5. Organize eating of meals with others, record amount of food eaten, and monitor activity for 2 hours after eating.
6. Promote the individual's sense of responsibility and involvement in recovery and treatment.
7. Participate on interdisciplinary team that uses multiple modalities such as individual and group psychotherapy, assertiveness training, music and/or art therapy, and nutritional education.
8. Support involvement of family members who are vital to recovery.

♠ Discharge Planning and Home Care

1. Recommend psychotherapy for treatment of distorted body image and self-concept.
2. Refer adolescent and family to community resources, that is, support groups and mental health professionals.

CLIENT OUTCOMES

1. The individual's physical health status improves without symptoms with steady, reasonable weight gain (about 1 lb every 4 days).
2. The individual establishes a healthy pattern of nutritional intake.
3. The individual establishes increased self-esteem and improvement in psychologic functioning.

REFERENCES

American Psychological Association: *Diagnostic and statistical manual of mental disorders*, ed 4, Washington, DC, 1994, The Association.

Atkins D, Silber T: Clinical spectrum of anorexia nervosa in children, *J Dev Behav Pediatr* 14(4):211, 1993.

Carpenito L: *Handbook of nursing diagnosis,* ed 5, Philadelphia, 1993, JB Lippincott.

Garfinkle P, Garner D, editors: *The role of drug treatments for eating disorders,* New York, 1987, Brunner/Mazel.

Gillberg C, Rastam M, Gillberg I: Anorexia nervosa: physical health and neurodevelopment at 16 and 21 years, *Dev Med Child Neurol* 36(7):567, 1994.

Irwin E: A focused overview of anorexia nervosa and bulimia. I. Etiological issues, *Arch Psychiatr Nurs* 7(6):342, 1993.

Irwin E: A focused overview of anorexia nervosa and bulimia. II. Challenges to the practice of psychiatric nursing, *Arch Psychiatr Nurs* 7(6):347, 1993.

Nussbausm M: Nutritional conditions: anorexia nervosa. In McArnarney E et al, editors: *Textbook of adolescent medicine,* Philadelphia, 1994, WB Saunders.

Sharp C, Freeman C: The medical complications of anorexia nervosa, *Br J Psychiatry* 162:452, 1993.

Solanto M et al: Rate of weight gain of inpatients with anorexia nervosa under two behavioral contracts, *Pediatrics* 93(6):989, 1994.

Touyz S, Kopee-Schraeder E, Beumont P: Anorexia nervosa in males: a report of 12 cases, *Aust N Z J Psychiatry* 27:512, 1993.

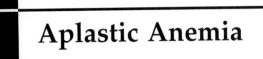

2

Aplastic Anemia

PATHOPHYSIOLOGY

Aplastic anemia is a disorder of bone marrow failure resulting in the depletion of all marrow elements. The production of blood cells is decreased or lacking. Pancytopenia and hypocellularity of the marrow occur. The manifestation of symptoms is dependent on the extent of the thrombocytopenia (hemorrhagic symptoms), neutropenia (bacterial infections, fever), and anemia (pallor, fatigue, congestive heart failure, tachycardia). Severe aplastic anemia is characterized by a granulocyte count of less than 500 per mm^3, a platelet count of less than 20,000 per mm^3, and a reticulocyte count of less than 1. Aplastic anemia can be acquired or inherited. Acquired forms can be caused by drugs (chloramphenicol), chemicals (benzene), radiation, or viral infection (hepatitis, Epstein-Barr) and, in rare instances, are associated with paroxysmal nocturnal hemoglobinuria. Fanconi's anemia is the most common inherited type. Prognosis is grave. Fifty percent of patients die within 6 months of diagnosis. With more than 70% nonhematopoietic cells, the patient's prognosis is poor.

INCIDENCE

1. Aplastic anemia may occur at any age.
2. Fifty percent of cases are idiopathic.
3. Long-term survival rate with bone marrow transplant (BMT) from histocompatible donors is as high as 70% to 90% in children.

4. Acquired aplastic anemia's incidence is one in 1 million, its male-female ratio is 1:1, and it may occur at any age.
5. In 75% of children with Fanconi's anemia the condition is diagnosed between the ages of 3 and 14 years; the male-female ratio of Fanconi's anemia is 1.3:1.

CLINICAL MANIFESTATIONS

1. Petechiae, ecchymoses, epistaxis (occur first)
2. Oral ulcerations, bacterial infections, fever (occur later in course)
3. Anemia, pallor, fatigue, tachycardia (late signs)
4. Café-au-lait spots, melanin-like hyperpigmentation, absent thumbs (Fanconi's anemia)

COMPLICATIONS

1. Sepsis
2. Sensitization to cross-reacting donor antigens resulting in uncontrollable bleeding
3. Graft vs. host disease (occurs after bone marrow transplant)
4. Failure of marrow graft (occurs after bone marrow transplant)
5. Acute myelogenous leukemia (AML)—associated with Fanconi's anemia

LABORATORY AND DIAGNOSTIC TESTS

1. Complete blood count with differential—macrocytic anemia; decreased granulocytes, monocytes, and lymphocytes
2. Platelet count—decreased
3. Reticulocyte count—decreased
4. Bone marrow aspiration and biopsy—hypocellular
5. Hemoglobin electrophoresis—elevated fetal hemoglobin level
6. Red cell i antigen titer—elevated
7. Sugar water test—positive
8. Ham's test—positive
9. Serum folate and B_{12} levels—normal or elevated
10. Chromosome breakage test—positive for Fanconi's anemia

MEDICAL MANAGEMENT

The first-choice treatment for aplastic anemia is bone marrow transplant with a sibling donor who is human lymphocyte antigens (HLA) matched. In more than 70% of cases there will be no sibling match. However, there is an increased chance that there will be a match between one parent and the child with aplastic anemia. If bone marrow transplant is to be done, HLA typing of the family is done immediately and blood products are used as little as possible to avoid sensitization. Also to avoid sensitization, blood should not be donated by the child's family. Blood products should always be irradiated and filtered to remove white blood cells before being given to a child who is a candidate for bone marrow transplant.

Immunotherapy with either antithymocyte globulin (ATG) or antilymphocyte globulin (ALG) is the primary treatment for those children not candidates for bone marrow transplant. The child will respond within 3 months or not at all to this therapy. Cyclosporine A is also an effective immunosuppressant that can be used in the treatment of aplastic anemia. Androgens are rarely used unless no other treatment is available.

Supportive therapy includes use of antibiotics and administration of blood products. Antibiotics are used to treat fever and neutropenia; prophylactic antibiotics are not indicated for the asymptomatic child. Blood product administration may include the following:

1. Platelets—to maintain platelet count greater than 20,000 per mm^3. Use single-donor platelet pheresis to decrease number of human lymphocyte antigens to which the child is exposed.
2. Packed red blood cells—to maintain hemoglobin (Hb) level higher than g/dl (chronic anemia is often well tolerated). For long-term therapy, use deferoxamine as chelating agent to prevent complications of iron overload.
3. Granulocytes—to transfuse to patient who has gram-negative sepsis.

NURSING ASSESSMENT

1. See the section on hematologic assessment in Appendix A.
2. Assess for sites of bleeding and hemorrhagic symptoms.

3. Assess for signs of infection.
4. Assess activity level.
5. Assess developmental level.

NURSING DIAGNOSES

- High risk for injury
- High risk for infection
- Activity intolerance
- Fatigue
- Altered growth and development

NURSING INTERVENTIONS

1. Identify and report signs and symptoms of hemorrhage.
   a. Vital signs (increased apical pulse, thready pulse, decreased blood pressure)
   b. Bleeding sites
   c. Skin color (pallor) and signs of diaphoresis
   d. Weakness
   e. Decreased level of consciousness
   f. Decreased platelet count
2. Protect from trauma.
   a. Do not administer aspirin or nonsteroidal antiinflammatory drugs (NSAIDs).
   b. Avoid use of intramuscular (IM) injection and suppositories.
   c. Administer contraceptive to decrease excessive menstruation.
   d. Provide good oral hygiene with soft toothbrush.
3. Protect from infection.
   a. Limit contact with potential source of infection.
   b. Use strict isolation precautions (refer to institution's policies and procedures).
4. Administer blood products and monitor child's response to their infusion (after bone marrow transplant to avoid sensitization to donor transplantation antigen).
   a. Observe for side effects or untoward response (transfusion reaction).
   b. Observe for signs of fluid overload.
   c. Monitor vital signs before infusion; monitor every 15 minutes during first hour and then hourly during infusion.

5. Provide frequent rest periods. Organize nursing care to increase activity tolerance and prevent fatigue.
6. Monitor child's therapeutic and untoward response to medications; monitor the action and side effects of administered medications.
7. Prepare child and family for bone marrow transplant.
8. Monitor for signs of bone marrow transplant complications (see section on complications, this chapter).
9. Provide age-appropriate diversional and recreational activities (see section on growth and development, Appendix B).
10. Provide age-appropriate explanation before procedures.

♠ Discharge Planning and Home Care

1. Instruct parents about measures to protect child from infection.
   a. Limit contact with infectious agents.
   b. Identify signs and symptoms of infection.
2. Instruct parents to monitor for signs of complications (see section on complications, this chapter).
3. Instruct parents about the administration of medication.
   a. Monitor child's therapeutic response.
   b. Monitor for untoward responses.
4. Provide child and family with information about community support systems for long-term adaptation.
   a. School reintegration
   b. Parent groups
   c. Child and sibling groups
   d. Financial advice

CLIENT OUTCOMES

1. Child will have gradual increase in red blood cells, white blood cells, and eventually platelets.
2. Child will have fewer infections.
3. Child will have minimal bleeding episodes.
4. Child and family understand home care and follow-up needs.

REFERENCES

Alter BP, Young NS: The bone marrow failure syndromes. In Nathan DG, Oski FA, editors: *Hematology of infancy and childhood*, ed 4, Philadelphia, 1993, WB Saunders.

Billett HH: Aplastic anemia: the role of immunosuppression, *Hosp Pract (Off Ed)* 27(8):35, 1992.

Nissen C: The pathophysiology of aplastic anemia, *Semin Hematol* 28(4):313, 1991.

Speck B: Allogeneic bone marrow transplantation for severe aplastic anemia, *Semin Hematol* 28(4):319, 1991.

3

Apparent Life-Threatening Event

PATHOPHYSIOLOGY

Apparent life-threatening event (ALTE) is an episode that may affect infants and that is characterized by some combination of the following: apnea (usually central, but occasionally obstructive), color change (cyanosis or pallor, or sometimes plethora), marked change in muscle tone (usually marked hypotonia or limpness), and choking or gagging. In some cases the infant appears to have died. Previously used terminology such as "near-miss sudden infant death syndrome" should be avoided. Many causes for ALTE have been identified. These causes include pathologic apnea, sepsis, seizures, gastroesophageal reflux, upper airway obstruction, hypoglycemia, and inborn error of metabolism or other metabolic problem. Only in approximately 50% of the cases of ALTE can a specific cause be determined.

INCIDENCE

1. ALTE affects 0.5% to 6.0% of all infants in the general public.
2. Peak age of incidence is 8 to 14 weeks.
3. Incidence is higher in male individuals.
4. Incidence is higher in premature infants (less than 34 weeks).
5. Infants who have had a previous ALTE are at increased risk for sudden infant death syndrome (SIDS); however, they constitute less than 7% of all SIDS victims.

15

Numerous studies with different designs, particularly in their inclusion and exclusion criteria, make it very difficult to determine the exact incidence.

CLINICAL MANIFESTATIONS

1. Apnea—respiratory pause greater than 20 seconds
2. Marked color change—particularly cyanosis or pallor
3. Hypotonia
4. Choking or gagging
5. Often, need for cardiopulmonary resuscitation (CPR) and/or "vigorous" stimulation to illicit a response

LABORATORY AND DIAGNOSTIC TESTS

1. Complete blood count with differential and platelet count (CBC d/p)—to rule out anemia and infection
2. Arterial blood gas (ABG)—to assess respiratory status and for evidence of metabolic acidosis
3. Blood chemistries (electrolytes, serum glucose, phosphorus, magnesium, blood urea nitrogen, and creatinine)—to assess for metabolic abnormalities
4. Chest x-ray—for evidence of a respiratory infection
5. Continuous cardiorespiratory monitoring

Further laboratory and diagnostic tests, such as an upper gastrointestinal tract study, a 12-lead electrocardiogram, or a lumbar puncture, can be performed if the initial tests suggest a specific diagnosis.

MEDICAL MANAGEMENT

Medical management focuses on care of the immediate problem and appropriate identification and evaluation of the specific cause. Initial management includes checking airway, breathing, and circulation (ABC), with restoration of cardiorespiratory function. Once stabilized, the infant should be admitted to the hospital for careful observation and further evaluation. A meticulous history and physical examination is performed, laboratory and diagnostic test results are obtained, and the infant is observed for 24 to 48 hours. These are essential in determining the specific cause of the ALTE. Further evaluation of the infant is performed as indicated by the initial assessment and test results.

Therapeutic interventions consist of the treatment of any underlying disorder and the education of the primary caregivers (e.g., the parents).

NURSING ASSESSMENT

1. See the section on cardiac and respiratory assessment in Appendix A.
2. Assess complete history—in particular, the infant's state before, during, and after the spell; duration of the episode; and associated changes of color, muscle tone, movements, and respiratory efforts during the episode.

NURSING DIAGNOSES

- High risk for altered respiratory function
- High risk for ineffective breathing patterns
- High risk for impaired gas exchange
- High risk for infection
- High risk for injury
- Anxiety
- Knowledge deficit
- High risk for ineffective management of therapeutic regimen
- Altered family processes

NURSING INTERVENTIONS

1. Assist in resuscitative efforts.
   a. Provide CPR, bag or mask breathing, or medication administration as directed by the team leader.
   b. Provide a neutral thermal environment.
   c. Ensure proper documentation of all resuscitative events.
2. Assess infant's cardiovascular and respiratory status.
   a. Ensure continuous cardiorespiratory monitoring.
   b. Monitor and record vital signs, including blood pressure in the four extremities.
   c. Check peripheral pulses, mucous membrane color, and capillary refill.
   d. Administer oxygen therapy or other respiratory treatments as ordered.
3. Ensure that proper diagnostic tests are ordered and results are obtained (see section on laboratory and diagnostic tests, this chapter).

4. If specific diagnosis is confirmed, administer therapeutic interventions as ordered.
5. Assess ability of family members to participate in home apnea monitoring program (if applicable).
6. Teach family about home apnea monitoring.
   a. Assess the need for monitoring.
   b. Teach family about use of the monitor.
   c. Instruct parents on the duration of monitoring.
   d. Provide 24-hour support, both medical and technical, for home monitoring.
   e. Teach parents infant CPR.
   f. Reinforce family's knowledge of medical condition.

🏠 Discharge Planning and Home Care

1. Teach parents to administer any medications.
2. Teach parents to administer any therapeutic interventions that may be prescribed based on the diagnosis (e.g., seizure interventions if a neurologic disorder is diagnosed).
3. Teach parents the signs of ALTE and how to perform infant CPR.
4. Provide training in home apnea monitoring if needed.
5. Refer family to community resources (e.g., home care specialists, early intervention programs, and parent support groups).
6. Stress the importance of follow-up care.

CLIENT OUTCOMES

1. Infant will be episode free.
2. Parents understand the reason for monitoring, how to use the monitor, and the required duration of monitoring.
3. Parents will be able to perform infant CPR if needed.

REFERENCES

Barron T: The child with spells, *Pediatr Clin North Am* 38: 1991.
Brooks J: Apparent life-threatening events and apnea of infancy, *Clin Perinatol* 19(4): 1992.
Burchfield D, Rawlings J: Sudden deaths and apparent life-threatening events in hospitalized neonates presumed to be healthy, *Am J Dis Child* 145: 1991.

Kahn A et al: Long term development of children monitored as infants for an apparent life-threatening event during sleep: a 10 year follow-up study, *Pediatrics* 80:1989.

Steinschneider A, Santos V: Parental reports of apnea and brady-cardia: temporal characteristics and accuracy, *Pediatrics* 88:1991.

4

Appendicitis and Appendectomy

PATHOPHYSIOLOGY

Appendicitis is the most common disease that requires surgical intervention during childhood. Appendicitis is caused by the obstruction of the appendiceal lumen and results in edema, inflammation, venous engorgement, and increased intralumenal pressure. It may lead to bacterial invasion, necrosis, and perforation, resulting in peritonitis.

Causes for obstruction of the lumen include hyperplasia of the submucosal lymphoid tissue, appendiceal fecaliths, and intestinal parasites. The prognosis is excellent, especially when surgery is performed before perforation occurs.

INCIDENCE

1. Incidence is slightly greater in male individuals.
2. Incidence is highest in later childhood.
3. Occurrence is unusual in children less than 2 years of age and is rare in children less than 1 year old.
4. Perforation is associated with age—it occurs more frequently in younger children.

CLINICAL MANIFESTATIONS

1. Pain—cramping located in periumbilical area migrating to the right lower quadrant
2. Anorexia
3. Nausea

4. Vomiting (common early sign; less common in older children)
5. Fever—low-grade early in disease; can rise sharply with peritonitis
6. Rebound tenderness
7. Decreased or absent bowel sounds
8. Constipation
9. Diarrhea
10. Dysuria
11. Irritability
12. Rapid progression of symptoms; condition may be diagnosed within 4 to 6 hours after initial occurrence of symptoms

COMPLICATIONS (IF NOT DIAGNOSED)

1. Perforation
2. Peritonitis

LABORATORY AND DIAGNOSTIC TESTS

1. Complete blood count (CBC)—leukocytosis, neutrophilia, absence of eosinophils
2. Ultrasound—noncalcified fecaliths, nonperforated appendix, appendiceal abscess
3. Abdominal x-ray examination—calcified fecaliths
4. Barium enema—nonfilling of appendix

SURGICAL MANAGEMENT

Children with suspected appendicitis are admitted, given intravenous (IV) fluids, and observed; the rapid progression of symptoms will make the diagnosis obvious. A nasogastric tube is inserted if the child is vomiting. The appendix is removed through an incision in the right lower quadrant. Perioperative antibiotics are given to reduce the incidence of wound infection. If the appendix has perforated, the abdominal cavity is irrigated and a drain may be inserted. In some cases a small catheter may be left in place to instill antibiotics. Postoperatively the child is in a semi-Fowler's position for the first 24 hours. Gastric drainage and administration of IV fluids and antibiotics are continued. Narcotic/analgesic medications are used for pain. Oral feedings are started within 2 or 3 days.

NURSING ASSESSMENT

1. See the section on gastrointestinal assessment in Appendix A.
2. Assess for rapid progression in severity of symptoms.
3. Assess for preoperative and postoperative pain.
4. Assess for bowel sounds and abdominal distention postoperatively.
5. Assess wound for drainage and signs of infection.

NURSING DIAGNOSES

- High risk for fluid volume deficit
- High risk for infection
- Pain
- Anxiety
- Knowledge deficit

NURSING INTERVENTIONS
Preoperative Care

1. Monitor child's status for progression of symptoms and complications.
   a. Shock—decreased blood pressure, decreased respiratory rate, pallor, diaphoresis, rapid thready pulse
   b. Perforation or peritonitis—absent bowel sounds, increased apical pulse, increased temperature, increased respiratory rate, abdominal splinting, diffuse abdominal pain followed by sudden relief from pain
   c. Intestinal obstruction—decreased or absent bowel sounds, abdominal distention, pain, vomiting, no stools
2. Maintain fluid and electrolyte balance.
   a. Monitor infusion of intravenous solution at maintenance rate.
   b. Monitor and record output of vomitus, urine, stool, and nasogastric drainage.
3. Provide pain relief and comfort measures.
   a. Position of comfort
   b. Avoidance of unnecessary movements and unnecessary palpation of abdomen
   c. Pain medications if ordered

4. Prepare child for surgery.
   a. Give nothing by mouth.
   b. Collect specimens for analysis preoperatively.
   c. Prepare child for and support during radiographic tests.
   d. Explain anticipated preoperative and postoperative events (e.g., dressing, nasogastric tube).

Postoperative Care

1. Prevent and monitor for abdominal distention.
   a. Provide nothing by mouth.
   b. Maintain patency of nasogastric tube.
   c. Assess abdominal tenseness (firm, soft).
2. Prevent spread of infection.
   a. Perform wound care as indicated and appropriate disposal of dressings.
   b. Provide universal isolation.
3. Monitor for signs of infection.
   a. Monitor vital signs as ordered.
   b. Observe wound for signs of infection—warmth, drainage, pain, swelling, and redness.
   c. Administer antibiotics; monitor child's response.
   d. Monitor IV site.
   e. Have child ambulate when able.
4. Promote wound healing.
   a. Perform wound care—maintain site, keeping it clean and dry.
   b. Position child in semi-Fowler's position to promote drainage if drain is present.
5. Assess pain and provide pain relief measures as needed.
   a. Administer analgesics as needed.
   b. Use distraction to alleviate pain.
   c. Use comfort measures such as massage and positioning.
6. Support child and parents to help them deal with emotional stresses of hospitalization and surgery.
   a. Provide age-appropriate information before procedures.
   b. Encourage activities.
   c. Promote contacts and visits with peers.
   d. Incorporate child's home routine into daily activities.

♠ Discharge Planning and Home Care

1. Instruct parents to observe for and report signs of complications.
   a. Infection
   b. Obstruction
2. Instruct parents regarding wound care.
3. Instruct parents about follow-up appointment.
   a. Name and phone number of physician
   b. Date and time of follow-up appointment

CLIENT OUTCOMES

1. Child will have return to normal gastrointestinal function.
2. Child will have minimal pain.
3. Child and family understand home care and follow-up needs.

REFERENCES

Raffensperger J, editor: *Swenson's pediatric surgery,* ed 5, East Norwalk, Conn, 1990, Appleton & Lange.

Stewart RJ et al: Peritoneal cytology for suspected acute appendicitis: an economic evaluation, *Health Econ* 3(5):321, 1994.

Wong ML et al: Sonographic diagnosis of acute appendicitis in children, *J Pediatr Surg* 29(10):1356, 1994.

5

Asthma

PATHOPHYSIOLOGY

Asthma is a lung disease in which there is airway obstruction, airway inflammation, and airway hyperresponsiveness or spasm of the bronchial smooth muscle. An exacerbation of asthma may be precipitated by specific allergens (e.g., pollen, mold, animal dander, dust, or foods) or by other factors such as weather changes, respiratory infections, exercise, or emotional factors. Asthma results from complex interactions among the inflammatory cells and mediators in the airways and autonomic neural regulation of the airway, where the following occurs:

1. Bronchial smooth muscle contraction
2. Bronchospasm
3. Mucosal edema from inflammatory cells in the airways with injury to the epithelium
4. Increased mucus production
5. Mucus plugging
6. Air trapped behind occluded or narrowed airways
7. Insufficient oxygenation and ventilation
8. Air hunger responses, resulting in anxious behavior

INCIDENCE

1. Asthma affects 5% to 10% of all children.
2. Asthma accounts for 25% of school absences caused by chronic illness (leading cause of absenteeism).
3. Asthma mortality rates are increasing by 6% per year.

CLINICAL MANIFESTATIONS

1. Clinical evidence of airway obstruction—obstruction may be gradual or acute, and estimation of severity of acute exacerbations is termed mild, moderate, or severe
2. Dyspnea with prolonged expiration
3. Expiratory wheeze, progressing to inspiratory and expiratory wheezing, progressing to breath sounds becoming inaudible
4. Grunting respirations in infancy
5. Nasal flaring
6. Cough
7. Accessory muscle use
8. Anxiety, irritability, to decreasing level of consciousness
9. Cyanosis
10. A drop in $PaCO_2$ initially, from hyperventilation; then a rise in $PaCO_2$ as obstructive process worsens

COMPLICATIONS

1. Status asthmaticus
2. Chronic persistent bronchitis, bronchiolitis, pneumonia
3. Chronic emphysema
4. Cor pulmonale with right-sided heart failure
5. Atelectasis
6. Pneumothorax
7. Death

LABORATORY AND DIAGNOSTIC TESTS

1. White blood count—increased with infection
2. Arterial blood gas (for severe cases)—initially increased pH, decreased PaO_2, and decreased $PaCO_2$ (mild respiratory alkalosis from hyperventilation); subsequently: decreased pH, decreased PaO_2, and increased $PaCO_2$ (respiratory acidosis)
3. Eosinophil count—increased in blood, sputum
4. Chest x-ray—to rule out infection or other cause of worsening respiratory status
5. Pulmonary function tests—decreased tidal volume, decreased vital capacity, decreased maximal breathing capacity

MEDICAL MANAGEMENT

Medical management is targeted at preventing asthma exacerbations by avoiding asthma triggers and by decreasing airway obstruction, inflammation, and reactivity with medications. Systemically acting B adrenergic agonists, such as epinephrine HCL (1:1000) and terbutaline, are administered subcutaneously; however, inhaled B adrenergic agonists, such as albuterol administered with oxygen, are preferred. Intravenous corticosteroids such as Solu-Medrol or Solu-Cortef may be added to decrease mucosal edema. Aminophylline or theophylline is sometimes added as an additional bronchodilator.

NURSING ASSESSMENT

1. See the section on respiratory assessment in Appendix A.
2. Assess breathing pattern.
3. Assess for anxiety/agitation.
4. Assess fluid volume status.
5. Assess child and family coping strategies.

NURSING DIAGNOSES

- Ineffective airway clearance
- Impaired gas exchange
- High risk for fluid volume deficit
- Anxiety
- High risk for ineffective family coping

NURSING INTERVENTIONS

1. Promote pulmonary function.
   a. Administer and assess response to oxygen for respiratory distress.
   b. Administer and assess response to aerosolized bronchodilators and antiinflammatory agents.
   c. Elevate head of bed.
   d. *Never* use sedatives for a child with asthma experiencing respiratory distress.
2. Assess and monitor child's hydration status.
   a. Monitor intake and output.
   b. Assess for signs of dehydration.
   c. Monitor infusion of intravenous solution.
   d. Monitor urine specific gravity.

3. Alleviate or minimize child's and parents' anxiety, using developmental level.
4. Assess child's and parents' feelings about having asthma and taking medications.
5. Assess willingness to participate in education programs and refer family to support groups as needed.

🏠 Discharge Planning and Home Care

Patient education should begin at the time of diagnosis and is integrated with continuing care.

1. Reinforce understanding of asthma.
2. Provide specific instructions about medications and adverse effects.
3. Instruct on monitoring signs and symptoms and peak expiratory flow rate, and indications for treatment modifications.
4. List steps in managing an acute episode of asthma and instruct on when to seek emergency medical care.
5. Identify asthma triggers and how to avoid, eliminate, or control.
6. Discuss fears and misconceptions concerning treatments.

CLIENT OUTCOMES

1. Child will have optimal pulmonary function.
2. Child is able to perform daily activities.
3. Child will participate in endurance activities (e.g., swimming, tennis).

REFERENCES

Bechler-Karsch A: Assessment and management of status asthmaticus, *Pediatr Nurs* 20(3):217, 1994.

Betz CL, Hunsberger MM, Wright S: *Family-centered nursing care of children,* ed 2, Philadelphia, 1994, WB Saunders.

Guidelines for the diagnosis and management of asthma: national asthma education program—expert panel report, *NIH Publication,* No 91-3042, August 1991.

Larter NL, Kieckhefer G, Paeth ST: Content validation of standards of nursing care for the child with asthma, *J Pediatr Nurs* 8(1):15, 1993.

Ryan-Wenger NM, Walsh M: Children's perspectives on coping with asthma, *Pediatr Nurs* 20(3):224, 1994.

6

Attention-Deficit/ Hyperactivity Disorder

PATHOPHYSIOLOGY

Attention-deficit/hyperactivity disorder (ADHD) is characterized by disturbance of attention, impulsivity, and hyperactivity. The *Diagnostic and Statistical Manual of Mental Disorders*, fourth edition (DSM IV), outlines specific observable behavioral symptoms in these three areas (see box). Most often, both inattention and hyperactive-impulsive behaviors are present. However, some children exhibit one predominant pattern of either hyperactivity-impulsivity or inattention.

Although symptoms of inattention and hyperactive-impulsive disorder are present before age 7, a diagnosis is not usually made until the child begins school, when behavior interferes with academic and social functioning. As the child enters adolescence, observable symptoms are less obvious. Restlessness and jitteriness replace the excessive activity seen during childhood. Adolescents with ADHD have difficulty complying with behavioral expectations or rules normally observed in educational and work settings. Conflicts with authority figures are also noted. Symptoms may persist into adulthood. These individuals may be described as "on the go," always busy, and unable to "sit still."

Children with ADHD may demonstrate deficits in sensorimotor coordination; clumsiness, or problems with spatial orientation, may be observed. Difficulties are noted

Diagnostic Criteria for Attention-Deficit/ Hyperactivity Disorder

A. Either (1) or (2):
  (1) Six (or more) of the following symptoms of **inattention** have persisted for at least 6 months to a degree that is maladaptive and inconsistent with developmental level:
  Inattention
    (a) Often fails to give close attention to details or makes careless mistakes in schoolwork, work, or other activities
    (b) Often has difficulty sustaining attention in tasks or play activities
    (c) Often does not seem to listen when spoken to directly
    (d) Often does not follow through on instructions and fails to finish schoolwork, chores, or duties in the workplace (not due to oppositional behavior or failure to understand instructions)
    (e) Often has difficulty organizing tasks and activities
    (f) Often avoids, dislikes, or is reluctant to engage in tasks that require sustained mental effort (such as schoolwork or homework)
    (g) Often loses things necessary for tasks or activities (e.g., toys, school assignments, pencils, books, or tools)
    (h) Is often easily distracted by extraneous stimuli
    (i) Is often forgetful in daily activities

(2) Six (or more) of the following symptoms of **hyperactivity-impulsivity** have persisted for at least 6 months to a degree that is maladaptive and inconsistent with developmental level:

Hyperactivity

- (a) Often fidgets with hands or feet or squirms in seat
- (b) Often leaves seat in classroom or in other situations in which remaining seated is expected
- (c) Often runs about or climbs excessively in situations in which it is inappropriate (in adolescents or adults, may be limited to subjective feelings of restlessness)
- (d) Often has difficulty playing or engaging in leisure activities quietly
- (e) Is often "on the go" or often acts as if "driven by a motor"
- (f) Often talks excessively

Impulsivity

- (g) Often blurts out answers before questions have been completed
- (h) Often has difficulty awaiting turn
- (i) Often interrupts or intrudes on others (e.g., butts into conversations or games)

B. Some hyperactive-impulsive or inattentive symptoms that caused impairment were present before age 7 years.

C. Some impairment from the symptoms is present in two or more settings (e.g., at school [or work] and at home).

D. There must be clear evidence of clinically significant impairment in social, academic, or occupational functioning.

Continued

31

E. The symptoms do not occur exclusively during the course of a pervasive developmental disorder, schizophrenia, or other psychotic disorder and are not better accounted for by another mental disorder (e.g., mood disorder, anxiety disorder, dissociative disorder, or a personality disorder).

Code based on type:

314.01 Attention-deficit/hyperactivity disorder, combined type: if both criteria A1 and A2 are met for the past 6 months

314.00 Attention-deficit/hyperactivity disorder, predominantly inattentive type: if criterion A1 is met but criterion A2 is not met for the past 6 months

314.01 Attention-deficit/hyperactivity disorder, predominantly hyperactive-impulsive type: if criterion A2 is met but criterion A1 is not met for the past 6 months

Coding note: For individuals (especially adolescents and adults) who currently have symptoms that no longer meet full criteria, "in partial remission" should be specified.

Modified from American Psychiatric Association: *Diagnostic and statistical manual of mental disorders,* ed 4, Washington, DC, 1994, The Association.

both at home and at school. Disruptiveness, temper outbursts, and aimless motor activity often irritate peers and family members. As a result, secondary problems such as oppositionalism, mood and anxiety disorders, and communication problems frequently emerge. Learning may be delayed due to chronic inability in attending to educational tasks.

Although there is no single etiologic factor that accounts for this complex disturbance of behavior, medical history reveals higher incidence of child abuse and/or neglect, prenatal drug exposure, low birth weight, lead poisoning, encephalitis, and mental retardation in affected children.

INCIDENCE

1. Studies suggest a higher incidence of ADHD in children with first-degree biologic relatives with diagnosed ADHD.
2. The incidence rate among school-age children is 3% to 5%.
3. Incidence is higher in male individuals than female individuals, by a ratio of 9:1.

CLINICAL MANIFESTATIONS

These are listed in the box on pp. 30-32.

COMPLICATIONS

1. Secondary diagnoses—conduct disorder, depression, and anxiety disorder
2. Academic underachievement, school failure, reading and/or arithmetic difficulties (frequently resulting from attentional abnormalities)
3. Poor peer relationships (frequently due to aggressive behavior and verbal outbursts)

LABORATORY AND DIAGNOSTIC TESTS

1. Behavioral history—Obtain historical data from parents and teachers. This is the most important method of gathering information.
2. To accurately diagnose ADHD, symptoms must meet specific criteria outlined in the DSM IV (see box).
3. Wechsler Intelligence Scale for Children, third edition (WISC-III), is often administered. Difficulty in copying block designs is often observed.
4. The following tools have been used to identify children with ADHD:
   a. Freedom from Distractibility (arithmetic, digit span, and coding)

b. ADHD checklist (i.e., Copeland Symptom Checklist for Attention-Deficit Disorders, Attention-Deficit Disorders Evaluation Scale)

MEDICAL MANAGEMENT

The treatment plan for the child with ADHD consists of use of psychostimulants, behavior modification, parent education, and family counseling. Parents may express concern about using medication. Risks and benefits of medication must be explained to parents, including prevention of potential ongoing scholastic and social impairment through the use of psychostimulant medications. The Conners rating scales may be used as a baseline and for monitoring the effectiveness of treatment.

Psychostimulants—methlyphenidate (Ritalin), amphetamine sulfate (Benzedrine), and dextroamphetamine sulfate (Dexedrine)—improve measures of attention and concentration by exerting a paradoxical effect on most children and some adults with ADHD.

NURSING ASSESSMENT

1. Assess family history via interview or genogram.
2. Assess the child's behavioral history.

NURSING DIAGNOSES

- Impaired social interactions
- Self-concept disturbance
- High risk for ineffective management of treatment regimen
- High risk for altered parenting
- High risk for violence
- High risk for self-injury

NURSING INTERVENTIONS

Nursing interventions are generally implemented in outpatient and community settings.
1. Assist parents in implementing a behavior program to include positive reinforcement.
2. Provide daily structure.
3. Administer stimulant medication as ordered.

  a. Stimulants may be temporarily discontinued on weekends and holidays.
  b. Stimulants are not given after 3 or 4 P.M.

♠ Discharge Planning and Home Care

1. Educate and support parents and family members.
2. Collaborate with teachers and involve parents. Encourage parents to ensure that teacher and school nurse are aware of medication name, dosage, and times to be administered.
3. Ensure that the child receives necessary academic evaluation and tutoring. Placement in special education class is often required.
4. Monitor child's progress and response to medication.
5. Refer to behavioral and parenting specialists to develop and implement a behavior plan.

CLIENT OUTCOMES

1. School performance improves, as evidenced by classroom grades and work completed.
2. Improvement of child's behavior according to teacher and parent rating is noted.
3. Child displays positive peer relationships.

REFERENCES

American Psychiatric Association: *Diagnostic and statistical manual of mental disorders,* ed 4, Washington, DC, 1994, The Association.

Chess S, Hassibi M: *Principles and practice of child psychiatry,* ed 2, New York, 1986, Plenum Press.

Faraone S et al: Intellectual performance and school failure in children with attention deficit hyperactivity disorder and in their siblings, *J Abnorm Psychol* 102(4):616, 1993.

Johnston C, Fine S: Methods of evaluating methylphenidate in children with attention deficit hyperactivity disorder: acceptability, satisfaction, and compliance, *J Pediatr Psychol* 18(6):717, 1993.

Niebuhr V, Smith L: The school nurse's role in attention deficit hyperactivity disorder, *J Sch Health* 63(2):112, 1993.

Risser M, Bowers T: Cognitive and neuropsychological characteristics of attention deficit hyperactivity disorder children receiving stimulant medications, *Percept Mot Skills* 77:1023, 1993.

7

Bronchiolitis

PATHOPHYSIOLOGY

Bronchiolitis is a lower respiratory tract viral illness characterized by inflammation of the smaller bronchioles. Edema of the mucous membranes lining the walls of the bronchioles plus cellular infiltrates and increased mucus production result in obstruction. The obstruction causes hyperinflation of the affected areas as expired air is trapped distally, resulting in hypoxemia. The obstructions do not occur uniformly throughout the lung. Symptoms are more severe in infants because the diameter of their bronchiole lumina is smaller. The infection is most commonly caused by the respiratory syncytial virus (RSV). RSV is transmitted by way of droplets. Other causative agents include adenovirus, parainfluenza, and rhinovirus. Prognosis is generally good.

INCIDENCE

1. Bronchiolitis is one of the most frequent reasons for hospitalization of infants less than 1 year old.
2. Mortality rate is determined by the presence of underlying disease; the rate is higher if RSV is present.
3. Bronchiolitis occurs most frequently in winter and early spring.

CLINICAL MANIFESTATIONS

1. Upper respiratory tract infection for 1 to 4 days; then acute phase for 2 to 6 days; resolution in 7 to 14 days

2. Labored respirations (rapid and shallow with nasal flaring and retractions)
3. Expiratory wheezing of acute onset
4. Anorexia or being difficult to feed
5. Coryza
6. Hacking, harsh paroxysmal cough
7. Cyanosis
8. Audible and palpable rhonchi
9. Temperature range: normal to as high as 40.6° C (105.4° F)
10. Malaise
11. Increased mucus production
12. Irritability
13. Tachypnea and/or restless sleep (above normal limits for age)

COMPLICATIONS

1. Atelectasis (acute)
2. Apnea (acute)
3. Respiratory fatigue or failure (acute)
4. Recurrent pulmonary infection (long term)

LABORATORY AND DIAGNOSTIC TESTS

1. Chest x-ray study (hyperinflation with air trapping, atelectasis, slight perihilar infiltrate)—widely varied diagnostic criteria
2. Rapid fluorescent antibody test for RSV—to diagnose RSV
3. Arterial blood gas—to assess gas exchange
4. White blood cell count—normal or a mild elevation

MEDICAL MANAGEMENT

Mild cases of bronchiolitis can usually be managed at home with fluids and humidification. Progressive respiratory distress and apnea are common indicators for inpatient admission and possible admission to the intensive care unit and might indicate the use of mechanical ventilation. Supportive therapy includes administration of humidified oxygen, intravenous (IV) hydration, and rest. The only specific pharmacologic therapy involves the use of ribavirin for RSV infection. Antibiotics are not indicated unless a bacterial infection is detected.

NURSING ASSESSMENT

1. See the section on respiratory assessment in Appendix A.
2. Assess respiratory status.
3. Assess for signs and symptoms of dehydration.
4. Assess for signs and symptoms of fluid overload.

NURSING DIAGNOSES

- Ineffective airway clearance
- Ineffective breathing pattern
- Impaired gas exchange
- High risk for hyperthermia
- High risk for fluid volume deficit
- Altered nutrition: less than body requirements
- Anxiety
- Knowledge deficit

NURSING INTERVENTIONS

1. Monitor respiratory status (including vital signs).
   a. Assess vital signs initially every 2 hours, until stable, then every 4 hours during acute episode.
   b. Assess for and report signs of increased respiratory distress and changes in respiratory status.
   c. Apnea monitoring may be indicated in acute phase.
2. Monitor child's response to oxygen therapy and humidified oxygen through hood, tent, or nasal cannulae.
   a. Assess for therapeutic response—improving respiratory status.
   b. Assess for signs of oxygen toxicity—increase in P_{CO_2} levels, increase in hypoventilation, decrease in level of consciousness.
   c. Monitor oxygen status with pulse oximetry.
3. Promote respiratory function.
   a. Semiprone or side-lying position; avoidance of neck hyperextension
   b. Opportunities for rest

4. Monitor hydration status.
   a. Monitor intake and output and urine specific gravity.
   b. Assess for signs of dehydration or fluid overload.
5. Assess child for untoward therapeutic response to medications if indicated.
6. Encourage intake of diet high in calories and protein.
   a. Serve favorite foods if possible.
   b. Arrange food attractively on tray (for the older child).
   c. Encourage use of routine feeding practices (e.g., usual mealtimes, presence of parents, or favorite cup).
7. Encourage age-appropriate quiet play (see section on growth and development, Appendix B).
8. Alleviate or minimize the child's and parents' anxiety during hospitalization (see Appendix J).
9. Provide consistent nursing care to promote trust and to alleviate anxiety.

♠ Discharge Planning and Home Care

Instruct parents about the following for home care of the child:
1. Use of humidifiers (may use moisture from hot shower)—cold vs. warm mists
2. Rationale for treatments (medication administration)
3. Signs of secondary infection
4. Infection control and prevention measures
5. Providing adequate fluid intake

CLIENT OUTCOMES

1. Infant or child will maintain patent airway with easy respiratory effort.
2. Infant or child exhibits appropriate weight gain and hydration status.
3. Infant or child exhibits no signs of anxiety or apprehension.

REFERENCES

Hanson IC, Shearer WT: Bronchiolitis. In Oski F et al, editors: *Principles and practice of pediatrics*, ed 2, Philadelphia, 1994, JB Lippincott.

Horst PS: Bronchiolitis, *Am Fam Physician* 49(6): 1449, 1994.

Larsen GL et al: Respiratory tract and mediastinum. In Hay WW et al, editors: *Current pediatric diagnosis and treatment,* ed 12, East Norwalk, Conn, 1995, Appleton & Lange.

Welliver RC, Cherry JD: Bronchiolitis and infectious asthma. In Feigen RD, Cherry JD, editors: *Textbook of pediatric infectious diseases,* ed 3, Philadelphia, 1992, WB Saunders.

Zander J, Hazinski MF: Pulmonary disorders. In Hazinski MF editor: *Nursing care of the critically ill child,* ed 2, St Louis, 1992, Mosby.

8

Bronchopulmonary Dysplasia

PATHOPHYSIOLOGY

Bronchopulmonary dysplasia (BPD) is the chronic lung disease that occurs in both full-term and preterm infants after prolonged ventilator and/or oxygen therapy. Clinical presentation is characterized by ongoing respiratory distress, persistent oxygen requirement (with or without ventilatory support), and a classically abnormal chest x-ray film, after 1 month of life.

The four major risk factors that contribute to the development of BPD are respiratory distress or failure, prematurity, exposure to high levels of oxygen, and exposure to mechanical ventilation. Other potential risk factors are pulmonary edema, pulmonary infections, and/or pulmonary air leaks. Pulmonary changes typical of infants with BPD include alterations in lung structure, increased airway resistance, increased airway reactivity, decreased lung compliance, increased mucus production, and increased work of breathing. Although pulmonary function often improves significantly in early childhood, recent research demonstrates that some pulmonary problems may persist into adult life.

INCIDENCE

1. Incidence varies among neonatal intensive care units (NICUs) because of differences in diagnostic criteria, patient populations, and patient management.

2. It is estimated that 3000 to 7000 infants are affected in the United States.
3. It is suggested that there is an increase in incidence due to improved survival rates.

CLINICAL MANIFESTATIONS

1. Hypoxia
2. Hypercapnia
3. Tachypnea
4. Retractions
5. "Seesaw" breathing (due to decreased lung compliance)
6. Wheezing
7. Rhonchi
8. Cough

COMPLICATIONS

1. Persistent changes in pulmonary function
2. Respiratory infections
3. Pulmonary hypertension
4. Cor pulmonale
5. Systemic hypertension
6. Altered growth and nutrient needs
7. Delayed development
8. Activity intolerance

LABORATORY AND DIAGNOSTIC TESTS

1. Chest x-ray studies—may include a spectrum of findings, including bilateral diffuse interstitial thickening (mild to very severe) and normal to increased lung expansion
2. Arterial and venous blood gases—hypercapnia and compensated respiratory acidosis are common findings
3. Pulmonary function testing
4. Serum electrolytes—useful when monitoring the effects of long-term diuretic therapy
5. Serial electrocardiograms (ECGs)—useful to monitor for cor pulmonale

MEDICAL MANAGEMENT

The goals of medical management for infants with BPD are (1) treatment of the complications and symptoms with oxygen and medication and (2) enhancement of lung healing through adequate nutrition and promotion of respiratory stability (stable oxygenation and prevention of infection).

Therapies commonly used include the following:

1. Oxygen
2. Bronchodilators—decrease pulmonary resistance and increase lung compliance
3. Diuretics—prevent fluid overload and pulmonary edema
4. Corticosteroids—decrease inflammatory responses and promote lung healing
5. Nutrition—adequate nutrition promotes lung and total body healing, growth, and development

NURSING ASSESSMENT

1. See the section on respiratory assessment in Appendix A.
2. Assess infant's cardiorespiratory status.
3. Assess for signs and symptoms of fluid overload.
4. Assess infant's oral intake and growth.
5. Assess developmental level.
6. Assess infant-parent interactions.
7. Assess parents' discharge readiness and ability to manage home care.

NURSING DIAGNOSES

- Impaired gas exchange
- Fluid volume excess
- Altered nutrition: less than body requirements
- Altered growth and development
- Activity intolerance
- Altered family processes
- Altered parenting
- Knowledge deficit
- High risk for ineffective management of treatment regimen

NURSING INTERVENTIONS

1. Maintain cardiorespiratory stability.
   a. Establish infant's baseline respiratory assessment and monitor for changes.
   b. Monitor responsiveness to medical interventions.

    c. Monitor trends in oxygenation through oximetry.

    d. Monitor action and side effects of medications.

       (1) bronchodilators

       (2) corticosteroids

       (3) diuretics

2. Evaluate for signs and symptoms of fluid overload.

    a. Monitor intake (ml/kg/day) and output (ml/kg/hr).

    b. Administer diuretic and/or fluid restrictive therapy as ordered.

3. Monitor for adequate caloric intake and growth over time.

    a. Weight gain should be approximately 20 to 30 grams per day.

    b. Monitor infant's ability to maintain adequate oral intake. (Infants who are tachypneic and have increased work of breathing may not be able to take in food orally because of the risk of aspiration.)

    c. Monitor for increased oxygen requirements during and immediately after oral feedings; provide increased oxygen as needed.

    d. Provide supplementation to oral feedings through gavage or gastrostomy tube feedings.

4. Promote growth and development through integration of play and positive stimulation into care routine.

    a. Provide opportunities for developmentally appropriate visual, auditory, tactile, and kinesthetic stimulation—when infant is alert and stable.

    b. Integrate pattern and routine into care, including undisturbed night sleep and predictable daytime activities.

5. Monitor infant's response to caregiving and developmental activities.

    a. Assess for increased oxygen requirements during and immediately following activity.

    b. Assess for patterns of response to activities and caregivers.

    c. Develop a list of likes, dislikes, and comfort measures from assessed patterns of response.

    d. Decrease environmental and caregiver stimulation during periods of agitation and/or stress.

6. Facilitate integration of infant into his or her family.

    a. Assist parents in recognizing infant's responses to activity.

b. Teach parents how they can best interact with and provide care for their child.

c. Develop parents' confidence in caring for their child.

d. Promote visitation and caregiving by other key family members, including siblings, as soon as appropriate.

♠ Discharge Planning and Home Care

1. Evaluate readiness for discharge. Factors to assess include the following:
   a. Stable respiratory status
   b. Adequate nutritional intake and growth
   c. Stable medication needs
   d. Medical treatment plan that is realistic for home
      (1) Parents or other caregivers can provide needed care.
      (2) Needed home equipment and monitoring is provided.
      (3) Parents have needed social and/or financial supports.
      (4) Respite or home nursing needs are provided for.

2. Provide discharge instruction for parents covering the following:
   a. Explanation of BPD
   b. How to monitor for signs of respiratory distress and other medical problems
   c. Individualized feeding needs
   d. Well-baby needs
   e. When to call the doctor
   f. How to perform cardiopulmonary resuscitation (CPR)
   g. Use of home equipment and monitoring
   h. How to administer and monitor effects of medications
   i. Infection prevention
   j. Importance of a smoke-free environment
   k. Appropriate developmental activities
   l. Recognition of infant's stress and interaction cues
   m. Available community resources and supportive services

3. Provide follow-up to monitor ongoing respiratory, nutritional, developmental, and other specialized needs.

a. Help parents make first follow-up appointments; provide written documentation of when the appointments are.
b. Make referral for in-home nursing visits or care based on needs of the infant and family.

CLIENT OUTCOMES

1. Infant will have optimal lung functioning, with gas exchange and oxygenation, sufficient for tissue perfusion, growth, and healing.
2. Infant will reach maximum potential for growth and development.
3. Parents will be competent in the care of their child.

REFERENCES

Abman SH, Groothius JR: Pathophysiology and treatment of bronchopulmonary dysplasia: current issues, *Pediatr Clin North Am* 41(2):277, 1994.

American Lung Association: *BPD: parent guide to bronchopulmonary dysplasia,* New York, 1987, The Association.

Howard G: Transition to home: discharge planning for the oxygen-dependent infant with bronchopulmonary dysplasia, *J Perinat Neonat Nurs* 6(2):85, 1992.

Northway WH: Bronchopulmonary dysplasia: twenty-five years later, *Pediatrics* 89(5):969, 1992.

Southwell SM: Complications of respiratory management. In Kenner, Breuggemeyer, Gunderson, editors: *Comprehensive neonatal nursing: a physiologic perspective,* Philadelphia, 1993, WB Saunders.

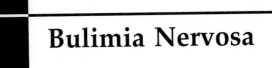

9

Bulimia Nervosa

PATHOPHYSIOLOGY

Bulimia nervosa is a nutritional and psychologic disorder characterized by excessive eating. The person with bulimia may consume as much as 6000 calories of food followed by one or more of the following behaviors to avoid the consequences of overeating: vomiting, and use of laxatives, enemas, and diuretics. Bulimia nervosa was identified as a diagnostic condition separate from anorexia nervosa in 1979. The *Diagnostic and Statistical Manual of Mental Disorders,* fourth edition (DSM IV), criteria are presented in the box on pp. 48-49.

Etiologic factors cited as contributing to bulimia nervosa include familial, sociocultural, physiologic, cognitive-behavioral, and psychologic factors. The affected adolescent may report difficulty with impulse control and have a history of self-destructive behaviors.

INCIDENCE

1. Bulimia nervosa affects about 3% of female adolescents and less than 1% of male adolescents.
2. Female-male ratio is 10:1.
3. Incidence is greater in higher socioeconomic groups.
4. Fifty percent of bulimic individuals have an alcoholic relative.

CLINICAL MANIFESTATIONS

1. Binge eating done in secret as a means of dealing with anxiety and stress

47

Diagnostic Criteria for Bulimia Nervosa

A. Recurrent episodes of binge eating. An episode of binge eating is characterized by both of the following:

   (1) Eating, in a discrete period of time (e.g., within any 2-hour period), an amount of food that is definitely larger than most people would eat during a similar period of time and under similar circumstances

   (2) A sense of lack of control over eating during the episode (e.g., a feeling that one cannot stop eating or control what or how much one is eating)

B. Recurrent inappropriate compensatory behavior in order to prevent weight gain, such as self-induced vomiting; misuse of laxatives, diuretics, enemas, or other medications; fasting; or excessive exercise.

C. The binge eating and inappropriate compensatory behaviors both occur, on average, at least twice a week for 3 months.

D. Self-evaluation is unduly influenced by body shape and weight.

E. The disturbance does not occur exclusively during episodes of anorexia nervosa.

Specify type:

  Purging type: during the current episode of bulimia nervosa, the person has regularly engaged in self-induced vomiting or the misuse of laxatives, diuretics, or enemas

Continued

Nonpurging type: during the current
episode of bulimia nervosa, the person
has used other inappropriate compensatory behaviors, such as fasting or excessive exercise, but has not regularly engaged in self-induced vomiting or the
misuse of laxatives, diuretics, or enemas

Modified from American Psychiatric Association: *Diagnostic and statistical manual of mental disorders*, Washington, DC, 1994, The Association, pp. 544-545.

2. Hiding or stealing food
3. Excusing self to use bathroom during or after meals
4. Compulsive dieting and exercise
5. Preoccupation with weight and physical appearance
6. Impaired body image and self-concept
7. Depression and dysthymia
8. Food cravings

COMPLICATIONS

1. Parotid and submaxillary gland swelling (sialadenosis)
2. Facial fullness
3. Russell's sign—scarring of and callus formation on
   knuckles
4. Enamel erosion of teeth
5. Abdominal tenderness or pain
6. Esophagitis, gastritis

LABORATORY AND DIAGNOSTIC TESTS

1. Thorough physical examination
2. Serum electrolytes—hypokalemia, hyponatremia, hypochloremic metabolic alkalosis
3. Serum amylase—may be elevated
4. Psychologic diagnostic evaluation—may include these
   psychologic inventories: Eating Attitudes Test (EAT), Eating Disorders Inventory (EDI), Beck Depression Inventory

MEDICAL MANAGEMENT

Treatment is provided on an outpatient basis unless severe medical problems emerge. An interdisciplinary approach is needed to ensure optimal outcomes. Outpatient treatment includes medical monitoring, dietary plan initiated to restore nutritional state, and psychotherapy. Psychopharmacologic treatment (i.e., antidepressants) may be initiated.

The following medications may be used:

1. Antidepressant medications—imipramine
2. Monoamine oxidase (MAO) inhibitors

NURSING ASSESSMENT

Thorough nursing history and assessment includes history of bulimic episodes, family psychodynamics, and psychosocial functioning.

NURSING DIAGNOSES

- Altered nutrition: less than body requirements
- Self-concept disturbance
- High risk for fluid volume deficit
- Ineffective individual coping
- Altered family process
- Impaired social interactions

NURSING INTERVENTIONS

1. Provide information about adequate nutritional intake and the impact inadequate intake has on energy level and psychologic well-being.
2. Establish trusting relationship that promotes disclosure of feelings and emotions.
3. Promote the individual's sense of responsibility and involvement in recovery and treatment.
4. Promote cognitive restructuring and self-esteem through counseling.
5. Incorporate a family-centered approach in providing services.

♠ Discharge Planning and Home Care

Discharge planning and home care should concentrate on psychotherapy for treatment of distorted body image and self-concept.

CLIENT OUTCOMES

1. The adolescent will maintain weight within the normal range for age.
2. The adolescent will cope more effectively.

REFERENCES

American Psychological Association: *Diagnostic and statistical manual of mental disorders,* ed 4, Washington, DC, 1994, The Association.

Boumann CE, Yates WR: Risk factors for bulimia nervosa: a controlled study of parental psychiatric illness and divorce, *Addict Behav* 19(6):667, 1994.

Heebink DM, Sunday SR, Halmi KA: Anorexia nervosa and bulimia nervosa in adolescence: effects of age and menstrual status on psychological variables, *J Am Acad Child Adolesc Psychiatry* 34(3):378, 1995.

Irwin EG: A focused overview of anorexia nervosa and bulimia. I. Etiological issues, *Arch Psychiatr Nurs* 7(6):342, 1993.

Position of the American Dietetic Association: nutrition intervention in the treatment of anorexia nervosa, bulimia nervosa, and binge eating, *J Am Diet Assoc* 94(8):902, 1994.

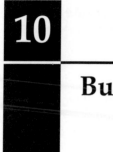

10

Burns

PATHOPHYSIOLOGY

Burns are the tissue damage that results from contact with thermal, chemical, or electrical agents. The severity of the burn is assessed by determining (1) the type of burn (flame, liquid, chemical, or electrical); (2) the duration of contact, which affects the depth of burn injury (first, second, or third degree); (3) the areas affected, including both the body surface and the location (vital anatomic areas); (4) related injuries; and (5) any preexisting illness or condition. See the box on p. 53 and Figure 1 for further descriptions of burn severity.

The severity of the burn determines the degree of change seen in all of the body's organs and systems. A thermal injury creates an open wound as a result of destruction of the skin. Following the burn, skin perfusion is decreased as blood vessels are occluded and vasoconstriction occurs. Intravascular volume decreases as fluids are leaked from the intravascular to interstitial space as a result of increased capillary permeability. Pulmonary injury may occur as a result of inhalation of smoke, steam, or irritants. With a major burn, cardiac output decreases and blood flow to the liver, kidney, and gastrointestinal tract is compromised. The child with a major burn is in a hypermetabolic state, consuming oxygen and calories at a rapid rate.

Prognosis is dependent on the severity of the burn that is sustained.

Burn Classification According to Depth

First Degree (Superficial)

- Superficial; involves only superficial epidermis (e.g., sunburn)
- Symptoms: pain, redness, no tissue or nerve damage

Second Degree (Partial Thickness)

- Superficial to deep dermal; involves entire epidermis and varying amounts of dermis (e.g., scald)
- Symptoms: pain, red edematous skin, vesicles

Third Degree (Full Thickness)

- Epidermis and dermis destroyed; involves subcutaneous adipose tissue, fascia, muscle, and bone (e.g., fire)
- Symptoms: no pain; white, red, or black skin; edematous skin

INCIDENCE

1. Burns are the second leading cause of accidental injury and death in children under 14 years of age.
2. Burns caused by thermal agents are the most common and usually occur in the kitchen or bathroom.
3. Electrical and chemical burns are uncommon in children.
4. Three fourths of all burns are thought to be preventable.

CLINICAL MANIFESTATIONS

The following are initial manifestations for moderate to severe burn:

1. Tachycardia
2. Decreased blood pressure
3. Cold extremities
4. Change in level of consciousness
5. Dehydration (decreased skin turgor, decreased urinary output, dry tongue and skin)
6. Increased rate of respirations
7. Pale (not present with second- and third-degree burn)

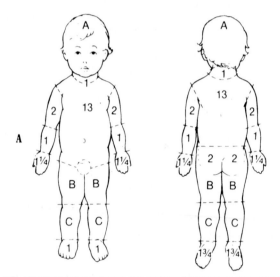

RELATIVE PERCENTAGES OF AREAS AFFECTED BY GROWTH

AREA	BIRTH	AGE 1 YR	AGE 5 YR
A = ½ of head	9½	8½	6½
B = ½ of one thigh	2¾	3¼	4
C = ½ of one leg	2½	2½	2¾

Figure 1. Estimated distribution of burns in children. **A,** Children from birth to age 5 years.
(From Whaley LF, Wong DL: *Nursing care of infants and children,* ed 5, St Louis, 1995, Mosby.)

Continued

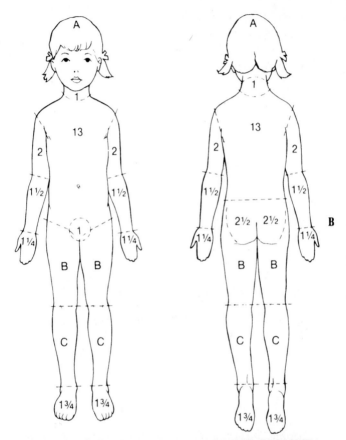

RELATIVE PERCENTAGES OF AREAS AFFECTED BY GROWTH

AREA	AGE 10 YR	AGE 15 YR	ADULT
A = ½ of head	5½	4½	3½
B = ½ of one thigh	4½	4½	4¾
C = ½ of one leg	3	3¼	3½

Figure 1, **cont'd. B,** Older children.

COMPLICATIONS

1. Renal failure
2. Metabolic acidosis
3. Hyperkalemia
4. Hyponatremia
5. Hypocalcemia
6. Pulmonary problems
   a. Pulmonary edema
   b. Pulmonary insufficiency
   c. Pulmonary embolus
   d. Bacterial pneumonia
7. Infection
8. Curling's ulcer

LABORATORY AND DIAGNOSTIC TESTS

1. Complete blood count (CBC)—decreased
2. Arterial blood gas values—metabolic acidosis (decreased pH, increased partial pressure of carbon dioxide [P_{CO_2}], and decreased partial pressure of oxygen [P_{O_2}])
3. Serum electrolytes—decreased because of loss to traumatized areas and interstitial spaces
4. Serum glucose—increased because of stress-invoked glycogen breakdown or glyconeogenesis
5. Blood urea nitrogen (BUN)—increased because of tissue breakdown and oliguria
6. Creatinine—increased because of tissue breakdown and oliguria
7. Serum protein levels—decreased because of protein breakdown for massive energy needs
8. Chest x-ray

MEDICAL MANAGEMENT

Burn treatment is based on the size and severity of the burn along with consideration as to its cause. Fluid resuscitation is critical in remedying intravascular fluid losses. Oxygen is delivered by mask or artificial ventilation. The burn itself may be covered with topical medications and is either left open to air or covered with gauze. Severe burns require debridement of the wound and grafting. The child will receive analgesics or narcotics for pain. With severe burns, nutritional requirements are met with either a high-calorie diet or intravenous nutritional support.

NURSING ASSESSMENT

1. See the section on nursing assessments in Appendix A.
2. Assess fluid volume status.
3. Assess for adequate oxygenation and tissue perfusion.
4. Assess for pain.
5. Assess cause, extent, and depth of burns.

NURSING DIAGNOSES

- Impaired gas exchange
- Fluid volume deficit
- Pain
- High risk for infection
- Impaired skin integrity
- Altered nutrition: less than body requirements
- High risk for disuse syndrome
- Anxiety
- Altered growth and development
- Altered family processes

NURSING INTERVENTIONS
First Aid and Emergency Care

Prevent further injury.

1. Scald burn—douse with water; remove individual's clothing.
2. Flame burn—have individual drop and roll to extinguish; douse with cool liquid; remove nonadherent clothing.
3. Chemical burn—flush eyes and skin for 20 minutes with water.
4. Electrical burn—turn off power sources; initiate cardiopulmonary resuscitation.

Hospitalization

1. Maintain patent airway.
   a. Monitor and report signs of respiratory distress (dyspnea, increased respiratory rate, air hunger, nasal flaring).

Electrolyte Imbalances

Hyperkalemia

Oliguria or anuria
Diarrhea
Muscle weakness
Arrhythmias
Intestinal colic

Hyponatremia

Abdominal cramps
Diarrhea
Apprehension

Hypocalcemia

Tingling in fingers
Muscle cramps
Tetany
Convulsions

b. Perform pulmonary toilet.
c. Monitor use of respirator and oxygen as ordered.
d. Provide tracheostomy care as ordered.
2. Monitor child for signs and symptoms of hypovolemic shock.
a. Monitor vital signs every hour or more frequently until stable.
b. Monitor input and output hourly (output—20 to 30 ml/hr, >2 years; 10 to 20 ml/hr, <2 years).
3. Monitor child for signs and symptoms of electrolyte imbalances (see the box above).
4. Monitor child for signs and symptoms of hemorrhage.
a. Vital signs (every hour or more frequently when first admitted [during critical period], then every 2 hours until stable, then every 4 hours)

    b. Bleeding

    c. Rapid, thready pulse

    d. Decreased blood pressure

5. Provide pain relief measures to alleviate or control child's pain (see section on pain, Appendix I).

    a. Use comfort measures (pillow, bed, cradle).

    b. Position for comfort.

    c. Medicate before wound care or dressing changes.

    d. Use distraction, guided imagery, hypnosis.

    e. Monitor child's therapeutic response to medications.

6. Protect child from potential infections.

    a. Administer tetanus booster as ordered.

    b. Monitor child's therapeutic and untoward response to antibiotics.

    c. Maintain and monitor use of protective isolation.

    d. Use sterile technique during wound care.

    e. Monitor for wound infections (offensive odor, redness at site, increased temperature, warmth, purulent drainage).

7. Promote adequate nutritional intake to counteract nitrogen loss and potential gastrointestinal complications.

    a. Provide diet high in calories and protein (total caloric requirement equals 60 calories times weight in kilograms plus calories times percentage of burn).

    b. Monitor for signs of Curling's ulcer (decreased hemoglobin level, decreased red blood cell count [anemia], coffee-ground emesis, abdominal distention).

    c. Administer antacids as needed.

    d. Monitor bowel sounds for ileus.

8. Promote optimal healing of wounds (see section on medical management, this chapter).

    a. Use sterile technique when dressing wound.

    b. Observe for cellulitus or area that is trapping pus.

9. Promote maximal function of joints.

    a. Use splints appropriately to prevent contractures.

    b. Check splints every 4 hours for pressure sores.

    c. Perform range of motion exercises and passive range of motion exercises for extremities.

    d. Encourage ambulation when child is able.

    e. Encourage participation in self-care activities.

10. Encourage verbalization of feelings regarding altered body image.
    a. Depression (associated with injury and pain)
    b. Anxiety (associated with treatments)
    c. Shame (associated with appearance)
11. Provide for child's developmental needs during hospitalization.
    a. Encourage use of age-appropriate toys (see section on growth and development, Appendix B); modify according to child's condition (e.g., use passive coloring—child directs nurse in coloring pictures).
    b. Encourage contact with peers (as appropriate).
    c. Provide age-appropriate roommate as dictated by condition.
    d. Encourage academic pursuits.
12. Provide emotional support to family.
    a. Encourage ventilation of concerns.
    b. Refer to social service as necessary.
    c. Refer to other parents in comparable situation as appropriate.
    d. Provide for physical comforts (e.g., place to sleep and bathe).
    e. Refer to support group (e.g., parent, religious) as needed.

♠ Discharge Planning and Home Care

1. Instruct child and/or parents in wound care.
2. Provide burn prevention education.
3. Make referrals for outpatient physical and occupational therapies as indicated.

CLIENT OUTCOMES

1. The child will be free from infection.
2. The child will have adequate intravascular fluid volume.
3. The child will demonstrate adequate respiratory function.
4. The child will experience little to no pain.

REFERENCES

Conway EE Jr, Sockolow R: Hydrofluoric acid burn in a child, *Pediatr Emerg Care* 7(6):345, 1991.

Cooper RL, Brown D: Pretransfer tissue expansion of a scalp free flap for burn alopecia reconstruction in a child: a case report, *J Reconstr Microsurg* 6(4):339, 1990.

Hazinski MF: *Nursing care of the critically ill child,* ed 3, St Louis, 1996, Mosby.

Whaley LF, Wong DL: *Nursing care of infants and children,* ed 5, St Louis, 1995, Mosby.

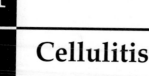

Cellulitis

PATHOPHYSIOLOGY

Cellulitis is an infection that affects the skin and subcutaneous tissue. The site of involvement is most commonly an extremity, but cellulitis may also occur on the scalp, head, and neck. Organisms causing cellulitis include *Staphylococcus aureus,* group A streptococci, *Haemophilus influenzae* (in young children), and *Streptococcus pneumoniae* (in infants). A history of trauma or, in young children, an upper respiratory tract infection is often reported. The site of infection is characterized by a swelling with indistinct margins that are tender and warm. Infection may extend to deeper tissues or spread systemically. See the box on p. 63 for orbital and periorbital cellulitis symptoms. Outcome is excellent with treatment.

INCIDENCE

1. Cellulitis occurs more frequently in boys than girls.
2. Five percent to 14% of cases of cellulitis in children are caused by *H. influenzae* type B.
3. More than 85% of children with *H. influenzae* type B cellulitis are under 2 years of age; the role of *H. influenzae* type B should significantly decrease as infants routinely receive the conjugate vaccine.

Orbital and Periorbital Symptoms

Orbital Cellulitis

- Infection easily spreads from sinuses because orbit shares common wall with ethmoid, maxillary, and frontal sinuses (caused by group A streptococci, *S. aureus*, *H. influenzae*, and *S. pneumoniae*)
- *Symptoms:* exophthalmos, ophthalmoplegia, and loss of visual acuity

Periorbital Cellulitis

- Caused by trauma, infected wound, or insect bite
- *Symptoms:* rapid onset of fever and swelling; area is warm, indurated, and tender

CLINICAL MANIFESTATIONS
Local Reaction

1. Lesion with indistinct margins
2. Usually red, warm, and painful site of involvement
3. Indurated tissue

For orbital and periorbital reactions, see the box above.

Systemic Reaction

1. Fever
2. Malaise
3. Chills
4. Red streak along lymphatic drainage path
5. Enlarged and painful lymph glands

COMPLICATIONS

1. Systemic involvement, septicemia
2. Osteomyelitis
3. Septic arthritis
4. Meningitis
5. Loss of visual acuity (periorbital cellulitis)
6. Potential for brain abscess (orbital, periorbital cellulitis)

LABORATORY AND DIAGNOSTIC TESTS

1. Complete blood count (CBC)—elevated white blood count (WBC)
2. Blood cultures—positive
3. Tissue aspirate culture—positive
4. X-ray study of paranasal sinuses (periorbital cellulitis)—opacification of sinuses
5. Computed tomographic scan of orbit and paranasal sinuses—to rule out orbital involvement

MEDICAL MANAGEMENT

Children with cellulitis may be treated with oral antibiotics as outpatients if they have localized symptoms without fever. When systemic symptoms are present, the child is admitted to the hospital for a course of intravenous (IV) antibiotics. Warm compresses are applied to the site. The site is elevated and immobilized whenever possible. Acetaminophen is given as needed to manage fever and pain. For the first 24 to 36 hours after effective antibiotics are begun, it is not unusual for the cellulitis to appear to progress. Antibiotic administration may be changed from IV to oral administration when symptoms of redness, warmth, and swelling have significantly improved. A total 10- to 14-day course of antibiotics is given. Incision and drainage may be performed if the area becomes suppurative.

NURSING ASSESSMENT

1. Assess for local and systemic reactions.
2. Assess for pain.

NURSING DIAGNOSES

- Impaired tissue integrity
- Pain
- Anxiety

NURSING INTERVENTIONS

1. Monitor child's status for progression of symptoms and complications.
   a. Assess skin locally for changes; minimize palpation because of pain.
   b. Assess for signs of systemic infection.
   c. Monitor therapeutic and untoward responses to antibiotics.
2. Provide pain relief and comfort measures.
   a. Bed rest; immobilization and elevation of affected extremity
   b. Warm compresses to site for 10 to 20 minutes daily or more frequently
   c. Pain medications as needed
3. Provide emotional support to child and family.
   a. Provide age-appropriate explanations before procedures.
   b. Incorporate home routine into care.
   c. Encourage parental ventilation of concerns.
   d. Refer to social service as needed.

♠ Discharge Planning and Home Care

1. Instruct parents about importance of continuing the full course of antibiotics even though symptoms have resolved.
2. Instruct parents about follow-up appointment.
3. Instruct parents to observe for and report signs of infection spread.

CLIENT OUTCOMES

1. Child will have decreased redness, swelling, and warmth at cellulitis site.
2. Child will be free of pain.
3. Child and family understand home care and follow-up needs.

REFERENCES

Ben-Amitai D, Ashkenazi S: Common bacterial skin infections in childhood, *Pediatr Ann* 22(4):225, 1993.

Malinow I, Powell KR: Periorbital cellulitis, *Pediatr Ann* 22(4):241, 1993.

12

Child Abuse and Neglect

PATHOPHYSIOLOGY

Child abuse is a nonaccidental act that (1) inflicts or allows another to inflict physical or emotional pain or injury; (2) creates or allows another to create a significant risk of serious physical or emotional pain or injury; or (3) is or allows an act of sexual abuse, as defined by law, against a child. There are four major types of abuse: physical abuse, emotional abuse, sexual abuse, and neglect.

Child abuse crosses all cultural, religious, socioeconomic, and professional groups. Risk factors associated with abuse include low socioeconomic status, parents who were abused as children, parental substance abuse, parental social isolation, poor parenting skills, children born prematurely, and children with chronic conditions such as mental retardation or cerebral palsy.

INCIDENCE

1. Nearly 3 million cases of physical and sexual child abuse were reported in 1992.
2. As many as 45 of every 1000 children may be abused.
3. More than 1000 children die annually as a result of abuse and neglect.
4. Sexual abuse is most common among girls, stepfamilies, and children living with one parent or a primary caregiver that is an unrelated male.

5. Incidence of physical and sexual abuse is four times greater, and neglect eight times greater, in families with incomes under $15,000 per year than in other families.

CLINICAL MANIFESTATIONS

See the box on pp. 69-71 for a list of the clinical manifestations.

LABORATORY AND DIAGNOSTIC TESTS

1. X-ray studies of affected areas
2. Computed tomography/magnetic resonance imaging of affected areas
3. Bone survey—to detect extent of traumatic injuries (fractures in various stages of healing may be identified)
4. Ophthalmology examination—to detect retinal hemorrhages (results from severe shaking or slamming of head)
5. Color photographs of injuries
6. Head circumference, abdominal circumference
7. Examination of cerebrospinal fluid
8. Pregnancy test
9. Screen for sexually transmitted diseases/human immunodeficiency virus (HIV)
10. Evidentiary examination (specimens and examination should be obtained to comply with recommendations of child protection services or local coroner or medical examiner)

MEDICAL MANAGEMENT

The first priority in the care of the abused child is resuscitation and stabilization as deemed necessary according to the injuries sustained. Confirmation of the abuse is achieved through thorough history taking, complete physical examination with detailed inspection of the child's entire body, and collection of laboratory specimens. All injuries should be documented with color photographs and recorded carefully in the written medical record.

Every state has a child abuse law that specifies legal responsibilities for reporting suspected abuse. Suspected abuse must be reported to the local child protective service agency. Mandated reporters include nurses, physicians, dentists, podiatrists, psychologists, speech pathologists,

Clinical Manifestations of Child Abuse and Neglect

Skin Injuries

Skin injuries are the most common and easily recognized signs of maltreatment in children. Human bite marks appear as ovoid areas with tooth imprints, suck marks, or tongue thrust marks. Multiple bruises or bruises in inaccessible places are indications that the child has been abused. Bruises in different stages of healing may indicate repeated trauma. Bruises that take the shape of a recognizable object are generally not accidental.

Traumatic Hair Loss

Traumatic hair loss occurs when the child's hair is pulled, or used to drag or jerk the child. The result of the pulling on the scalp can cause the blood vessels under the skin to break. An accumulation of blood can help differentiate between abusive and nonabusive loss of hair.

Falls

If a child is reported to have had a routine fall but has what appear to be severe injuries, the inconsistency of the history with the trauma sustained indicates suspected child abuse.

External Head, Facial, and Oral Injuries

Cuts, bleeding, redness, or swelling of the external ear canal; tears of the lip;

Continued

loosened or fractured teeth; tongue lacerations; and bilateral black eyes without trauma to the nose may all indicate abuse.

Deliberate or Unexplained Thermal Injuries

Immersion burns, with clear line of demarcation; multiple small circular burns, in varying stages of healing; iron burns (show iron pattern); diaper area burns; and rope burns suggest intentional harm.

Shaken Infant Syndrome

Shaking produces an acceleration-deceleration injury to the brain, causing stretching and breaking of blood vessels. Serious insult to the central nervous system may result, without evidence of external injury.

Unexplained Fractures and Dislocations

Posterior rib fractures in different stages of healing, spiral fractures, or dislocation from twisting of an extremity may provide evidence of nonaccidental injury in children.

Sexual Abuse

Lacerations or irritation of external genitalia, repeated urinary tract infections, sexually transmitted disease, nonspecific vaginitis, pregnancy in the young adolescent, penile discharge, and sexual promiscuity may provide evidence of sexual abuse.

Neglect

The symptoms of neglect reflect a lack of both physical and medical care. Manifestations include failure to thrive without a medical explanation, multiple cat or dog bites and scratches, feces and dirt in the skin folds, severe diaper rash with the presence of ammonia burns, feeding disorders, and developmental delays.

coroners, medical examiners, child day care center employees, children's services workers, social workers, and schoolteachers. Failure to report suspected child abuse can result in a fine or other punishment, according to individual statutes.

NURSING ASSESSMENT

1. Comprehensive history and parent (or caregiver) interview
2. Comprehensive physical examination, including social, emotional, and cognitive assessment
3. Observation of parent-child interactions, including frequency of contact, and length of time the parent visits the child
4. Emotional status of parents

NURSING DIAGNOSES

- High risk for injury
- Pain
- Fear
- Altered growth and development
- Ineffective family coping

NURSING INTERVENTIONS

1. Resuscitate and stabilize as necessary.
2. Protect from further injury.

3. Assist with diagnosis of abuse.
4. Report suspected abuse.
5. Provide supportive care.
6. Document assessment of physical findings, parent inter-actions, and child's verbal disclosures.
7. Serve as role model for positive parenting skills.
8. Make appropriate referrals (child life specialist, child protection services, social worker, home visiting nurse, parenting classes, Parents Anonymous).

♠ Discharge Planning and Home Care

1. Refer parents to multidisciplinary community resources that will assist with improving impulse control, increasing knowledge of growth and development, setting realistic expectations, and providing alternatives to physical abuse.
2. Refer family to support groups, family therapy, or parenting effectiveness classes.

CLIENT OUTCOMES

1. Child will be protected from further injury or harm.
2. Child will demonstrate minimal long-term sequelae as a result of abuse.
3. Parents will develop effective parenting skills.

REFERENCES

Chadwick D: Child abuse. In Rudolph A, editor: *Rudolph's pediatrics,* ed 19, Norwalk, Conn, 1991, Appleton & Lange.

Devlin B, Reynolds R: Child abuse, *Am J Nurs* 94(3):26, 1994.

Krugman R, Jones D: The assessment process of a child protection team. In Helfer R, Kempe R, editors: *The battered child,* Chicago, 1987, University of Chicago Press.

Monteleone J: *Recognition of child abuse for the mandated report,* St Louis, 1994, GW Medical.

Schmitt B: The child with nonaccidental trauma. In Helfer R, Kempe R, editors: *The battered child,* Chicago, 1987, University of Chicago Press.

US Department of Health and Human Services: *Child health '93,* Washington, DC, 1995, US Government Printing Office.

13

Cleft Lip, Cleft Palate, and Repair

PATHOPHYSIOLOGY

Cleft lip and cleft palate are the outcomes of the failure of the soft tissue and/or bony structure to fuse during embryonic development. They may occur on one or both sides of the palate's midline and may occur separately or together. Cleft lip results from failure of the maxillary and median nasal processes to fuse. Cleft palate is a midline fissure of the palate that results from the failure of the two sides to fuse. The exact etiology is unknown, but several drugs (e.g., cortisone, anticonvulsants, chlorcyclizine), environmental factors, and genetic disorders must be considered as causes of these defects. The child initially seen with cleft lip and/or cleft palate defects must also be assessed for other anomalies, including spina bifida, anencephalic hydrocephalus, and cardiac abnormalities. These children should also be examined for chromosomal abnormalities.

INCIDENCE

1. Cleft lip with or without cleft palate occurs once in 1000 births.
2. Cleft palate alone occurs once in 2500 births.
3. Highest incidence is associated with Asians; lowest with African Americans.
4. Occurrence of cleft lip predominates in male individuals.
5. Occurrence of cleft palate predominates in female individuals.

CLINICAL MANIFESTATIONS

1. Visible unilateral or bilateral cleft lip
2. Palpable and/or visible cleft palate
3. Nasal distortion
4. Feeding difficulties

COMPLICATIONS

1. Speech difficulties—hypernasality, compensatory articulation
2. Malocclusion—abnormal tooth eruption pattern
3. Hearing problems—caused by recurrent otitis media secondary to eustachian tube dysfunction
4. Altered self-esteem and body image—affected by degree of disfigurement and scarring

LABORATORY AND DIAGNOSTIC TESTS

1. Routine preoperative workup (i.e., complete blood count)
2. Additional laboratory and diagnostic tests if other anomalies exist

SURGICAL MANAGEMENT: CLEFT LIP AND CLEFT PALATE REPAIR

Cleft lip is repaired either immediately after birth or within 3 months. It has been suggested that early surgical repair facilitates parent-infant attachment because of the infant's resultant aesthetic appearance. Repairs are performed at 2 to 3 months of age if the infant demonstrates steady weight gain and a hemoglobin level greater than 10 g/dl. Several types of surgery are performed to correct the cleft lip: (1) a straight-line operation, (2) a lower one-third flap repair, (3) an upper one-third flap operation, and (4) a combined upper and lower one-third flap operation. In each of the surgeries, closure of the lip is usually performed with a Z-plasty procedure to avoid the risk of contracture and elevation of the lip.

Cleft palate surgery is usually performed when the child is 9 to 12 months of age. Palatoplasty involves closure of the mucous membrane and restoration of the anatomic structure. Several types of surgical repairs are used because of the many different forms of cleft palates. With a severe defect, staged procedures may continue until the patient is 4 to 5 years of age.

NURSING ASSESSMENT

1. See the section on gastrointestinal assessment in Appendix A.
2. Assess parents' interactions with infant.
3. Assess parents' reactions to upcoming surgery.
4. Assess infant's fluid and nutritional intake.
5. Assess respiratory status.
6. Assess for signs of infection.
7. Assess infant's level of pain.
8. Assess parents' readiness for discharge and ability to manage home care.

NURSING DIAGNOSES

- High risk for altered parenting
- Knowledge deficit
- Altered nutrition: less than body requirements
- Pain
- High risk for aspiration
- High risk for infection
- High risk for ineffective management of treatment regimen

NURSING INTERVENTIONS
Preoperative Care

1. Facilitate parents' positive adjustment to infant.
   a. Assist parents in dealing with phasic reactions—shock, denial, grief, and mourning.
   b. Encourage expression of negative feelings.
   c. Discuss surgery with parents and role-play the behavioral strategies for coping with the reactions of family and friends.

   d. Provide information that instills hope and positive
      feelings for infant (e.g., comment on infant's positive
      features, note positive aspects of parent-child interac-
      tions).
   e. Convey attitude of acceptance of infant.
   f. Arrange meeting with other parents who have had a
      similar experience.
2. Provide and reinforce information to parents about infant's prognosis and treatment.
   a. Stages of surgical intervention
   b. Feeding techniques
   c. Cause of cleft
3. Promote and maintain adequate fluid and nutritional intake.
   a. Facilitate breast or bottle feeding using appropriate
      bottle and nipple—regular nipple with enlarged hole,
      Breck feeder (syringe adapted with 2-inch tubing), or
      other special feeding appliances.
   b. Place infant in upright position and direct the flow of
      milk to the side of the mouth, avoiding the cleft in
      the palate.
   c. Direct fluids inside the gums near tongue (Breck
      feeder).
   d. Burp infant frequently during feeding, because infant
      will swallow excessive air.
   e. Assess infant's response to feeding, and proceed at
      rate suitable to needs.
   f. Follow feeding with water to cleanse formula from
      mouth.
4. Promote and maintain clear airway.
   a. Monitor respiratory status (respiratory effort, breath
      sounds, vital signs).
   b. Position infant on right side with some elevation.
   c. Place suction bulb near infant at all times.
   d. Feed infant in upright position and burp frequently.

Preoperative home care

1. Instruct parents about care and maintenance of presurgical orthodontic device, if used (promotes alignment of
   maxilla and proper lateral arch position).
   a. Remove and clean every day.

    b. Replace after cleaning.
    c. Monitor for white pressure areas in palate.
    d. Apply elbow restraints to child to prevent removal of plate.
2. Instruct parents about care of cleft lip and cleft palate.
    a. Cleanse lip and oral cavity with water before and after feedings.
    b. Cleanse affected nostril before and after meals.
3. Instruct parents about preparing infant for surgery.
    a. Provide nothing by mouth after midnight (water may be given 3 to 4 hours before surgery).
    b. Refer to institutional regimen for preoperative procedure.
    c. Monitor reactions to preoperative medications.

Postoperative Care

1. Promote adequate nutritional fluid intake.
    a. Offer clear liquid (when recovered from anesthesia) with Breck feeder.
    b. Advance to formula as tolerated (cleft lip).
    c. Advance to blenderized or soft diet as tolerated (cleft palate).
    d. Burp infant frequently during feeding.
2. Promote healing and maintain integrity of child's incision site.
    a. Cleanse suture line gently per institutional protocol (cleft lip).
    b. Apply antibiotic ointment to suture line (cleft lip).
    c. Rinse mouth with water before and after feedings.
    d. Maintain lip protective device (cleft lip)—that is, Logan's bow.
    e. Avoid placing objects in child's mouth following both cleft lip and cleft palate repair (suction catheters, tongue depressors, straws, pacifier, spoon, ice chips).
    f. Remove toys with pointed objects.
    g. Use elbow restraints to prevent child from injuring surgical site (use jacket restraints on older child); remove at least once every 2 hours.
    h. Place infant on right side after feedings to decrease incidence of aspiration.

 i. Monitor for signs of infection both at surgical site and systemically.
 j. Monitor infant's level of pain and need for pain medication.

♠ Discharge Planning and Home Care

1. Instruct parents about care of surgical site.
2. Instruct parents about feeding practices.
3. Instruct parents about restraints.
4. Encourage parents to ventilate feelings of insecurity and concerns about caring for child at home, as well as about long-term management and prognosis.
5. Reinforce to parents the importance of long-term management to prevent development of speech and language, hearing loss, and dentition problems.
6. Discuss with parents the possibility of long-term consequences and outcomes.
 a. Secondary lip deformity
 b. Excessive nasality
 c. Problems with articulation
 d. Crossbite
 e. Malocclusion
 f. Underdeveloped mandible

CLIENT OUTCOMES

1. Infant's or child's wound heals properly without complications.
2. Infant or child has appropriate weight gain.
3. Infant or child experiences no signs of aspiration.
4. Parents demonstrate understanding of feeding techniques and home care instructions.
5. Parents demonstrate acceptance of infant's or child's condition.

REFERENCES

Curtin G: The infant with cleft lip or palate: more than a surgical problem, *J Perinat Neonat Nurs* 3(3):80, 1990.
Sauter S: Cleft lips and palate: types, repairs, nursing care, *AORN J* 50(4):813, 1989.

Stewart JM, Manchester DK, Sujansky E: Genetics and dysmorphia. In Hay WW et al, editors: *Current pediatric diagnosis and treatment,* ed 12, East Norwalk, Conn, 1995, Appleton & Lange.

Wellman C, Coughlin S: Preoperative and postoperative nutritional management of the infant with cleft palate, *J Pediatr Nurs* 6(3):154, 1991.

14

Coarctation of the Aorta and Coarctectomy

PATHOPHYSIOLOGY

Coarctation of the aorta is a localized narrowing of the aortic lumen. This narrowing increases pressures in the ascending aorta, leading to higher pressures in the coronary arteries and vessels that arise from the aortic arch. There are three basic types of coarctation: (1) juxtaductal—narrowing at the level of the ductus arteriosus; (2) preductal—narrowing proximal to the ductus arteriosus; and (3) postductal—narrowing distal to the ductus arteriosus. Coarctation of the aorta is associated with several other defects, including anomalies of the left side of the heart, bicuspid aortic valve defect, and ventricular septal defect. Two thirds of children with this defect are asymptomatic. Severe cases can become apparent in infancy; many cases are discovered during a physical examination when hypertension of the upper extremity is noted. Prognosis is excellent with surgical intervention.

INCIDENCE

1. Coarctation of the aorta accounts for 10% of congenital cardiac defects.
2. Electrocardiogram (ECG) is normal in 50% of cases.

CLINICAL MANIFESTATIONS
Infants

Most infants are asymptomatic; initially, symptoms may be associated with severe sudden onset of congestive heart failure.

Children

1. Absent or diminished lower-extremity pulses
2. Hypertension of upper extremities, with bounding pulses
3. Systolic, or systolic and diastolic murmurs
4. Leg muscle cramps during exercise (tissue anoxia)
5. Headache
6. Epistaxis
7. Cool feet

COMPLICATIONS

1. Heart failure
2. Cerebrovascular accident
3. Hypertensive encephalopathy
4. Dissecting aortic aneurysm
5. Bacterial endocarditis

LABORATORY AND DIAGNOSTIC TESTS

1. ECG—normal or may reveal left-ventricular hypertrophy and ST and T wave abnormalities
2. Chest x-ray examination—to determine cardiac size or pulmonary venous congestion (in infants, consistent with clinical findings; in older patient, normal)
3. Cardiac catheterization—to diagnose associated defects and abnormal pressure gradient
4. Echocardiogram—to examine size, shape, and motion of heart structures; may reveal reduced ejection fraction
5. Preoperative laboratory data:
   a. Complete blood count, urinalysis, serum glucose, blood urea nitrogen

b. Baseline electrolytes—sodium, potassium, chloride, carbon dioxide
c. Blood coagulation studies—prothrombin time (PT), partial thromboplastin time (PTT), platelet count
d. Type and cross match for 6 U of blood, with 2 U drawn first day of surgery

SURGICAL MANAGEMENT: COARCTECTOMY

Repair of a coarctation may be accomplished through several methods, depending on the age of the child and the degree of constriction. Elective repair in early childhood is generally preferred; infants with congestive heart failure who do not respond to medical treatment have surgical correction in infancy.

Repair is designed to reduce risks of restenosis. The left subclavian artery may be ligated distally and sutured over an opening in the aorta to provide for a patch enlargement of the aorta. This subclavian flap aortoplasty reduces the number of cases of restenosis because the natural tissue will grow with the child, causing less tension than an end-to-end anastomosis. By 4 to 8 years of age the aorta is nearly adult size, and hypertension is still reversible. Many surgeons prefer this age for repair; other physicians believe performing the procedure in 1- to 4-year-olds has results that are just as good and include fewer later complications. Postoperative complications increase if surgery is delayed until the child is more than 8 to 10 years old.

The area of coarctation is patched with Teflon material, leaving some natural material to grow with the child. Some surgeons excise the area of coarctation, but that procedure may lead to repeat coarctation. Entry to the thoracic cavity for both age groups is performed through a left posterolateral thoracotomy incision. Bypass is not necessary, although adequate flow to the lower extremities must be maintained through collateral circulation, hypothermia, a temporary shunt or grafts connecting the ascending and descending aorta, or a partial cardiopulmonary bypass.

Complications

1. Chylothorax as a result of injury to thoracic duct or lymphatics
2. Congestive heart failure
3. Hemothorax caused by bleeding from the collateral network or aortic anastomosis
4. Repeat coarctation, especially in infants
5. Vomiting resulting from increased circulation to the gastrointestinal tract
6. An increased incidence of cardiovascular disease 11 to 25 years after surgery
7. Mortality rate ranging from 4% to 25%, depending on the age of the child, degree of constriction, other associated defects, skill of the cardiac team, and the medical center used for the surgery

Medications: Antihypertensives

1. Sodium nitroprusside (Nipride)—used to treat postoperative hypertension; acts on the smooth muscle to produce peripheral vasodilation, causing decreased arterial pressures
2. Propranolol (Inderal)—used to treat postoperative hypertension; acts as a beta blocker of cardiac and bronchial adrenoreceptors, resulting in decreasing heart rate and myocardial irritability and potentiating contraction and conduction pathway
3. Reserpine—used to treat postoperative hypertension; acts as a sympathetic inhibitor, resulting in decreased blood pressure and cardiac output
4. Captopril (Capoten)—used to treat postoperative hypertension; works on the renin-angiotensin system to reduce afterload

NURSING ASSESSMENT

1. See the section on cardiovascular assessment in Appendix A.
2. Assess for paradoxical hypertension.
3. Perform frequent assessment for bowel sounds, abdominal tenderness, distention, and vomiting; notify physician immediately if any changes occur.

NURSING DIAGNOSES

- Activity intolerance
- Decreased cardiac output
- High risk for injury
- High risk for fluid volume excess
- High risk for impaired gas exchange
- Altered family processes
- Knowledge deficit

NURSING INTERVENTIONS
Preoperative Care

1. Monitor infant's or child's cardiac status.
   a. Color of mucous membranes and nail beds
   b. Quality and intensity of peripheral pulses
   c. Capillary refill time
   d. Temperatures of extremities
   e. Apical pulse
   f. Blood pressure
   g. Respiratory rate
2. Assist child in understanding in age-appropriate ways (see Appendix J).
3. Provide information and assist parents in understanding child's condition.

Postoperative Care

1. Monitor infant's or child's cardiac status every hour for first 24 to 48 hours, then every 2 to 4 hours.
   a. Apical pulse, respiratory rate, temperature
   b. Arterial blood pressure
   c. Capillary refill time
   d. Blood pressure—hypertension often present initially (no blood pressure present in left arm if subclavian artery used for surgery)
   e. Cardiac arrhythmias
2. Monitor for signs and symptoms of hemorrhage.
   a. Measure chest tube output every hour—greater than 3 to 5 ml indicates problems.
   b. Assess for clot formation in chest tube (increased output of blood followed by an abrupt decrease).

    c. Assess bowel sounds and monitor for abdominal distention.

    d. Assess for bleeding from other sites (e.g., nose, mouth, gastrointestinal tract).

    e. Record strict input and output (refer to institutional procedure manual).

3. Monitor infant's or child's hydration status.

    a. Mucous membranes

    b. Bulging or depressed fontanels

    c. Decreased tearing; dry mouth

    d. Poor skin turgor

    e. Specific gravity (urine will be concentrated immediately after surgery)

    f. Daily weights

    g. Input and output

    h. Fluids—intravenous (IV) at 50% to 75% of maintenance fluids first 24 hours postoperatively

4. Promote optimal respiratory status.

    a. Have child turn, cough, and deep breathe.

    b. Perform chest physiotherapy.

    c. Humidify air.

    d. Monitor for chylothorax (assess breath sounds; note chest tube drainage).

    e. Keep thoracotomy tray at bedside for emergency use.

    f. Monitor chest tube for patency to prevent pneumothorax; keep two chest tube clamps at bedside to prevent pneumothorax if tubing separates.

5. Monitor child's response to medications and blood products.

    a. See the section on medications, this chapter.

    b. Assist with collection of laboratory data.

6. Use no cuff pressure or arterial punctures in left arm if left subclavian flap was performed, because only collateral vessels are providing the arterial circulation.

7. Resume by-mouth feedings slowly; monitor abdominal status.

8. Control hypertension through medications and anxiety relief measures.

9. Relieve postoperative pain: pain adds stress to the suture lines (see Appendix I).

10. Provide age-appropriate diversional activities (see section on growth and development, Appendix B).
11. Provide age-appropriate explanations before treatments and painful procedures (see Appendix J, section on preparation for procedure/surgery).

🏠 Discharge Planning and Home Care

Stress importance of follow-up to screen for residual or premature cardiovascular problems, including the development of calcific aortic stenosis. Antibiotic prophylaxis may be required during infectious periods.

CLIENT OUTCOMES

1. Child will be free of postoperative complications.
2. Child will demonstrate sense of mastery of the surgical experience as evidenced by expression of feelings and resumption of normal activity level.
3. Child will participate in physical activities appropriate for age.

REFERENCES

Foldy S et al: Preoperative nursing care for congenital cardiac defects, *Crit Care Nurs Clin North Am* 1(2):289, 1989.

Gerraughty A: Caring for patients with lesions obstructing systemic blood flow, *Crit Care Nurs Clin North Am* 1(2):231, 1989.

Greenberg S, Balsara R, Faerber E: Coarctation of the aorta: diagnostic imaging after corrective surgery, *J Thorac Imaging* 10(1):36, 1995.

Hazinski M: *Nursing care of the critically ill child,* ed 2, St Louis, 1992, Mosby.

Hellman G, Coaley D, Gutgsell H: *Surgical treatment of congenital heart disease,* Philadelphia, 1987, Lea & Febiger.

O'Brien P et al: Discharge planning for children with heart disease, *Crit Care Nurs Clin North Am* 1(2):297, 1989.

Park M: *Pediatric cardiology for practitioners,* St Louis, 1984, Mosby.

Trinquet F et al: Coarctation of the aorta in infants: which operation? *Ann Thorac Surg* 45(2):186, 1988.

Uzark K et al: Health education needs of adolescents with congenital heart disease, *J Pediatr Health Care* 3(3):137, 1989.

Zehr K et al: Repair of coarctation of the aorta in neonates and infants: a thirty-year experience, *Ann Thorac Surg* 59(1):33, 1995.

15

Congenital Dislocation of the Hip

PATHOPHYSIOLOGY

Congenital dislocation of the hip is an orthopedic deformity that is acquired immediately before or at birth.

The condition ranges from minimal lateral displacement to complete dislocation of the femoral head out of the acetabulum.

There are three patterns seen: (1) subluxation—femoral head rests in acetabulum and can be partially dislocated by examination; (2) dislocatable—hip can be dislocated fully with manipulation but is located normally when infant is at rest; and (3) dislocated—hip rests in a dislocated position (most severe).

In newborns, the condition is not evident because the deformity of both the femoral head and the acetabulum is minimal and the soft tissue is not contracted. Most dislocated hips in the newborn are minimally unstable; 60% spontaneously stabilize during the first few weeks of life.

INCIDENCE

1. Congenital dislocation of the hip occurs once in 1000 births.
2. Female-male ratio is 7:1.
3. Incidence increases with breech delivery.
4. Increased incidence is evident among siblings of affected children.
5. Left hip is affected more often than right hip.

6. There is frequent association with other conditions, such as spina bifida.
7. Increased incidence occurs in Canadian Eskimos and certain American Indian groups that swaddle children in cradle boards during first few months of life.

CLINICAL MANIFESTATIONS
Infants

1. Possibly no symptoms evident because infant may have minimal displacement of femur
2. Asymmetrical gluteal folds (prone position)
3. Shortening of limb on affected side
4. Restricted abduction of hip on affected side
5. Positive Galeazzi's sign (see box)
6. Positive Barlow's maneuver (see box)
7. Positive Ortolani's maneuver (see box)

Toddlers and Older Children

1. Waddling gait (bilateral dislocation of the hip)
2. Leaning to side of body that bears weight
3. Increased lumbar lordosis during standing (bilateral dislocation of hip)
4. Affected leg shorter than other
5. Trendelenburg sign (see box)

COMPLICATIONS

1. Persistent dysplasia
2. Recurrent dislocation
3. Iatrogenic avascular necrosis of femoral head

LABORATORY AND DIAGNOSTIC TESTS

An anteroposterior pelvic roentgenogram is obtained (assesses extent of femoral displacement or dislocation; not useful for infants less than 1 month old).

MEDICAL MANAGEMENT

Treatment varies with the severity of the clinical manifestations and the child's age. If the dislocation is corrected in the first few days to weeks of life, the dysplasia is com-

Assessment Criteria

Ortolani's Maneuver

Fingers are placed over greater trochanter as thigh is abducted and lifted toward acetabulum. A click is heard in infants less than 3 months of age, and a jerk is felt in older infants and children.

Barlow's Maneuver

Hand is placed over knee. Leg is adducted past midline and outward. Positive sign is a sensation of abnormal movement.

Galeazzi's Sign

Flexing both hips at 90-degree angle results in one knee being below the level of the other.

Trendelenburg Test

When child stands on leg of affected side, the opposite hip slants downward instead of remaining level.

pletely reversible and a normal hip will develop. During the neonatal period, positioning and maintaining the hip in flexion and abduction is achieved with the use of a corrective device. Between the ages of 2 months and 12 to 18 months, traction followed by either open or closed reduction (depending upon whether or not contracture of the adductor muscles and displacement of the femoral head have occurred) and hip spica casting is used.

NURSING ASSESSMENT

1. See the section on musculoskeletal assessment in Appendix A.
2. See the assessment criteria in the box on p. 89.
3. Assess for signs of skin irritation.
4. Assess child's response to traction and immobilization in spica cast.
5. Postoperatively, assess vital signs and signs of wound drainage.
6. Assess child's developmental level.
7. Assess parents' ability to manage home care for spica cast.

NURSING DIAGNOSES

- Impaired physical mobility
- High risk for injury
- High risk for impaired skin integrity
- High risk for altered growth and development
- Knowledge deficit

NURSING INTERVENTIONS

Instruct parents on maintenance and care of corrective device.

1. Pavlik harness (maintains hip flexion)
   a. Maintain harness (on continuously for 3 to 6 months).
   b. Perform skin care (lubricant and sponge bath).
   c. Change diapers frequently.
2. Abduction brace (maintains hip in abducted and fixed position)
   a. Perform skin care.
   b. Monitor for signs of skin irritation.
   c. Change diapers frequently (to prevent skin breakdown and to maintain clean brace).

   If conservative treatment is unsuccessful or if condition is diagnosed after infant is 3 months of age, he or she may be treated first with traction (4 to 6 months) followed by open or closed reduction (as indicated) and then a spica cast.

1. Monitor child's response to traction (2 to 3 weeks).
2. Monitor child's response to spica cast immobilization.

If open reduction is performed, do the following:

1. Prepare child and parents for surgery (see Appendix J, section on preparation for procedure/surgery).
   a. Provide information about presurgical routine.
   b. Reinforce information given about surgery and open reduction.
2. Monitor child's response postoperatively.
   a. Monitor vital signs every 2 hours until stable, then every 4 hours.
   b. Monitor for signs of drainage on cast.
   c. Perform circulation checks every hour during the immediate postoperative period, then every 4 hours.
3. Provide pain relief measures as necessary.
   a. Provide tactile comfort and holding.
   b. Administer analgesics.

♠ Discharge Planning and Home Care

1. Instruct parents on applying and maintaining the correction device (see section on nursing interventions this chapter).
2. Instruct parents on care of spica cast.
   a. Apply waterproof material to cast edges (pedal cast edges) in perineal area; change diaper often.
   b. Keep skin clean and dry under cast every day.
   c. Check for signs of infection and pressure (e.g., musty odor and reddened area).
   d. Monitor for small items placed in cast (e.g., food and small toys).
3. Instruct parents on appropriate feeding techniques.
   a. Feed infant in supine position.
   b. Child can be held in parent's arm or propped with pillows.
4. Instruct parents to provide age-appropriate stimulating activities (see section on growth and development, Appendix B).
5. Instruct parents on needed car seat modifications.

CLIENT OUTCOMES

1. Infant's or child's hip remains in desired position.
2. Infant or child has intact skin without redness or breakdowns.

3. Parents demonstrate care activities to accommodate the infant's or child's corrective device or hip spica cast.

REFERENCES

Corbett D: Information needs of parents of a child in a Pavlik harness, *Othopaed Nurs* 7(2):20, 1988.

Eilert RE, Georgopoulos G: Orthopedics. In Hay WW et al, editors: *Current pediatric diagnosis and treatment,* ed 12, East Norwalk, Conn, 1995, Appleton & Lange.

Mott SR, James SR, Sperhac AR: *Nursing care of children and families,* ed 2, Menlo Park, Calif, 1990, Addison-Wesley.

Sponsuler P: Bone, joint, and muscle problems. In Oske F et al, editors: *Principles and practice of pediatrics,* ed 2, Philadelphia, 1994, JB Lippincott.

16

Congestive Heart Failure

PATHOPHYSIOLOGY

Congestive heart failure (CHF) occurs when the heart cannot pump the blood returning to the right side of the heart, or provide adequate circulation to meet the needs of organs and tissues in the body. The components of CHF include preload and circulating volume, afterload, and contractility. Causes include the following:

1. High output state, usually related to congenital heart diseases where there is increased pulmonary blood flow returning to the right side of the heart and, subsequently, lungs; common defects producing this volume overload are patent ductus arteriosus and ventricular septal defect.

2. Low output state, related to (1) congenital heart diseases where there are left-side heart obstructions causing the heart to pump harder to bypass the restrictive area, such as with coarctation of the aorta or aortic valve stenosis, (2) a primary heart muscle disease, as in the cardiomyopathies, or (3) rhythm disturbances, either tachycardia or bradycardia dysrhythmias.

If the heart fails for any reason and cardiac output is not sufficient to respond to the metabolic needs of the body, the sympathetic nervous system responds by trying to increase circulating blood volume by diverting blood from nonessential organs, which decreases renal blood flow, activates the renin-angiotensin-aldosterone mechanism, and increases sodium and water retention. Catecholamine release with decreased cardiac output causes increased heart rate, increased vascular tone, and sweating. These initial compensatory mechanisms (increased circulating blood volume, increased heart rate, and vascular tone) for maintaining cardiac output eventually lead to clinical manifestations of CHF.

INCIDENCE

1. Ninety percent of infants with congenital heart defects develop CHF within the first year of life.
2. The majority of affected infants manifest symptoms within the first few months of life.

CLINICAL MANIFESTATIONS

1. Tachycardia
2. Cardiomegaly
3. Increased respiratory effort
4. Tachypnea
5. Hepatomegaly
6. Edema
7. Diaphoresis
8. Feeding difficulty and poor weight gain
9. Irritability

COMPLICATIONS

Low cardiac output syndrome refractory to the use of medications may develop.

LABORATORY AND DIAGNOSTIC TESTS

Diagnosis is made on the basis of physical examination with manifestation of signs and symptoms previously noted. The following can assist in further evaluation:

1. Electrocardiogram (ECG)—for diagnosis of tachycardia or bradycardia dysrhythmias (a 12-lead ECG may show ventricular hypertrophy)
2. Chest x-ray—heart size will be enlarged and pulmonary infiltrates will be present
3. Echocardiogram
4. Cardiac catheterization

MEDICAL MANAGEMENT

The initial management of CHF is accomplished by the use of pharmacologic agents that act to improve the function of the heart muscle and/or reduce the work load on the heart. Digitalis is given to increase cardiac output by slowing the A-V note to make each contraction stronger. Diuretics decrease preload volume as their actions result in decreased extracellular fluid volume. Venous, arteriolar, and mixed dilators may be given to decrease preload volume by reducing systemic or pulmonary vascular resistance. Fluids are usually restricted to two thirds of maintenance levels, and attention is given to nutrition and rest. Medical management continues with the plan for interventional cardiac catheterization or surgical intervention if indicated.

NURSING ASSESSMENT

1. See the section on cardiovascular and respiratory assessment in Appendix A.
2. Assess activity level.
3. Assess extremities for edema.
4. Assess feeding pattern and weight gain history.
5. Assess family coping patterns.

NURSING DIAGNOSES

- Decreased cardiac output
- Ineffective breathing pattern
- Activity intolerance
- Fluid volume excess
- Altered nutrition: less than body requirements
- Knowledge deficit
- Altered family processes

NURSING INTERVENTIONS

1. Promote cardiac output.
   a. Continue cardiovascular assessments, including vital signs, pulses, color, capillary refill, and lung sounds.
   b. Administer medications with assessment and recording of effects.

2. Promote oxygenation and ventilation.
    a. Maintain patent airway and assess effect of oxygen if provided.
    b. Elevate head of bed or place infant in infant seat to prevent systemic venous return.
3. Provide rest and comfort measures.
    a. Maintain a quiet environment with quick response to crying infant or child.
    b. Swaddle infants.
    c. Provide a neutral thermal environment, maintaining constant temperature for least oxygen consumption.
    d. Schedule activities to provide extended rest periods.
4. Promote and maintain child's fluid and electrolyte balance.
    a. Assess intake and output.
    b. Assess edema.
    c. Measure and record child's daily weight.
    d. Restrict fluids, usually, to two thirds of maintenance fluid levels.
    e. Follow potassium levels closely if child is on diuretics.
5. Promote child's nutritional status.
    a. Assess and record infant's tolerance of and response to feedings.
    b. Provide small frequent feedings for conservation of energy.
    c. Collaborate with nutrition services for optimal diet for maximal calories and minimal fluids.
6. Assist family in understanding, accepting, and working through emotions of having a child with a chronic condition.

♠ Discharge Planning and Home Care
1. Educate on specific condition.
2. Provide specific instructions about medications and adverse effects.
3. Although caregivers of infants with chronic CHF are usually quite skilled in assessing for signs and symptoms of CHF, reinforce as necessary.

4. Instruct in feeding techniques and nutritional requirements.
5. Refer as indicated for infant stimulation programs or parent support groups.

CLIENT OUTCOMES

1. Child will have adequate cardiac output.
2. Child will have normal growth and development.
3. Caregivers will demonstrate ability to handle all facets of infant's home care.

REFERENCES

Baker LK, Alyn IB: Pharmacologic manipulation of preload, afterload, and contractility in the young, *J Cardiovasc Nurs* 6(3):12, 1992.

Hazinski MF: *Nursing care of the critically ill child,* ed 3, St Louis, 1996, Mosby.

Jensen C, Hill CS: Mechanical support for congestive heart failure in infants and children, *Crit Care Nurs Clin North Am* 6(1):165, 1994.

Monaco MP, Gay WM: *Moller and Neals' fetal, neonatal, and infant cardiac disease,* East Norwalk, Conn, 1990, Appleton & Lange.

Werner NP: Congestive heart failure: pathophysiology and management throughout infancy, *J Perinat Neonat Nurs* 7(3):59, 1993.

17

Croup

PATHOPHYSIOLOGY

Croup, or acute laryngotracheobronchitis, is a viral infection that affects the larynx and the trachea. Subglottic edema with upper respiratory tract obstruction results, accompanied by thick secretions. Children are susceptible to airway obstruction because the diameter of the subglottic area is narrow. Croup is caused by any virus associated with upper respiratory tract infection. Causative agents include parainfluenza virus types 1, 2, and 3; respiratory syncytial virus (RSV); influenza virus types A_1, A_2, and B; adenovirus; and rhinovirus. Onset occurs after 12 to 72 hours of coughing. Coryza is often accompanied by a low-grade fever.

Spasmodic croup is a sudden attack of croup, which usually occurs during the night and can be associated with an upper respiratory tract infection, fever, or allergies. This type of attack is of a recurrent nature. Mortality rate is 1%.

INCIDENCE

1. Incidence is seasonal—higher in late fall and early winter.
2. Incidence is higher in boys.
3. Age range of occurrence is 3 months to 3 years; peak age of onset is 9 to 18 months.
4. Significant airway obstruction develops in one of every 20 children.

5. Incidence is higher in areas with increased atmospheric pollution and/or rapid atmospheric changes in humidity.
6. There is reoccurrence in 5% of affected children.

CLINICAL MANIFESTATIONS
Initial Phase

1. Persistent, brassy, barking cough that worsens
2. A cold that lasts for 1 to 2 days
3. Rhinorrhea accompanied by low-grade fever
4. Stridor (progression of stridor is an indicator of the severity of the disease)
5. Hoarse cry

Acute Phase

1. Stridor at rest
2. Retractions at rest
3. Nasal flaring
4. Tachypnea (respiratory rate greater than 60 breaths per minute)
5. Often, dehydration
6. Agitation and restlessness
7. Listlessness
8. Decrease in stridor and retractions without clinical improvement
9. Cyanosis (rare)

COMPLICATION

Potential respiratory failure resulting from airway obstruction is the main complication of croup.

LABORATORY AND DIAGNOSTIC TESTS

1. Arterial blood gas values—normal to decreased pH, decreased PaO_2, increased $PaCO_2$
2. Throat culture
3. Chest x-ray
4. Lateral neck x-ray examination—pencil/steeple sign; also to rule out epiglottitis and foreign bodies
5. Complete blood count—normal

MEDICAL MANAGEMENT

When a child with suspected croup is presented at the hospital, supplemental humidified oxygen is given as indicated by the child's appearance and results of blood gases, vital signs, and pulse oximetry. A mixture of helium and oxygen (usually 70:30) might also be used because helium is a light gas and can move more easily through the narrowed airways carrying the oxygen along. The child can be treated with bronchodilators, usually racemic epinephrine. The use of corticosteroids and antibiotics is controversial in the treatment of croup but not uncommon. The treatment of croup is mostly supportive, but if the child does not respond, an artificial airway may be indicated to support the child until the airway inflammation subsides. Intravenous fluids may also be indicated, depending on the child's hydration status.

NURSING ASSESSMENT

1. See the section on respiratory assessment in Appendix A.
2. Assess oxygenation status—blood gas values, pulse oximetry, increased respiratory distress.
3. Assess hydration status.
4. Assess child and parent anxiety level.

NURSING DIAGNOSES

- Potential for ineffective breathing pattern
- Potential for ineffective airway clearance
- Fluid volume deficit
- Anxiety

NURSING INTERVENTIONS

1. Monitor respiratory status (vital signs—use of accessory muscles, position, arterial blood gas values, color, pulse oximetry).
2. Report signs of increased respiratory distress such as increased respiratory rate, labored breathing, wheezing, stridor, intercostal retractions, and circumoral cyanosis.
3. Allow child to maintain a position of comfort.

4. Monitor and observe effects of oxygen therapy (intermittent positive pressure breathing [IPPB] with racemic epinephrine, mist tent with humidified oxygen).
    a. Quality of respiratory effort (see number 2)
    b. Arterial blood gas values—within normal limits
5. Encourage oral feedings.
6. Monitor action and side effects of medications.
    a. Bronchodilators (i.e., racemic epinephrine)
    b. Corticosteroids—for antiinflammatory properties
    c. Antibiotics—if a secondary bacterial infection is present
7. Provide age-appropriate quiet play and recreational activities (see section on growth and development, Appendix B).
8. Provide for child's developmental needs during hospitalization.
    a. Encourage contact with siblings and parents.
    b. Incorporate home routines into hospital stay (e.g., feeding practices, night routine).
9. Provide emotional support to family.
    a. Encourage ventilation of concerns.
    b. Refer to social service person.
    c. Provide for physical comforts (e.g., place to sleep and bathe).
    d. Provide explanations before performing procedures.

♠ Discharge Planning and Home Care

Instruct parents about home management.
1. Use of humidifiers (including use of shower)
2. Signs of secondary infection (increased temperature, signs of a cold or respiratory infection)
3. Administration of medications (see section on medical management, this chapter)
4. Infection control
    a. Avoid large groups of people.
    b. Avoid cold temperatures.

CLIENT OUTCOMES

1. Child will return to normal respiratory function.
2. Child will be hydrated adequately.

3. Child and/or family demonstrate understanding of home care and follow-up.

REFERENCES

Gomberg SM: Mistaken identity . . . is it epiglottitis or croup? *Pediatr Nurs* 16(6):567, 1990.

Hazinski MF, editor: *Nursing care of the critically ill child*, St Louis, 1992, Mosby.

Soler M, Eldadah M: Croup in older children, *Clin Pediatr* 29(10):581, 1990.

Wong DL, editor: *Essentials of pediatric nursing*, St Louis, 1993, Mosby.

18

Cystic Fibrosis

PATHOPHYSIOLOGY

Cystic fibrosis (CF) is inherited as an autosomal-recessive trait due to a mutation of the CF gene on chromosome 7. The disorder affects the exocrine glands, causing the production of viscous mucus leading to obstruction of the small passageways of the bronchi, the small intestine, and the pancreatic and bile ducts. The effects of this biochemical defect on the involved organs are as follows:

1. Pancreas
   a. Degeneration and fibrosis of acini occur.
   b. Secretion of pancreatic enzymes is inhibited, causing impaired absorption of fats, proteins, and, to a limited degree, carbohydrates.
2. Small intestine—absence of pancreatic enzymes (trypsin, amylase, lipase) causes impaired absorption of fats and proteins, resulting in steatorrhea and azotorrhea
3. Liver—biliary obstruction, fibrosis
4. Lungs
   a. Bronchial and bronchiolar obstruction from excessive pooling of secretions causes generalized hyperinflation and atelectasis.
   b. Pooled mucous secretions increase the susceptibility to bacterial infections (*Pseudomonas aeruginosa* and *Staphylococcus aureus* are the predominant organisms found in sputum and lungs).

    c. Altered oxygen and carbon dioxide exchange can cause varying degrees of hypoxia, hypercapnia, and acidosis.

    d. Fibrotic lung changes occur, and, in severe cases, pulmonary hypertension and cor pulmonale can occur.

5. Skeleton
   a. Growth and onset of puberty are retarded.
   b. Retardation of skeletal maturation results in delayed bone aging and shortness of stature (38% to 42% of children with cystic fibrosis).

6. Reproductive organs
   a. Female—late menses; possible infertility because of thickness of cervical mucus
   b. Male—vas deferens often absent; sterility but not impotency

INCIDENCE

1. Cystic fibrosis affects one in 2000 white infants each year.
2. It affects one in 17,000 African American infants each year.
3. It rarely affects infants of Asian descent.
4. Odds are one in four (25%) that each subsequent pregnancy after birth of child with cystic fibrosis will result in child with cystic fibrosis.
5. Cystic fibrosis affects male and female individuals equally.
6. Symptoms vary greatly, resulting in variable life span—95% survival rate to age 16, 50% to age 28.
7. Length and quality of life have greatly increased in recent years, but disease is ultimately terminal.

CLINICAL MANIFESTATIONS

1. Dry, nonproductive cough initially, changing to loose and productive
2. Viscous sputum, increasing in amount, with yellow-gray color normally and greenish color during infection
3. Wheezy respirations, moist crackles
4. Cyanosis (late sign)
5. Clubbed fingers and toes

6. Increased anteroposterior diameter of chest
7. Steatorrhea
8. Bulky, loose, foul-smelling stools
9. Distended abdomen
10. Thin extremities
11. Failure to thrive (below norms for height and weight despite large food intake)
12. Meconium ileus (infants)
13. Profuse sweating in warm temperature
14. Salty-tasting skin
15. Excessive loss of sodium and chloride

COMPLICATIONS

Pulmonary complications include emphysema, pneumothorax, pneumonia, bronchiectasis, hemoptysis, cor pulmonale, and respiratory failure.

Gastrointestinal complications include cirrhosis, portal hypertension, esophageal varices, fecal impactions, enlarged spleen, intussusception, cholelithiasis, pancreatitis, and rectal prolapse.

Endocrine complications include diabetes mellitus and heat prostration.

LABORATORY AND DIAGNOSTIC TESTS

1. Sweat test—to measure concentration of sodium and chloride in sweat; most definitive diagnostic test; not reliable for newborns less than 1 month old (two positive sweat tests are diagnostic; greater than 60 mEq/L, positive for CF)
2. Pulmonary function testing—used as diagnostic test to identify disease, to assess severity and degree of condition, and to determine therapy
3. Genetic blood testing for cystic fibrosis marker
4. Chest x-ray study—for evaluation of pulmonary complications

MEDICAL MANAGEMENT

The child with symptoms of CF is hospitalized for the diagnostic workup, initiation of treatment, clearing of any respiratory tract infection symptoms, and education of the child and family. The goal of this hospitalization is to stabilize the child's condition so that care can be managed for long periods at home.

Antibiotics are given based on the suspected organisms, sensitivity to antibiotics, severity of infection, and child's response to therapy. The course of therapy is usually at least 14 days. After the initial admission, when respiratory tract infections are not responsive to intensive home treatment measures or oral antibiotics, the child may either be readmitted for intravenous (IV) antibiotics or have home IV antibiotic therapy.

Pulmonary toilet includes adequate hydration to loosen secretions, and chest percussion and postural drainage to clear mucus from the small airways. Aerosol generators may be used to administer normal saline, bronchodilators (such as albuterol or other β-agonist drugs), antibiotics, and sometimes mucolytics. Some bronchodilators are administered through a metered dose inhaler with or without a spacer. Intermittent positive pressure breathing does not improve drug delivery and may aggravate the pulmonary status. Mist tents are no longer used because they may provide a medium for bacterial growth.

Pancreatic enzyme supplements are given with meals and snacks; dosages are individualized for the child and generally increase as the child gets older. Supplements of fat-soluble vitamins (A, D, and E) are needed in greater than the normal dose because they are not well absorbed. Vitamin K supplementation may be needed by the infant or if there is hemoptysis or surgery. Diet is modified to increase the number of calories provided (up to 150% more than the normal needs based on age, weight, and activity). High levels of protein and normal amounts of fat (about 30%) should be included in the child's diet.

Lung or heart-lung transplantation may be an option for the child with poor quality of life and decreasing exercise tolerance who has chronic respiratory failure and a life expectancy of less than a year. Specific criteria for transplantation vary from institution to institution. The child with CF who undergoes transplantation is at risk for the same complications as other children (effects of immunosuppression, infection, acute rejection, and bronchiolitis obliterans). In addition, due to cystic fibrosis, such a child may also have malabsorption of the immunosuppressive agents.

NURSING ASSESSMENT

1. See the section on respiratory and gastrointestinal tract assessment in Appendix A.
2. Assess amount of sputum production, and its color and characteristics.
3. Assess activity level.
4. Assess height and weight for age of child.

NURSING DIAGNOSES

- Ineffective airway clearance
- High risk for activity intolerance
- Altered nutrition: less than body requirements
- High risk for infection
- High risk for ineffective family coping
- Altered growth and development

NURSING INTERVENTIONS

1. Monitor respiratory status and report any significant changes (respiratory rate, presence of intercostal retractions, presence of cyanosis, and color and amount of sputum).
2. Monitor effects of aerosolized treatment (performed before postural drainage).
3. Administer and evaluate effects of postural drainage and percussion.
4. Administer and monitor side effects and actions of medications.
   a. Antibiotics
   b. Pancreatic enzymes
   c. Fat-soluble vitamins
   d. Bronchodilators
5. Teach and supervise breathing exercises (exhalation, inhalation, and coughing), although these are not a substitute for percussion and postural drainage.
6. Encourage physical activity as condition permits.

7. Obtain baseline information about dietary habits (food preferences, dislikes, eating attitudes, developmental abilities).
8. Monitor and record characteristics of stool (color, consistency, size, frequency).
9. Promote nutritional status.
   a. Administer high-protein, high-calorie, normal-fat diet.
   b. Administer supplemental fat-soluble vitamins.
   c. Administer pancreatic enzymes before meals and snacks.
   d. Assess need for supplemental protein formula.
10. Observe and report signs of complications (see section on complications, this chapter).
11. Provide emotional support to patient and parents during hospitalization.
12. Provide guidance related to independence, self-care, sexuality, and educational planning as the adolescent undergoes transition to adulthood.

🏠 Discharge Planning and Home Care

1. Instruct parents and child about techniques of home management.
   a. Dietary needs
   b. Postural drainage and percussion
   c. Aerosol treatments
   d. Breathing exercises
   e. Administration of medications
   f. Avoiding exposure to respiratory tract infections
   g. Management of constipation or diarrhea
2. Monitor family's compliance with home management.
   a. Monitor child's clinical course.
   b. Monitor frequency of hospital admissions.
   c. Assess family's level of knowledge.
3. Assist family in contacting support systems for financial, psychologic, and medical assistance (e.g., Cystic Fibrosis Foundation).
4. Provide genetic counseling.
5. Immunize annually against influenza.

CLIENT OUTCOMES

1. Child's ability to clear the airway will improve.
2. Child will gain weight.
3. Parents administer home care regimen and provide for medical follow-up.

REFERENCES

Baker KL, Coe LM: Growing up with a chronic condition: transition to young adulthood for the individual with cystic fibrosis, *Holist Nurs Pract* 8(1):8, 1993.

Browning I, D'Alonzo G, Tobin M: Importance of respiratory rate as an indicator of respiratory dysfunction in patients with cystic fibrosis, *Chest* 97(6):1317, 1990.

Fernbach SD, Thomson EJ: Molecular genetic technology in cystic fibrosis: implications for nursing practice, *J Pediatr Nurs* 7(1):20, 1992.

Kuhn RJ, Horn L: Pancreatic enzyme therapy in patients with cystic fibrosis: the high dose lipase issue, *Pediatr Nurs* 20(6):623, 1994.

Maynard LC: Pediatric heart-lung transplantation for cystic fibrosis, *Heart Lung* 23(4):279, 1994.

Rushton CH: Cystic fibrosis and the pediatric caregiver: benefits and burdens of genetic technology, *Pediatr Nurs* 21:57, 1995.

19

Cytomegaloviral Infection

PATHOPHYSIOLOGY

Cytomegalovirus (CMV) is the leading cause of congenital viral infections in North America. A number of related strains of CMV exist; the virus is a member of the herpes family. CMV is probably transmitted through direct person-to-person contact with body fluids or tissues, including urine, blood, saliva, cervical secretions, semen, and breast milk. The period of incubation is unknown; the following are estimated incubation periods: after delivery—3 to 12 weeks; after transfusion—3 to 12 weeks; and after transplant—4 weeks to 4 months. The urine often contains CMV from months to years after infection. The virus can remain dormant in individuals and be reactivated. Currently, no immunizations exist to prevent its occurrence.

Three types of CMV exist.

1. Congenital—acquired transplacentally in utero. Approximately 40% of infants born to women experiencing a primary (first) CMV illness during pregnancy will be infected. The most severe form of this infection is cytomegalic inclusion disease.
2. Acute-acquired—acquired anytime during or after birth through adulthood. Symptoms resemble those of mononucleosis (malaise, fever, pharyngitis, splenomegaly, petechial rash, respiratory symptoms). Infection is not without sequelae, especially in young children, and can result from transfusions.

3. Generalized systemic disease—occurs in individuals who are immunosuppressed, especially if they have undergone organ transplantation. Symptoms include pneumonitis, hepatitis, and leukopenia, which can occasionally be fatal. Previous infection does not produce immunity and may result in reactivation of the virus.

INCIDENCE

1. Of live births, 0.5% to 2% have congenital infection.
2. Premature infants are affected more often than full-term infants.
3. Ten percent of infected infants are symptomatic at birth; by 2 years of age another 10% develop serious sequelae (e.g., deafness or ocular abnormalities).
4. Twenty-five percent of infants are symptomatic at birth and die by 3 months of age; the remaining 60% to 75% will have some form of intellectual impairment or developmental delays. Approximately 10% will be normal in late childhood.
5. Sixty percent of adult women are seropositive.
6. Incidence is higher in lower socioeconomic groups.

CLINICAL MANIFESTATIONS

In the newborn period, an infant infected with the cytomegalovirus is usually asymptomatic. Onset of congenitally acquired infection can occur immediately after birth or at up to 12 weeks of age.

There are no predictable indicators, but the following symptoms are common:

1. Petechiae and ecchymoses
2. Hepatosplenomegaly
3. Neonatal jaundice; direct hyperbilirubinemia
4. Microcephaly with periventricular calcifications
5. Intrauterine growth retardation
6. Prematurity
7. Small size for gestational age

Other symptoms can occur in the newborn or older child:

1. Purpura
2. Hearing loss
3. Chorioretinitis; blindness

4. Fever
5. Pneumonia
6. Tachypnea and dyspnea
7. Brain damage

COMPLICATIONS

1. Variable hearing loss
2. Lower intelligence quotient (IQ)
3. Visual impairment
4. Microcephaly
5. Sensorineural handicaps

LABORATORY AND DIAGNOSTIC TESTS

1. Viral cultures from urine, pharyngeal secretions, and peripheral leukocytes
2. Microscopic examination of urinary sediment, body fluids, and tissues for the virus in large quantities (examining urine for intranuclear inclusions is not helpful; verification of congenital infection must be accomplished within the first 3 weeks of life)
3. Toxoplasmosis, other, rubella, cytomegalovirus, and herpes (TORCH) screen—used to assess presence of other viruses
4. Serologic tests
   a. IgG and IgM antibody titers (elevated IgM level indicates exposure to virus; elevated neonatal IgG indicates prenatally acquired infection; negative maternal IgG and positive neonatal IgG indicate postnatal acquisition)
   b. Positive rheumatoid factor test (is positive in 35% to 45% of cases)
5. Radiologic studies—skull x-ray films or computed tomography scans of the head used to reveal intracranial calcifications

MEDICAL MANAGEMENT

Only symptomatic relief is available at this time (e.g., fever management, transfusions for anemia, respiratory support). Some evidence exists that CMV-immune globulin given intravenously in combination with the drug ganciclovir can reduce the severity of an infection in immunocompromised individuals. A live CMV vaccine is being tested on renal transplant patients. Chemotherapy offers some promise, but toxicity and immunosuppression associated with these drugs raise concerns about their use in newborns. No special precautions are necessary. However, caregivers should wear gloves and employ good hand-washing techniques and use universal precautions.

NURSING ASSESSMENT

1. See the section on respiratory and neurologic assessment in Appendix A.
2. Assess nutritional status.
3. Assess developmental level.
4. Assess for history of impaired vision and hearing.

NURSING DIAGNOSES

- High risk for infection
- Altered nutrition: less than body requirements
- Altered growth and development
- Sensory/perceptual alteration
- High risk for impaired home maintenance management

NURSING INTERVENTIONS

1. Monitor action and side effects of medications.
2. Monitor response to and side effects of blood transfusions.
3. Assess age and developmental level.
4. Weigh child upon admission and daily.
5. Monitor urine and serum electrolytes and glucose as needed.
6. Provide age-appropriate stimulation.
7. Review and reinforce with parents the importance of maintaining adequate caloric intake.
8. Promote process of attachment between parents and infant.
9. Identify community resources that may be helpful in dealing with long-term sequelae.

🏠 Discharge Planning and Home Care

1. Instruct parents about methods to prevent spread of infection.
    a. Advise parents of possibility that virus is secreted for more than a year.

b. Pregnant friends should not perform child care (e.g., changing the child's diapers).

c. Care should be taken to perform thorough hand washing after each diaper change and to dispose of diapers properly.

2. Instruct parents about long-term management of condition.

a. Reinforce information about virus.

b. If neurologic, cognitive, or developmental sequelae are evident, refer to community-based services.

c. Emphasize importance of medical monitoring after acute episode.

Sequelae will necessitate further interventions beyond the scope of this section.

CLIENT OUTCOMES

1. Child will have consistent weight gain.
2. Child will have a maximized level of developmental functioning.
3. Parents will verbalize an understanding of the child's condition, home care, and follow-up needs.

REFERENCES

American Academy of Pediatrics: *Report of the committee on infectious diseases (the red book)*, Evanston, Ill, 1991, The Academy.

Boppanna SB et al: Symptomatic congenital cytomegalovirus infection: neonatal morbidity and mortality, *Pediatr Infect Dis J* 11:93, 1992.

Sessions CF: Viral infections of the fetus and newborn. In Taeusch H et al, editors: *Schaeffer's diseases of the newborn*, ed 6, Philadelphia, 1991, WB Saunders.

Stagno S: Cytomegalovirus. In Remington JS, Klein JO, editors: *Infectious diseases of the fetus and newborn infant*, ed 3, Philadelphia, 1990, WB Saunders.

20

Diabetes Mellitus: Insulin-Dependent (Type I)

PATHOPHYSIOLOGY

Insulin-dependent diabetes mellitus (IDDM), or juvenile-onset diabetes, is caused by a negligible or completely lacking secretory capacity of the beta cells of the pancreas, resulting in insulin deficiency. Complete insulin deficiency necessitates the use of exogenous insulin to promote appropriate glucose use and to prevent complications related to elevated glucose levels, such as diabetic ketoacidosis (DKA) and death. Insulin is necessary for the following physiologic functions: (1) to promote the use and storage of glucose in the liver, muscles, and adipose tissue for energy; (2) to inhibit and stimulate glycogenolysis or gluconeogenesis, depending on the body's requirements; and (3) to promote the use of fatty acids and ketones in cardiac and skeletal muscles. Insulin deficiency results in unrestricted glucose production without appropriate use, resulting in hyperglycemia and increased lipolysis and production of ketones, and, in turn, resulting in lipemia, ketonemia, and ketonuria. The insulin deficiency also heightens the effects of the counterregulatory hormones—epinephrine, glucagon, cortisol, and growth hormone (refer to the box on p. 116 for the hormones' functions). Diagnosis of insulin-dependent diabetes mellitus is based on the patient's clinical history, lab work, and initial symptoms. The cause is unknown, although it is widely accepted that the presence of human lymphocyte antigens (HLA) is associated with

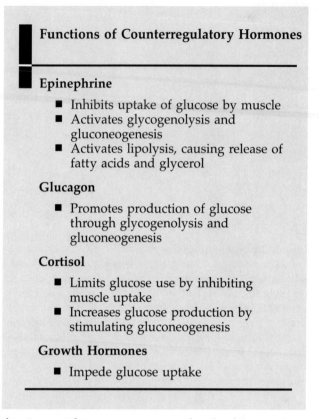

Functions of Counterregulatory Hormones

Epinephrine

- Inhibits uptake of glucose by muscle
- Activates glycogenolysis and gluconeogenesis
- Activates lipolysis, causing release of fatty acids and glycerol

Glucagon

- Promotes production of glucose through glycogenolysis and gluconeogenesis

Cortisol

- Limits glucose use by inhibiting muscle uptake
- Increases glucose production by stimulating gluconeogenesis

Growth Hormones

- Impede glucose uptake

this disease. This presence suggests that the child may have a predisposition to a genetic defect in his or her immunologic response system, resulting in the destruction of pancreatic beta cells. Another relationship suggests that infection serves as a trigger (e.g., Coxsackie virus).

INCIDENCE

1. Fifteen percent of all diabetic individuals have insulin-dependent diabetes mellitus.
2. Ninety-seven percent of newly diagnosed juvenile diabetic patients have insulin-dependent diabetes mellitus.
3. Mean age of onset is 11 years in girls and 12.5 years in boys.

4. Among preschool-age children, the disease is more commonly diagnosed in boys.
5. Among children 5 to 10 years of age, the disease is more commonly diagnosed in girls.
6. The disease is diagnosed more often in winter than in summer.
7. Diabetic ketoacidosis is a frequent cause of morbidity and sometimes of death.
8. Age ranges of peak incidence are 5 to 7 years and puberty.

CLINICAL MANIFESTATIONS
Initial Effects

1. Polyuria
2. Polydipsia
3. Polyphagia
4. Yeast infections in girls
5. Recent weight loss (during a period of less than 3 weeks)
6. Fruity breath odor
7. Dehydration (usually 10% dehydrated)
8. Diabetic ketoacidosis (see the box on p. 119)—hyperglycemia, ketonemia, ketonuria, metabolic acidosis, Kussmaul respirations
9. Abdominal pain
10. Change in level of consciousness (due to progressive dehydration, acidosis, and hyperosmolality resulting in decreased cerebral oxygenation)

Long-Term Effects

1. Failure to grow at normal rate and delayed maturation
2. Neuropathy
3. Recurrent infection
4. Retinal and/or renal microvascular disease
5. Ischemic heart disease or arterial obstruction

COMPLICATIONS

1. Diabetic ketoacidosis
2. Coma
3. Hypokalemia and hyperkalemia
4. Hypocalcemia

5. Hypoglycemia
6. Osteopenia
7. Limited joint mobility
8. Microvascular changes resulting in retinopathy (maintaining a high degree of metabolic control is associated with delay and possible prevention of microvascular changes)
9. Myocardial infarction
10. Thromboemboli
11. Overwhelming infections

LABORATORY AND DIAGNOSTIC TESTS

1. Initial serum blood glucose—300 mg/dl and higher
2. Serum ketones—greater than 3 mM/L
3. Serum pH—less than 7.3
4. Serum $NaHCO_3$—less than 15 mEq/L
5. Fasting blood glucose—venous plasma greater than or equal to 140 mg/dl; venous blood greater than or equal to 120 mg/dl; capillary blood greater than or equal to 120 mg/dl
6. Oral glucose tolerance—venous plasma greater than or equal to 200 mg/dl; venous blood greater than or equal to 180 mg/dl; capillary blood greater than or equal to 200 mg/dl
7. Glycosated hemoglobin (hemoglobin A_{1c})—reflects average hemoglobin level in the last 6 months
8. Blood urea nitrogen (BUN), creatinine—increased because of interference of ketones in measurement
9. Serum calcium, magnesium, phosphate—decreased as a result of diuresis
10. Serum electrolytes (potassium [K^+] and sodium [Na^+])—may be falsely elevated as a result of hyperosmolarity
11. White blood count—increased, with predominance of polymorphonuclear lymphocytes
12. Blood and urine cultures—positive culture
13. Lead II electrocardiogram (ECG)—increased T wave with hyperkalemia

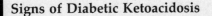

Signs of Diabetic Ketoacidosis

- Kussmaul respirations (deep sighing respirations)
- Hyperglycemia (serum glucose level greater than 300 mg/dl)
- Ketonuria (moderate to large amounts; positive ketostix)
- Metabolic acidosis (pH <7.3; increased partial pressure of carbon dioxide [Pco_2]; decreased partial pressure of oxygen [Po_2]; sodium bicarbonate [$NaHCO_3$] <15 mEq/L)
- Dehydration (as a result of polyuria and polydipsia)
- Fruity breath odor
- Electrolyte imbalance (falsely elevated potassium and sodium levels)
- Potential for life-threatening cardiac arrhythmias (as a result of electrolyte imbalance)
- Cerebral edema (caused by overzealous infusion of fluids)
- Coma (caused by electrolyte imbalance and acidosis)
- Death (infrequent)

14. Immunoassay—to measure level of C-peptides after glucose challenge (to verify endogenous insulin secretion)
15. Twenty four–hour urine analysis for glucose—considered a more reliable measure of urine glucose
16. Arterial blood gas values—to assess acidosis
17. Complete blood count

MEDICAL MANAGEMENT

Children with the initial diagnosis of IDDM are admitted to the hospital for stabilization and education. The management of these children requires a multidisciplinary approach. Medical management includes the regulation of serum glucose, fluid, and electrolyte levels. This is accomplished through monitoring of lab results, administration of insulin, and intravenous (IV) administration of fluids containing indicated additives. Secondary problems (i.e., infections) are also treated accordingly. Once glucose levels are stabilized, the child's insulin doses are typically dictated by a sliding scale based on the serum glucose level. Regulation of nutrition and exercise is also a key factor in managing diabetes.

NURSING ASSESSMENT

1. See the section on nursing assessments in Appendix A.
2. Assess for hyperglycemia.
3. Assess for hypoglycemia.
4. Assess hydration status.
5. Assess dietary patterns.
6. Assess activities and exercise patterns.
7. Assess self-administration of insulin.

NURSING DIAGNOSES

- Fluid volume deficit
- High risk for infection
- Altered nutrition: less than body requirements
- Knowledge deficit
- Impaired home maintenance management

NURSING INTERVENTIONS
Diabetic Ketoacidosis

1. Monitor and observe child for change in status of diabetic ketoacidosis (see the box on p. 119).
2. Promote child's hydration status.
   a. Record accurate intake, output, and specific gravity.
   b. Monitor for dehydration.
      (1) Dry or doughy skin
      (2) Increased specific gravity
      (3) Dry mucous membranes
      (4) Depressed fontanels (infants)

c. Monitor for fluid overload.
  (1) Decreased specific gravity
  (2) Peripheral edema
d. Administer and monitor IV solutions as ordered based on lab results and clinical appearance.

3. Monitor child's glucose level hourly.
  a. Blood glucose level should not fall below 250 mg/dl during the first 12 hours of treatment; the glucose level should not fall more than 100 mg/dl/hr because too rapid a decline in osmolarity predisposes the child to cerebral edema.
  b. Regular insulin is preferably administered intravenously for the treatment of DKA; typically a bolus dose (0.1 U/kg) is given, followed by a continuous infusion (0.1 U/kg/hr).
    (1) Prime tubing with the insulin solution before starting infusion.
    (2) Once the serum glucose level reaches 250 mg/dl and the serum pH is 7.35, insulin administration is switched to the subcutaneous route.
  c. Monitor urine for glucose and ketones with each voiding (dip stick).

4. Monitor for signs of complications.
  a. Acidosis
  b. Coma
  c. Hyperkalemia and hypokalemia
  d. Hypocalcemia
  e. Cerebral edema
  f. Hyponatremia

Recovery and Maintenance

1. Monitor and observe for signs of hypoglycemia and hyperglycemia.
2. Promote glucose control.
  a. Monitor urine and blood glucose levels as needed to assess effectiveness of insulin.
  b. Insulin dose is based on a sliding scale related to serum glucose level; typically, a total insulin dose of two thirds NPH and one third Regular is administered, two thirds of total dose ½ hour before dinner.
3. Promote adequate nutritional intake (see the box on pp. 123-124 for nutritional recommendations).

4. Monitor and establish appropriate relationship between insulin, dietary requirements, and exercise.
5. Provide emotional support to patient and family to promote psychosocial adaptation to diabetes.

🏠 Discharge Planning and Home Care

1. Instruct patient and parents about the management of diabetes.
   a. Insulin administration
   b. Dietary intake
   c. Blood glucose monitoring
   d. Glucose monitoring
   e. Prevention of complications
   f. Care of hypoglycemic and hyperglycemic states
   g. Skin care
   h. Activity regimen
   i. Illness management
2. Initiate a home care referral to assess adherence to diabetic regimen.
3. Promote resumption of normal activities.
4. Promote ventilation by patient and parents of concerns about diabetes as a chronic illness and its long-term management.
5. Promote interest in support groups.

CLIENT OUTCOMES

1. The child will achieve normal growth and development.
2. The child will maintain normal serum glucose levels.
3. The child and family will demonstrate the care required at home and have a support system in place.

REFERENCES

Betschart J: Children and adolescents with diabetes, *Nurs Clin North Am* 28(1):35, 1993.

Dickerman JD, Lucey JF: *Smith's: the critically ill child,* ed 3, Philadelphia, 1985, WB Saunders.

Hazinski MF, editor: *Nursing care of the critically ill child,* St Louis, 1992, Mosby.

Peterson A, Drass J: Managing acute complications of diabetes, *Nursing 91* 21(2):34, 1991.

Wong DL, editor: *Essentials of pediatric nursing,* St Louis, 1993, Mosby.

Diabetic Nutritional Requirements

Purpose of Dietary Plan

The dietary plan provides the necessary intake of calories for energy requirements and appropriate distribution of nutrients (carbohydrates, fats, and proteins).

Energy Requirements

Carbohydrates: 40%-60% of total calories
Fats: 25%-40% of total calories
Proteins: 15%-30% of total calories
Ratio of polyunsaturated to saturated fat should be at least 1:0. Total daily fat intake should be 420 g/day.

Dietary Plans

Two exchange systems are used by diabetic individuals: the American Diabetic Association (ADA) exchange group and the British Diabetic Association exchange system. The ADA exchange group has six exchange lists, which are for milk, fruit, vegetables, bread, meat, and fat. The exchange lists give the equivalent amounts of calories and nutrients.

The British Diabetic Association exchange focuses on carbohydrate intake only. A liberal intake of protein is allowed and fats are less restricted.

Continued

General Information

- Foods high in fiber retard carbohydrate absorption.
- Foods have different glycemic responses (glycemic index).
- Long delays between eating must be avoided.
- Extra food must be consumed for increased activity (10 to 15 g of carbohydrate for every 30 to 45 minutes of activity).
- Quantity of food needed between meals will vary according to increase or decrease in physical activity.

21

Disseminated Intravascular Coagulation

PATHOPHYSIOLOGY

Disseminated intravascular coagulation (DIC) is a defect in coagulation characterized by simultaneous hemorrhage and coagulation. DIC is the result of abnormal stimulation of the normal coagulation process with subsequent formation of widespread microvascular thrombi and depleted clotting factors. The syndrome is triggered by a variety of illnesses such as sepsis, multiple trauma, burns, or neoplasms. DIC can be described in terms of two precisely controlled coagulation processes that become accelerated and uncontrolled. Initially, the injury to tissue caused by the primary disorder (e.g., infection or trauma) activates a mechanism that releases thrombin, which is necessary for fibrin clot formation, into the circulation. Thrombin also activates the process that is necessary for the breakdown of fibrin and fibrinogen, resulting in fibrin and fibrinogen degradation products (FDP). FDPs in the circulation act as anticoagulants. DIC is characterized by the following three major symptoms: (1) generalized hemorrhage; (2) ischemia caused by thrombi, which results in organ ischemia; and (3) anemia. Prognosis is dependent on a variety of factors including the severity of the primary and secondary conditions.

INCIDENCE

1. Exact incidence is unknown.
2. DIC occurs in both children and adults.

3. DIC results from an underlying injury or illness.
4. Stress and steroids are possible precipitating factors.
5. Mortality rate is high.

CLINICAL MANIFESTATIONS

1. Spontaneous bleeding
2. Hypoxia
3. Cutaneous oozing
4. Petechiae
5. Ecchymoses
6. Pain
7. Symptoms based on severity and extent of organic involvement
   a. Renal: oliguria, anuria
   b. Central nervous system: altered mental status
   c. Skin: mottled, necrotic lesions; cyanosis

COMPLICATIONS

1. Gangrenous extremities
2. Shock
3. Hypoxia
4. Multiple organ dysfunction syndrome

LABORATORY AND DIAGNOSTIC TESTS

1. Platelet count—decreased
2. Red cell structure—altered due to widespread clotting
3. Hematocrit—decreased due to blood loss and breakdown of red blood cells
4. Fibrin degradation products—increased due to active fibrinolytic system
5. Protamine sulfate—strongly positive —(helps differentiate DIC from surgical or hepatic bleeding disorders)
6. Plasminogen levels—low
7. Prothrombin time—prolonged
8. Partial thromboplastin time—prolonged
9. Thrombin time—prolonged
10. Fibrinogen level—usually decreased
11. Factor assays—usually decreased

12. Blood typing and cross match—for replacement therapy

MEDICAL MANAGEMENT

The major focus in the medical management of DIC is the correction of the primary illness or injury that initiated the coagulopathy. Correcting the underlying problem may control the DIC so that normal coagulation can be restored. Treatment of infection, shock, acidosis, and hypoxia must be priorities. Fluid replacement therapy with crystalloids is essential in the early stages of shock. Although blood replacement therapy with whole blood, cryoprecipitate, red blood cells (RBCs), fresh frozen plasma, and platelet concentrates is often required, it is risky because these products enhance the clotting process. Heparin therapy has been advocated because it interferes with the coagulation cascade and antagonizes the production of thrombin. This therapy, however, remains very controversial, and its use may increase bleeding. Overall, therapy must be tailored to the clinical and laboratory data available.

NURSING ASSESSMENT

1. See the section on hemodynamic assessment in Appendix A.
2. Recognize conditions that predispose to DIC.
3. Assess for signs of bleeding.
4. Assess bleeding sites.
5. Assess oxygenation.
6. Assess for signs and symptoms of impaired tissue perfusion and organ failure.
7. Assess family coping skills.

NURSING DIAGNOSES

- High risk for fluid volume deficit
- High risk for altered tissue perfusion
- Impaired gas exchange
- Pain
- High risk for impaired skin integrity
- High risk for injury
- High risk for infection
- Anxiety

NURSING INTERVENTIONS

1. Monitor child's clinical status; report any significant changes.
   a. Monitor for signs of hemorrhage—bleeding, petechiae, cutaneous oozing, dyspnea, lethargy, pallor, increased apical pulse, decreased blood pressure, headache, dizziness, muscle weakness, restlessness.
   b. Monitor for signs of ischemia—changes in level of consciousness, decreased urine output, electrocardiogram (ECG) changes, gangrenous extremities, mottled skin, necrotic skin lesions, respiratory failure.
2. Control bleeding.
   a. Do not disturb clots.
   b. Use pressure to control bleeding when possible.
   c. Administer blood products safely.
   d. Monitor bleeding closely—inspect skin carefully.
   e. Measure blood loss.
   f. Monitor laboratory data.
   g. Test urine output for bleeding.
3. Promote adequate oxygenation.
   a. Position child for effective ventilation.
   b. Administer oxygen and monitor response.
   c. Perform frequent respiratory assessments.
   d. Reduce oxygen needs.
   e. Control environmental stimuli.
4. Provide measures to alleviate or control pain.
   a. Immobilize joints.
   b. Apply hot or cold compresses.
   c. Use bed cradle.
   d. Use an air mattress.
   e. Change child's position frequently.
   f. Provide mouth and skin care.
   g. Utilize pain scale to assess degree of pain.
   h. Administer pain medication.
5. Monitor child's therapeutic and untoward response to administration of blood products.
   a. Platelets—used to decrease bleeding
   b. Fresh frozen plasma—used to correct deficiencies of fibrinogen, prothrombin, factor II, factor VIII, and other deficient factors

   c. Fresh whole blood and packed red blood cells—used to maintain hematocrit
6. Monitor child's therapeutic and untoward response to administration of heparin.
7. Provide support for patient and family.
   a. Identify knowledge deficits.
   b. Provide accurate information.
   c. Give honest answers in clear, concise terms.
   d. Provide consistent caregivers.

♠ Discharge Planning and Home Care

1. Instruct parents to observe and report any signs of complications.
   a. Infection
   b. Organ dysfunction
   c. Abnormal bleeding
2. Instruct parents about follow-up appointments.
   a. Name and phone number of physician
   b. Date and time of follow-up appointment

CLIENT OUTCOMES

1. Child will have normal coagulation.
2. Child will have adequate perfusion.
3. Child will have minimal organ damage.

REFERENCES

Bailes BK: Disseminated intravascular coagulation: principles, treatment, nursing management, *AORN J* 55(2):515, 1992.
Bill TN: DIC: clinical complexities of aberrant coagulation, *Critical Care Nursing Clinics* 5(3):389, 1993.
Epstein C, Bakanauskas A: Clinical management of DIC: early nursing interventions, *Critical Care Nurse* 11(10):42, 1991.
Holland JA, Bryan S, Huff-Slankard J: Nursing care of the child with meningococcemia, *J Pediatr Nurs* 8(4):211, 1993.
Volker DL: Challenges of DIC, *Dimensions of Oncology Nursing* 5(2):26, 1991.

22

Drowning and Near-Drowning

PATHOPHYSIOLOGY

Each year between 4000 and 5000 people drown in the United States, and the number of near-drownings is estimated to be much higher. Drowning is defined as death from suffocation that results from submersion. Near-drowning is defined as survival, at least temporarily, from the lethal effects of hypoxia.

A variety of terms associated with drowning and near-drowning require clarification. *Dry drowning* (occurs in 10% to 15% of cases) consists of airway obstruction after the aspiration of little to no fluid. It produces reflux closure of the glottis, as well as apnea.

Wet drowning (majority of cases) consists of the initial aspiration of fluids, causing laryngospasm and vomiting. The resultant asphyxia causes the glottis to relax, allowing the lungs to be flooded with the immersion fluids.

Secondary drowning (edema in the lungs not due to the immediate drowning but to increased pulmonary capillary permeability) occurs in one out of five near-drowning cases. Increased intracranial pressure (ICP) and hypoxic brain cell injury may also develop. Secondary drowning symptoms may appear 24 to 72 hours after the near-drowning episode. The clinical manifestations include the following:

1. Coma
2. Increased pulmonary edema
3. Circulatory collapse

4. Hypoxemia
5. Respiratory acidosis
6. Development of hypercapnia

The physiologic events that occur after submersion are sequential. After the initial panic and struggle, victims will hold their breath and swallow large amounts of water. Laryngospasm occurs initially, but for most children, muscle relaxation follows and they aspirate large amounts of water. Cardiopulmonary arrest follows quickly and hypoxia develops. Hypoxia is the common pathophysiologic response that affects all organ systems in near-drowning. Hypoxia from dry drowning is the result of airway obstruction caused by laryngeal spasm. In wet drowning, hypoxia results from a combination of alveolar and interstitial pulmonary edema, protein deposits in the alveoli, damage to pulmonary capillaries, decreased surfactant production, and aspiration of foreign material.

The type of water aspirated will play a part in determining the pathophysiology of wet drowning. In *saltwater* drowning, the hypertonic fluid is drawn into the alveoli, diluting surfactant and causing hypovolemia, hemoconcentration, and increased serum electrolyte concentrations. In *freshwater* drowning, the aspirated fluid is rapidly drawn out of the alveoli into the intravascular space. This shift of fluids causes hypervolemia resulting in hemodilution and decreased serum electrolyte concentrations. Fresh water is thought to damage alveolar type II cells, which control pulmonary surfactant production.

Prognosis is affected by a variety of factors, such as length of time immersed, temperature of immersion fluid, and length of time until effective cardiopulmonary resuscitation is provided. Even though these factors affect prognosis and have multisystem effects, morbidity and death are directly related to the degree of neuronal damage. Only a small percentage of patients die as the result of other organ system failures.

INCIDENCE

1. Drowning is the third leading cause of death in children.
2. Children under 5 years of age and young adults between 15 and 24 years of age have the highest risk.

3. Forty percent of the victims are less than 4 years of age.
4. Male individuals are more likely to drown than female individuals.
5. Peak incidence occurs during summer months.
6. More than 50% of victims under 13 years of age drown in pools.
7. Younger children most often drown (1) in unprotected pools and ponds, (2) after falling through ice, or (3) in bathtubs after a fall.
8. Older children most often drown (1) while swimming, (2) during unsupervised water sports, (3) while boating, (4) after hyperventilating before diving, or (5) because of environmental hazards or associated alcohol ingestion.

CLINICAL MANIFESTATIONS

1. Respiratory rate—ranges from rapid, shallow breathing to apnea
2. Cyanosis
3. Pink, frothy sputum
4. Pulmonary edema
5. Flaccidity
6. Decorticate or decerebrate posturing
7. Coma with irreversible brain injury
8. Convulsions
9. Twitching
10. Disorientation
11. Agitation
12. Lethargy
13. Headaches
14. Hypotension or hypertension
15. Arrhythmias
16. Tachycardia
17. Metabolic or respiratory acidosis
18. Hypothermia

COMPLICATIONS

1. Hypoxic encephalopathy
2. Secondary drowning

3. Aspiration pneumonia
4. Pulmonary interstitial fibrosis
5. Ventricular dysrhythmias
6. Renal failure
7. Disseminated intravascular coagulation (DIC)
8. Pancreatic necrosis
9. Infection

LABORATORY AND DIAGNOSTIC TESTS

1. Chest x-ray examination—variable findings (from scattered parenchymal infiltrates to extensive pulmonary edema)
2. Arterial blood gas values—to determine respiratory and metabolic acidosis
3. ICP monitoring—to monitor cerebral perfusion
4. Computerized axial tomography (CAT) scan
5. Electroencephalogram (EEG)—to assess seizure activity and document brain death (seizure activity is decreased in freshwater drowning and is increased in saltwater drowning)
6. Serum osmolarity
7. Electrocardiogram (ECG)
8. Complete blood count (CBC), hematocrit (Hct), hemoglobin (Hb)—decreased values caused by hemodilution (freshwater drowning); increased values caused by hemoconcentration (saltwater drowning)
9. Serum electrolytes—decreased values caused by hemodilution except for an increase in serum potassium caused by hemolysis (freshwater drowning); increased values caused by hemoconcentration (saltwater drowning)
10. Blood urea nitrogen (BUN)—increased in freshwater drowning and decreased in saltwater drowning
11. Creatinine—increased in freshwater drowning and decreased in saltwater drowning
12. Culture and sensitivity—used to detect superimposed respiratory infection

MEDICAL MANAGEMENT

Aggressive basic and advanced life support at the scene are essential because the full extent of the central nervous system injury cannot be accurately assessed at the time of rescue. Ensure the adequacy of airway, breathing, and circulation. Other injuries must be considered, and the need for hospitalization is determined by the severity of the event and clinical evaluation. Patients with respiratory symptoms, decreased oxygen saturation, and altered level of consciousness must be admitted. Ongoing attention to oxygenation, ventilation, and cardiac function are priorities. Protecting the central nervous system and reducing cerebral edema are of paramount importance and directly relate to outcome.

Medications used include vecuronium for paralyzing skeletal muscles, furosemide (Lasix) for diuresis, and mannitol (Mannitor) for controlling intracranial hypertension and for sedation.

NURSING ASSESSMENT

1. See the section on nursing assessment in Appendix A.
2. Assess for spontaneous respirations.
3. Assess for level of consciousness.
4. Assess core temperature.
5. See sections on respiratory assessment and neuromuscular assessment in Appendix A.

NURSING DIAGNOSES

- Impaired gas exchange
- Ineffective airway clearance
- Altered cerebral tissue perfusion
- Ineffective breathing patterns
- Decreased cardiac output
- Fluid volume excess
- High risk for injury
- Altered nutrition: less than body requirements
- Knowledge deficit related to near-drowning

NURSING INTERVENTIONS

1. Establish and maintain patency of airway.
   a. Suction airway as needed.
   b. Insert nasogastric tube (to prevent aspiration of vomitus).

2. Monitor and record child's response to oxygen therapy.
   a. Perform respiratory assessment (frequency is dependent on status).
   b. Monitor use of ventilator and respiratory equipment.
   c. Monitor central venous pressure (CVP) and arterial lines.
   d. Monitor use of intermittent positive pressure breathing (IPPB) and/or positive end-expiratory pressure (PEEP).
3. Monitor and record child's level of neurologic functioning.
   a. Perform neurologic assessment (frequency is dependent on status).
   b. Observe and report signs of ICP (lethargy, increased blood pressure, decreased respiratory rate, increased apical pulse, dilated pupils).
4. Monitor and maintain fluid balance.
   a. Record intake and output.
   b. Maintain patency and care for Foley catheter.
   c. Maintain fluid restriction with presence of cerebral edema.
5. Monitor and maintain homeostatic temperature regulation (decreased oxygen requirements).
   a. Monitor temperature.
   b. Provide cooling mattress (prevent shivering).
   c. Administer antipyretics.
6. Provide and maintain adequate nutritional intake.
   a. Assess child's ability for nasogastric or oral nutritional intake (NG/po).
   b. Assess child's capacity to tolerate nasogastric or oral feedings (check for residuals and vomiting).
   c. Advance amount and type of nutritional intake.
7. Observe and report signs of complications (see section on complications, this chapter).
8. Monitor child's response to physical therapy regimen.
9. Monitor child's therapeutic response to and any side effects from medications.

♠ Discharge Planning and Home Care
Preventive Care

Instruct parents about instituting the following preventive measures: parents' learning cardiopulmonary resuscitation

(CPR); water safety and swimming lessons for child; water-proofing backyard (e.g., pool cover, fence enclosures); measures to raise awareness of environmental hazards; and appropriate supervision during use of pool.

Long-Term Care (as Indicated)

1. Instruct parents about the proper administration of medication to enhance compliance.
   a. Correct dose, route, time
   b. Observation for side effects
2. Promote and maintain patency of airway.
   a. Suction as needed.
   b. Perform percussion and postural drainage as needed.
   c. Change child's position frequently.
   d. Raise head of bed to semi-Fowler's position to increase lung expansion.
   e. Provide or teach tracheostomy care if appropriate.
3. Provide for child's nutritional needs.
   a. Nasogastric tube
      (1) Check placement before feeding.
      (2) Check for residual before feeding.
      (3) Monitor intake and output.
      (4) Provide oral care frequently.
      (5) Monitor for problems (e.g., aspiration, abdominal distention).
   b. Gastrostomy tube
      (1) Raise head of bed to semi-Fowler's position and place patient on right side before feeding.
      (2) Check for residual before feeding; feed residual again and subtract from amount of next feeding.
      (3) Provide oral care.
      (4) Monitor input and output.
4. Provide skin care to prevent skin breakdown and infection.
   a. Keep creases and folds of skin clean and dry.
   b. Change child's position frequently.
   c. Use sheepskin and/or waterbed.
   d. Lubricate skin with lotion.
   e. Change diapers frequently.
   f. Use lubricating ointment in perineal area.

5. Provide environmental stimulation (child may hear even though unresponsive).

CLIENT OUTCOMES

1. The child will return to optimal level of neurologic function.
2. Respiratory distress will be reduced or eliminated.
3. The child will maintain adequate perfusion, and vital signs will be within normal parameters.

REFERENCES

Glankler D: Caring for the victim of near-drowning, *Critical Care Nurse* 13(8):25, 1993.

Leach S: Continuing care for the near-drowning child, *Critical Care Nursing Clinics* 3(2):307, 1991.

Luttrell P: Care of the pediatric near-drowning victim, *Critical Care Nursing Clinics* 3(2):293, 1991.

McKinley M: Near-drowning: a nursing challenge, *Critical Care Nurse* 9(10):52, 1989.

Walsh EA: Childhood near-drowning: nursing care and primary prevention, *Pediatr Nurs* 20(3):292, 1994.

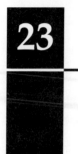

23

Epiglottitis

PATHOPHYSIOLOGY

Epiglottitis is an acute bacterial infection of the epiglottis and the surrounding areas (the aryepiglottic folds and the supraglottic area) that causes airway obstruction. The infection is caused by *Haemophilus influenzae* type B or, on rare occasions, streptococci or pneumococci. Onset is sudden and infection progresses rapidly, causing acute respiratory difficulty. This condition requires emergency airway stabilization and medical measures because a fatal outcome can occur. The child is extubated when the epiglottis appears normal and the child is able to breathe around the tube (usually 48 to 72 hours after antibiotic treatment is started).

INCIDENCE

1. Boys, ages 2 to 7 years, are most often affected.
2. Incidence is highest in winter, but infection can occur anytime.
3. Epiglottitis may be preceded by upper respiratory tract infection.

CLINICAL MANIFESTATIONS

1. Respiratory difficulty, which can progress to severe respiratory distress in a matter of minutes or hours (dyspnea)
2. Dysphagia, drooling

3. Absence of spontaneous cough
4. Edematous, cherry-red epiglottis
5. Red and inflamed oral cavity
6. Breathing in upright position with head extended forward
7. Complaining of intense sore throat
8. Sudden increase in temperature
9. Muffled voice
10. Pale color
11. Decreased breath sounds
12. Substernal or suprasternal and intercostal retractions
13. Bilateral cervical adenitis
14. Lethargy

COMPLICATIONS
1. Airway obstruction
2. Laryngospasm
3. Death

LABORATORY AND DIAGNOSTIC TESTS
1. Oxygen saturation—decrease in the amount of oxygen
2. Arterial blood gas values—decreased pH, decreased partial pressure of oxygen (Po_2), increased partial pressure of carbon dioxide (Pco_2)
3. Lateral neck radiograph—to confirm diagnosis
4. Throat culture—to rule out other bacterial infections
5. Blood culture—to rule out other bacterial infections
6. Direct laryngoscopy—performed in operating room to prevent complications; to confirm diagnosis

MEDICAL MANAGEMENT
Children suspected of having epiglottitis should be examined where personnel and equipment are available for an emergency tracheal intubation or tracheostomy. Visual examination of the throat is contraindicated until this requirement is met. Lateral neck x-ray studies may help confirm the diagnosis but should be performed in the least distressing manner possible, usually with the child being held in the parent's lap. Endotracheal intubation or tracheostomy is

performed in the operating room along with the placement of any invasive intravenous lines. The child is observed in the intensive care area until swelling of the epiglottis decreases, usually by the third day. Antibiotics are given for a total of 7 to 10 days.

NURSING ASSESSMENT

1. See the section on respiratory assessment in Appendix A.
2. Assess hydration status.
3. Assess anxiety level.

NURSING DIAGNOSES

- High risk for suffocation
- Ineffective airway clearance
- Ineffective breathing pattern
- Altered tissue perfusion
- High risk for fluid volume deficit
- Anxiety
- Altered family processes

NURSING INTERVENTIONS

1. Monitor respiratory status (including vital signs).
   a. Temperature, apical pulse, respiratory rate, blood pressure
   b. Presence of pulmonary congestion
   c. Presence of intercostal retractions
   d. Presence of circumoral cyanosis
   e. Use of accessory muscles
   f. Noninvasive oxygen saturation monitoring
   g. Arterial blood gas
2. Observe and report signs of increased respiratory distress or changes in respiratory status.
3. Maintain upright position (semi-Fowler's or high-Fowler's position) to facilitate breathing.
4. Prepare child preoperatively for airway insertion (endotracheal tube or a tracheostomy) if condition allows.
5. Assist and support physician during emergency procedure.
   a. Ventilate through bag and mask if child becomes obstructed before reaching operating room.

b. Observe and monitor respiratory status during intubation.
6. Maintain patency of airway and ventilator.
7. Provide tracheostomy care (if tracheostomy is performed).
   a. Maintain patent airway.
   b. Monitor cardiopulmonary status.
   c. Use aseptic technique when suctioning.
   d. Clean tracheostomy site.
   e. Observe tracheostomy for incrustation.
8. Monitor action and side effects of prescribed medications.
   a. Sedate as needed.
   b. Restrain as needed.
9. Assess hydration status: monitor input and output and specific gravity.
10. Provide for child's developmental needs during hospitalization.
    a. Provide age-appropriate toys (see section on growth and development, Appendix B).
    b. Incorporate home routines into hospital routine (e.g., feeding practices and bedtime rituals).
    c. Encourage ventilation of feelings through age-appropriate means.
11. Provide consistent nursing care to promote trust and to alleviate anxiety.

♠ Discharge Planning and Home Care

1. If child is discharged on a regimen of oral antibiotics, provide teaching regarding administration and side effects.
2. Educate family on the value of the *Haemophilus influenzae* type B vaccine.

CLIENT OUTCOMES

1. Child will return to normal respiratory status.
2. Child and family demonstrate understanding of home care and follow-up needs.

REFERENCES

American Academy of Pediatrics, Committee on Infectious Diseases: *Haemophilus influenzae* type b conjugate vaccine: immunization of children 2-13 months of age, *AAP News* 6(11):19, 1990.

Cressman WR, Myer CM III: Diagnosis and management of croup and epiglottitis, *Pediatr Clin North Am* 41(2):265, 1994.

Gomberg SM: Mistaken identity ... is it epiglottitis or croup? *Pediatr Nurs* 16(6):567, 1990.

Henry RL, Bingham AL, Halliday JA: The management of epiglottitis in a small paediatric intensive care unit, *J Qual Clin Pract* 14(1):17, 1994.

24

Foreign Body Aspiration

PATHOPHYSIOLOGY

Foreign body aspiration refers to the lodgment of an object or substance in the airway. The foreign body tends to lodge most often in the cricopharyngeal area because of the strong, propulsive pharyngeal muscles that move it to this location. Obstruction may be partial or complete. Complete airway obstruction usually occurs in the upper airway and is life threatening. Most objects aspirated by children are small enough to pass through the larynx and trachea and lodge in either of the main bronchi. The right main bronchus is a more common site in that it is larger, receives greater airflow, and has a straighter line of entry than the left bronchus. The mechanisms of airway obstruction depend on the site of obstruction and whether the foreign body is partially or completely obstructing an airway. Atelectasis occurs distal to the area where air can no longer enter. Air trapping or hyperinflation occurs when air is inhaled but can only be partially exhaled.

In many cases foreign bodies are spontaneously expelled from the tracheobronchial tree and symptoms that persist are from residual irritation and bronchial edema. When foreign body aspiration is diagnosed quickly and the object or substance is removed in a prompt manner, the condition follows a typically benign course. Aspiration of foreign bodies containing saturated fats such as peanuts is more problematic due to irritation and inflammation of mucosal tissue. The longer a foreign body remains lodged in place, the more complications—related to increasing edema, inflammation, and threat of infection—can develop.

INCIDENCE

1. Foreign body aspiration most commonly occurs in children 6 months to 6 years of age.
2. Foreign body aspiration is the leading cause of accidental death in children less than 1 year of age.
3. Peanuts and other nuts account for about half of all aspirated foreign bodies; hot dogs are also common culprits.

CLINICAL MANIFESTATIONS

Clinical manifestations vary according to the site in which the foreign body lodges and the degree of obstruction that occurs.

1. Initial coughing, gagging, or choking episode, which may or may not be observed
2. Acute coughing or wheezing
3. Subtle chronic cough or wheeze
4. Dyspnea
5. Retractions
6. Cyanosis
7. Decreased breath sounds over affected side
8. Possible quiet period or symptomless phase
9. Fever
10. Hoarseness (larynx)
11. Stridor (larynx)
12. Aphonia (larynx)
13. Audible slap with coughing as foreign body moves (in trachea)

COMPLICATIONS

Complications most often result from delayed diagnosis and removal.

1. Bronchospasm
2. Atelectasis
3. Bronchitis
4. Bronchiectasis

5. Pneumonia
6. Lung abscess
7. Bronchopulmonary fistula
8. Death

LABORATORY AND DIAGNOSTIC TESTS

1. Chest x-ray study—anterior, posterior, lateral, and oblique views, to evaluate for opaque foreign body location; for nonopaque foreign body, assess x-ray films for area of atelectasis, or with inspiratory and expiratory x-ray films, may assess for air trapping
2. Bronchoscopy—done with general anesthetic in the operating room, providing direct visualization into the upper trachea (a telescope can be used to locate the foreign body, and removal is accomplished by inserting an optical forcep)
3. Fluoroscopy—provides a dynamic moving image of the structures under x-ray examination, giving an advantage over x-ray examination alone in showing trapped air distal to the foreign body site
4. Xeroradiography (an x-ray technique using specially coated x-ray films)—provides greater resolution of images such as nonmetallic foreign bodies

MEDICAL MANAGEMENT

Emergency management of foreign body aspiration may begin prior to hospitalization for a life-threatening obstruction when attempts at relief via the Heimlich maneuver or blow to the back cannot be delayed. Once foreign body aspiration is suspected, immediate attention is warranted, with aggressive diagnostic workup including bronchoscopy for identification and removal to prevent complications.

Medications that may be used are as follows:

1. Inhaled bronchodilators for laryngospasm or bronchospasm
2. Corticosteroids to decrease airway edema
3. Systemically acting antibiotics in cases where retained fragments are suspected, purulent secretions are noted in the airway, or signs and symptoms of pneumonia are present

NURSING ASSESSMENT

1. See the section on respiratory assessment in Appendix A.
2. Assess level of anxiety.

NURSING DIAGNOSES

- Ineffective airway clearance
- Anxiety
- High risk for impaired gas exchange

NURSING INTERVENTIONS
Emergency Measures

For total airway obstruction or ineffective airway clearance, an airway must be established.

1. Deliver back blows followed by chest thrusts for infants 1 year and younger.
2. Perform the Heimlich maneuver (abdominal thrusts) in children older than 1 year.

Preoperative Care

1. Provide continuous respiratory monitoring; be prepared to assist with emergency airway management if partial obstruction becomes complete.
2. Provide position (of comfort) to ensure adequate airway.
3. Provide nothing by mouth before surgery.
4. Prepare child for bronchoscopy and/or thoracotomy.
5. Minimize anxiety.

Postoperative Care

1. Make respiratory assessments to detect signs and symptoms of respiratory distress from secondary airway edema.
2. Assess effects of administered medications.

🏠 Discharge Planning and Home Care

1. Instruct parents to observe for, and report immediately, signs of respiratory distress.
2. Provide list of resources for parents to call in case of emergency.

3. Instruct parents in foreign body airway obstruction removal and cardiopulmonary resuscitation (CPR).
4. Instruct in prevention of foreign body aspiration.
   a. Offer types and sizes or portions of food appropriate for age of child.
   b. Discourage child from eating during activities.
   c. Restrict access to small toys or objects.
5. Make referral for home safety assessment if indicated.

CLIENT OUTCOMES

1. Child will achieve and maintain a patent airway.
2. Child will return to a safe home environment.

REFERENCES

Betz CL, Hunsberger MM, Wright S: *Family-centered nursing care of children,* ed 2, Philadelphia, 1994, WB Saunders.

Drake AF, Smith TL, Fischer ND: Foreign body aspiration in North Carolina children, *N C Med J* 55(2):83, 1994.

Gatch G, Myre L, Black RE: Foreign body aspiration in children, *AORN J* 46(5):850, 1987.

Losek JD: Diagnostic difficulties of foreign body aspiration in children, *Am J Emerg Med* 8(4):348, 1990.

Thompson JE, Farrell E, McManus M: Neonatal and pediatric airway emergencies, *Respir Care* 37(6):582, 1992.

25

Fractures

PATHOPHYSIOLOGY

Fractures can have a variety of causes, including (1) a direct force applied to the bone; (2) a spontaneous fracturing secondary to an underlying pathologic condition such as rickets; (3) abrupt, intense muscle contractions; and (4) an indirect force (e.g., being hit by a flying object) applied from a distance. Other cause of fractures include child abuse, metastatic neuroblastoma, Ewing's sarcoma, osteogenic sarcoma, osteogenesis imperfecta, rickets, copper deficiency, osteomyelitis, overuse injuries, and immobilization.

There are a variety of fractures, which can be categorized using the Salter-Harris classification system (see the box on p. 149). The most common type seen in children less than 3 years of age is the greenstick fracture. It involves an incomplete break of the cortex, which occurs because the bone is softer and more pliable than bones in older children. Other fractures (with their related sites) include upper epiphyseal and supracondylar fractures, lateral condylar humeral fractures, medial epicondylar fractures (humerus); proximal radial physis and radial neck fractures, nursemaid's elbow (elbow); fractures of the shaft of the radius and ulna (forearm); and fractures of the femoral shaft and tibia (lower limb).

Salter-Harris Classifications

Type I

- Fracture passes through growth plate without involvement of metaphysis or epiphysis
- Occurs with mild traumatic injuries
- Seen most often in distal fibula

Type II

- Fracture extends through growth plate, involving metaphysis
- Occurs as result of severe trauma such as car accident, fall from skateboard
- Seen most often in distal radius and proximal humerus

Type III

- Fracture extends through growth plate, involving epiphysis and joint
- Occurs during moderately severe trauma
- Seen most often in distal tibia

Type IV

- Fracture involves metaphysis, extending through growth plate into epiphysis
- Occurs as result of falls, skateboard and bicycle accidents
- Seen most often in humerus
- Can result in serious damage

Type V (Rare)

- Growth plate is crushed
- Compression fracture, resulting from falling or projectile impact

INCIDENCE

1. Pelvic fracture constitutes a small portion of skeletal fractures in children; it ranks second in terms of morbidity and mortality.
2. Most fractures occur to pedestrians.
3. Skull fracture ranks first in terms of morbidity and mortality.
4. Injuries to the growth plate occur in one third of skeletal traumas.

CLINICAL MANIFESTATIONS

1. Pain, relieved with rest
2. Tenderness
3. Swelling
4. Impaired function, limping
5. Limited motion
6. Ecchymosis surrounding site
7. Crepitus at site of fracture
8. Decreased neurovascular status distal to site of fracture
9. Distal atrophy

COMPLICATIONS

1. Deformity of limb
2. Limb length discrepancy
3. Joint incongruity
4. Limitation of movement
5. Nerve injury resulting in numbness
6. Circulatory compromise
7. Volkmann's ischemic contracture
8. Gangrene
9. Compartment syndrome

LABORATORY AND DIAGNOSTIC TESTS

1. X-ray examination of injury site
2. Bone scan—done if roentgenograms are negative
3. Complete blood count (CBC)
4. Erythrocyte sedimentation rate

MEDICAL MANAGEMENT

Management varies according to the type of fracture. Management modalities include open reduction, traction, casting, and remodeling. Analgesics are used for pain relief. The dosage and type depend on the child's level of pain intensity.

NURSING ASSESSMENT

1. Assess site of injury for pain, swelling, skin color, neurovascular status.
2. Assess for cause of injury.
3. Assess child's need for pain relief.
4. Assess for signs and symptoms of infection.
5. Assess for wound healing (if open reduction done).
6. Assess for skin irritation (if casted).
7. Assess for cast or traction integrity.
8. Assess for hydration status.
9. Assess for signs and symptoms of complications such as fat emboli, compartment syndrome.
10. Assess child's and family's ability to adhere to treatment regimen.
11. Assess child's ability to participate in self-care activities.
12. Assess child's need for diversional activities.

NURSING DIAGNOSES

- High risk for injury
- Impaired mobility
- Impaired tissue integrity
- High risk for infection
- Pain
- Self-care deficit
- High risk for diversional activity deficit
- Knowledge deficit

NURSING INTERVENTIONS
Admission

1. Monitor and document condition and cause of injury.
   a. Amount of swelling
   b. Amount of pain
   c. Change in skin color

    d. Circulatory status of limb distal to injury (color, warmth, pulses)

    e. Neurologic status of limb distal to injury (tingling, numbness)

    f. Factors associated with injury

2. Apply splint or Jones dressing to affected limb to alleviate pain and prevent further injury (traction may be used).

    a. Apply to one side of affected limb.

    b. Immobilize fracture site and joints above and below it.

    c. Stabilize splints with bandages.

    d. Jones dressing—wrap extremity with two or three layers of cotton and cover with Ace bandage; repeat process three or four times.

3. Maintain nothing by mouth (NPO) diet until after treatment; child may have to be anesthetized.

4. Prepare child and family for selected treatment modality.

Later Treatment

1. Observe and report status of limb distal to fracture site.

    a. Neurovascular status

        (1) Upper limbs—radial and ulnar pulse

        (2) Lower limbs—dorsalis pedis and posterior tibial pulses

        (3) Motor function and sensation

    b. Edema and swelling

    c. Skin color and warmth

2. Alleviate edema and swelling of trauma site and area distal to it.

    a. Elevate limb for 24 to 48 hours.

    b. Apply ice if necessary.

    c. Monitor every hour immediately after treatment, then every 4 hours for 48 hours.

3. Promote skin integrity.

    a. Apply alcohol to reddened areas.

    b. Petal cast edges to prevent skin irritation.

    c. Reposition every 2 hours to alleviate increased pressure on bony prominences.

    d. Observe for reddened areas every 4 hours.

4. Observe and report signs of infection.

    a. Elevated temperature

    b. Offensive odors

    c. Drainage

5. Observe for and record bleeding; note and outline amount.
6. Provide cast care (as indicated).
7. Maintain traction (as indicated).
8. Provide age-appropriate diversional activities to alleviate and minimize effects of sensory deprivation and immobilization (see section on growth and development, Appendix B).
9. Promote adequate fluid and nutritional intake.
    a. Encourage fluid intake; maintenance fluids—0 to 10 kg: 100 ml/kg; 11 to 20 kg: 50 ml/kg (plus 100 ml/kg for the first 10 kg); greater than 20 kg: 20 ml/kg.
    b. Provide high-fiber and high-roughage diet to promote peristalsis.
    c. Provide well-balanced diet to promote healing.
10. Prevent complications of unaffected limb; provide daily exercises.
11. Refer case to child protection services if suspected child abuse (see Chapter 12, Child Abuse and Neglect).

♠ Discharge Planning and Home Care
1. Monitor child's and family's ability to keep follow-up appointments.
2. Instruct parents and child about care of cast, use of crutches, etc.
3. Instruct parents and child to monitor and report signs of complications.
    a. Skin breakdown
    b. Signs of infection
    c. Signs of bleeding
    d. Contractures

CLIENT OUTCOMES
1. Child's fracture will heal without complications.
2. Child's level of pain will be minimized or alleviated.
3. Child will participate in self-care activities as fully as possible.

REFERENCES

Huo MH et al: Traumatic fracture-dislocation of the hip in a 2-year-old child, *Orthopedics* 15(12):1430, 1992.

Leventhal JM et al: Fractures in young children: distinguishing child abuse from unintentional injuries, *Am J Dis Child* 147(1):87, 1993.

Meadows LL: Pediatric management problems: femoral fracture due to child abuse, *Pediatr Nurs* 20(2):168, 1994.

Mintzer C, Waters PM: Acute open reduction of a displaced scaphoid fracture in a child, *J Hand Surg* 19(5):760, 1994.

Ward WT, Levy J, Kaye A: Compression plating for child and adolescent femur fractures, *J Pediatr Orthop* 12(5):626, 1992.

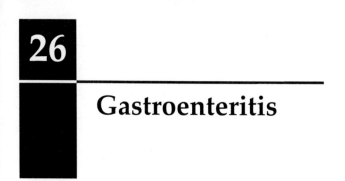

26

Gastroenteritis

PATHOPHYSIOLOGY

Gastroenteritis is defined as inflammation of the mucous membranes of the stomach and intestines. Acute gastroenteritis is characterized by vomiting and/or diarrhea resulting in fluid and electrolyte losses that lead to dehydration and electrolyte imbalances. The major causes of acute gastroenteritis include viruses (rotavirus, enteric adenovirus, Norwalk-virus, and others), bacteria or their toxins (*Campylobacter, Salmonella, Shigella, Escherichia coli, Yersinia,* and others), and parasites (*Giardia lamblia, Cryptosporidium*). (Refer to Table 1.) These pathogens cause illness by infecting the cells, producing enterotoxins or cytotoxins that damage the cells, or adhering to the walls of the intestines. In acute gastroenteritis, the small intestine is actually the most often affected.

Acute gastroenteritis is transmitted by the fecal-oral route from person to person. Some cases have been spread through contaminated water and food supplies. Exposure to day care facilities increases the risk for gastroenteritis, as does travel to developing countries. Most infections are self-limited and prognosis is favorable with treatment. Malnourished children may have more severe infections and take longer to recover.

Text continued on p. 160.

Table 1. Characteristics of Acute Gastroenteritis

Pathogen	Vomiting	Diarrhea	Fever	Stool Characteristics	Abdominal Cramps	Epidemiologic Features
Rotavirus	24-48 hr	2-7 days	Yes, abrupt onset	Profuse, watery; green, yellow, or clear color; no blood or pus	Some, with tenesmus	2-7 days incubation period; occurs during cooler months in temperate climates
Enteric adenovirus	24-48 hr	2-7 days	No	Watery		7-8 days incubation period; milder course than rotavirus
Norwalk-virus	Common for 24-48 hr	Less common (in <50% of patients) for 24-48 hr	Rare	Watery	Yes	Occurs in epidemics, primarily in school-age children and adolescents

Campylobacter jejuni	Starts 24 hr after fever	Starts 24 hr after fever	Yes	Profuse, watery and foul smelling initially; later with pus, mucus, and blood	Yes	Peaks worldwide during warm season
Escherichia coli—enterotoxigenic	None	Self-limited	No	Profuse, watery, no pus or blood	Sometimes	Common cause of "summer" diarrhea in developing countries and of traveler's diarrhea
E. coli—enteroinvasive	On occasion	Self-limited	Yes	Scanty; initially watery, later with pus and mucus; may become bloody	Tenesmus, cramping	
E. coli—enteropathogenic	On occasion	Self-limited but can become chronic	Yes	Profuse and watery	Tenesmus	Common cause of outbreaks in nurseries; usually occurs in summer

Continued

Table 1. Characteristics of Acute Gastroenteritis—cont'd

Pathogen	Vomiting	Diarrhea	Fever	Stool Characteristics	Abdominal Cramps	Epidemiologic Features
Salmonella	Present	3-7 days; may secrete organisms in stool for 3 wk or more	Yes	Watery, green with blood and pus, foul smelling	Tenesmus	12-72 hr incubation period; common cause of outbreaks in nurseries; bacteremia is common
Shigella	Mild	>7 days, range of illness; usually self-limited but can be severe	Yes, low grade	Bloody and green with mucus, pus, (dysentery form characterized by watery diarrhea, high fever, malaise followed in 24 hr by tenesmus and colitis)	Tenesmus	Prevalent in developing countries and Central America; as few as 10 organisms can cause disease

Yersinia enterocolitica	On occasion	Self-limited	Sometimes	Variable consistency, with pus and blood in 25% of cases	Some	Common in Canada and Europe; less common in the United States

Modified from San Joaquin V, Marks M: New agents in diarrhea, *Pediatric Infections Disease Journal* 1(1):53, 1982; Walker WA et al, editors: *Pediatric gastrointestinal disease: pathophysiology, diagnosis, management*, Philadelphia, 1991, BC Decker.

INCIDENCE

1. Acute gastroenteritis is the second most common condition affecting children (the cold is first).
2. Rotavirus causes approximately 35% to 50% of hospital admissions for acute gastroenteritis; between 7% and 17% of the admissions result from enteric adenoviruses; and another 15% result from bacterial causes.
3. Breast-fed infants have gastroenteritis less often than formula-fed infants; maternal antibodies to some enteric pathogens are transferred in breast milk.

CLINICAL MANIFESTATIONS

1. Loose consistency of stools (diarrhea) with increased frequency
2. Vomiting (usually short duration)
3. Fever (may or may not be present)
4. Abdominal cramping, tenesmus
5. Dry mucous membranes
6. Sunken fontanel (infant)
7. Weight loss
8. Malaise

COMPLICATIONS

1. Severe dehydration, electrolyte imbalance
2. Decompensated hypovolemic shock (hypotension, metabolic acidosis, poor systemic perfusion)
3. Febrile seizures
4. Bacteremia

LABORATORY AND DIAGNOSTIC TESTS

1. Hematest stool—to check for presence of blood (more common with bacterial origin)
2. Stool evaluation for volume, color, consistency, presence of mucus or pus
3. Complete blood count with differential
4. Enzyme immunoassay antigen tests—to confirm rotavirus
5. Stool culture (if hospitalized, pus in stool or course of diarrhea is prolonged)—to determine pathogen
6. Stool evaluation for ova and parasites
7. Duodenal aspirate (if *G. lamblia* is suspected)

8. Urinalysis and culture (specific gravity increases with dehydration; *Shigella* organisms are shed in urine)

MEDICAL MANAGEMENT

When the child is only mildly dehydrated, rehydration may be accomplished orally on an outpatient basis with commercially available oral rehydration solutions (Pedialyte, Ricelyte). Oral rehydration fluids are given frequently, in small volumes (5 to 15 ml), even in the event of vomiting. In the case of severe dehydration, the child is admitted for intravenous (IV) therapy to correct dehydration. The amount of dehydration is calculated and fluid is replaced over 24 hours, at the same time that maintenance fluids are given.

When shock is present, fluid resuscitation commences immediately (20 ml/kg of normal saline or lactated Ringer's solution; repeat if needed). In these cases, when rapid peripheral IV access is unsuccessful, the intraosseous route may be used for emergency fluid administration in the child less than 6 years of age. When systemic perfusion has been improved, correction of dehydration that is present is begun.

Once rehydration is completed, the diet may be advanced to regular easily digested foods such as bananas, rice and rice cereal, toast, dry cereal, and breast milk. Feeding and oral rehydration fluids have reportedly decreased the duration of diarrhea. Early return to normal oral feedings is important, especially in cases of preexisting malnutrition. Milk and juices are initially diluted when reintroduced.

Antiemetics and antispasmodics are generally not recommended. Neither are antibiotics indicated in most cases, because bacterial and viral gastroenteritis is self-limited. Antibiotics are, however, used in the treatment of diseases caused by *Shigella* organisms, *E. coli, Salmonella* organisms (with sepsis or localized infection present), and *G. lamblia.* Antibiotics may increase the length of the carrier state with salmonella infections.

NURSING ASSESSMENT

See the section on gastrointestinal assessment in Appendix A.

NURSING DIAGNOSES

- High risk for fluid volume deficit
- Diarrhea

- Potential for impaired skin integrity
- Knowledge deficit

NURSING INTERVENTIONS

1. Promote and monitor child's fluid and electrolyte balance.
   a. Monitor IV fluids.
   b. Assess intake and output (weigh diapers).
   c. Assess hydration status.
   d. Monitor daily weight.
   e. Assess child's ability to rehydrate by mouth.
2. Prevent further gastrointestinal (GI) tract irritability.
   a. Assess child's ability to take nourishment by mouth (i.e., first provide oral rehydration fluids [Pedialyte, Ricelyte], then advance to a regular diet of easily digested foods such as bananas, rice, toast, dry cereal, and breast milk).
   b. Avoid use of milk products; initially dilute milk or juices when gradually reintroducing.
   c. Consult with dietitian about selection of foods.
3. Prevent skin irritation and breakdown.
   a. Change diapers frequently, assessing skin condition each time.
   b. Wash perineum with mild soap and water, and expose perineum to air.
   c. Apply zinc oxide or lubricating ointment to rectum and perineum (acidic stools irritate skin).
4. Follow universal precautions and/or enteric precautions to prevent transmission of infection (refer to institution's policies and procedures).
5. Provide for child's developmental needs during hospitalization.
   a. Provide age-appropriate toys (see section on growth and development, Appendix B).
   b. Incorporate home routine into hospitalization (e.g., feeding practices, bedtime ritual).
   c. Encourage ventilation of feelings through age-appropriate means.
6. Provide emotional support to family.
   a. Encourage ventilation of concerns.
   b. Refer to social service as needed.

   c. Provide for physical comforts (e.g., place to sleep and bathe).

♠ Discharge Planning and Home Care

1. Instruct parents and child about personal and environmental hygiene.
   a. Safe drinking water
   b. Sanitary disposal of excreta
   c. Sanitary food preparation
   d. Toileting practices
2. Reinforce dietary information provided to parents about menu planning.
3. Instruct parents to observe for and report signs of dehydration or problems with oral rehydration and advancement of feedings.
4. Instruct parent about follow-up appointment.

CLIENT OUTCOMES

1. Child will have a return to normal gastrointestinal function.
2. Child will be well hydrated.
3. Parents and child understand home care and medical follow-up needed.

REFERENCES

Betz CL, Hunsberger MM, Wright S: *Family-centered nursing care of children,* ed 2, Philadelphia, 1994, WB Saunders.

Griffiths RI et al: Economic impact of immunization against rotavirus gastroenteritis: evidence from a clinical trial, *Arch Pediatr Adolesc Med* 149(4):407, 1995.

Imamura Y et al: Detection and typing of human rotavirus in reference to repeated acute gastroenteritis in infants, *Microbiol Immunol* 38(8):673, 1994.

San Joaquin V, Marks M: New agents in diarrhea, *Pediatric Infections Disease Journal* 1(1):53, 1982.

Snyder JD: Gastroenterology. In Graef JW, editor: *Manual of pediatric therapeutics,* ed 5, Boston, 1994, Little, Brown & Company.

Walker WA et al, editors: *Pediatric gastrointestinal disease: pathophysiology, diagnosis, management,* Philadelphia, 1991, BC Decker.

27

Gastroesophageal Reflux

PATHOPHYSIOLOGY

Gastroesophageal reflux is the presence of abnormal amounts of gastric contents in the esophagus, upper airways, and tracheobronchial area. The reflux of gastric contents can result in inflammation and stricture of the esophagus. Resultant effects include aspiration of the gastric contents, recurrent pneumonia, pulmonary disease, esophagitis, and esophageal stricture. Factors that can predispose the infant or child to gastroesophageal reflux are (1) lower-esophageal sphincter pressure, (2) volume of reflux material in the esophagus, (3) rate of gastric secretion, and (4) inability of the stomach to empty. A child may require surgery if he or she does not respond to medical management.

INCIDENCE

1. Vomiting occurs in two thirds of children with gastroesophageal reflux.
2. Failure to thrive occurs in 34% of these children.
3. Bleeding occurs in 28% of these children.
4. Pulmonary complications occur in 12% of these children.

CLINICAL MANIFESTATIONS

1. Chronic vomiting (most common)
2. Weight loss, failure to thrive

3. Apnea (in infants) due to aspiration
4. Hematemesis or melena due to esophageal bleeding

COMPLICATIONS

1. Aspiration pneumonia
2. Apnea and cyanosis
3. Esophagitis
4. Chest pain
5. Gastric fistula
6. Herniation

LABORATORY AND DIAGNOSTIC TESTS

1. Esophageal sphincter pressure (less than 6 mm Hg is diagnostic)
2. Measure of pH in esophagus (lower pH is direct measure of reflux)
3. Radionuclide gastroesophagraphy (noninvasive test for gastroesophageal reflux)
4. Barium esophagram (often fails to detect intermittent reflux)
5. Acid reflux test (detects acid regurgitation)
6. Endoscopy (detects presence of gross and microscopic esophagitis)

MEDICAL MANAGEMENT

The treatment of gastroesophageal reflux is reflective of the severity of symptoms. Thickened feedings are given, and the child is placed in a prone position after feedings with the head of the bed elevated to prevent aspiration. Infant seats are contraindicated because they increase intraabdominal pressure. A small infant may be placed in a cholasia harness to keep the infant from sliding to the foot of the crib. Medications that may be used include antacids. Medications such as cisapride, metaclopramide, and cimetidine may also be given.

Fundoplication is the surgical procedure performed for gastroesophageal reflux. The upper end of the stomach is wrapped around the lower portion of the esophagus, and the fundus is sutured in front of the esophagus, creating a circular acute-angle valve mechanism. Fundoplication results in complete relief of symptoms—the reflux is treated, vomiting ceases, and failure to thrive is resolved. The child retains feedings and regains weight. A gastrostomy tube is often put in place for feedings with the fundoplication.

NURSING ASSESSMENT

1. See the section on gastrointestinal assessment in Appendix A.
2. Assess feeding history.
3. Assess hydration status.
4. Assess frequency and volume of emesis and length of time between feedings and emesis.
5. Assess weight gain.

NURSING DIAGNOSES

- Fluid volume deficit
- Pain
- Altered nutrition: less than body requirements
- High risk for impaired gas exchange
- Knowledge deficit
- High risk for impaired home maintenance management

NURSING INTERVENTIONS

1. Promote adequate nutritional and fluid intake.
   a. Maintain head of bed in 60-degree position for 30 to 40 minutes after feeding.
   b. Raise head of bed with 6-inch blocks.
   c. Provide small, frequent feedings every 2 to 3 hours.
   d. Thicken formula with cereal.
   e. Provide last meal of day several hours before bedtime.
   f. Weigh patient daily.
   g. Monitor intake and output.
2. Observe, monitor, and report signs of respiratory distress; assess for changes in respiratory status.
3. Preoperatively, prepare child and family for surgery.
4. Monitor surgical site for intactness.
5. Prevent abdominal distention.
   a. Maintain patency of nasogastric (NG) or gastrostomy tube if placed.
   b. Check position of NG tube.
   c. Auscultate for bowel sounds.

6. Monitor for signs and symptoms of postoperative hemorrhage.
   a. Decreased blood pressure and increased apical pulse
   b. Gross blood in NG drainage
   c. Coffee-ground NG drainage expected for first 24 hours
7. Assist parents in expression of feelings—may express anger, guilt, or frustration because they feel inadequate or responsible.
8. Provide developmentally appropriate stimulation activities (see section on growth and development, Appendix B).

♠ Discharge Planning and Home Care

1. Instruct parents about medication administration.
2. Instruct parents about feeding techniques.
3. Instruct parents to report any vomiting or presence of frank blood.

CLIENT OUTCOMES

1. The child will have consistent weight gain.
2. The child will have decreased frequency and volume of emesis.
3. The child will have decreased pain ("heartburn").
4. The child will not aspirate.

REFERENCES

Feranchak AP, Orenstein SR, Cohen JF: Behaviors associated with onset of gastroesophageal reflux episodes in infants: prospective study using split-screen video and pH probe, *Clin Pediatr* 33(11):654, 1994.

Glassman M, George D, Grill B: Gastroesophageal reflux in children: clinical manifestations, diagnosis, and therapy, *Gastroenterol Clin North Am* 24(1):71, 1995.

Hyman PE: Gastroesophageal reflux: one reason why baby won't eat, *J Pediatr* 125(6):103, 1994.

Nagaya M, Akatsuka H, Kato J: Gastroesophageal reflux occurring after repair of congenital diaphragmatic hernia, *J Pediatr Surg* 29(11):1447, 1994.

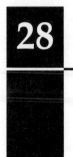

28

Glomerulonephritis

PATHOPHYSIOLOGY

Glomerulonephritis is a term used for a collection of disorders that involve the renal glomeruli (the renal glomeruli are responsible for filtering body fluids and wastes). There are two types of this disease: acute and chronic, with chronic being the progressive form. Acute glomerulonephritis is the most common form of nephritis in children. It is an inflammation of the glomeruli that usually follows an upper respiratory tract, streptococcal infection. It is considered an immune complex disease. The glomerular injury is induced by antigen-antibody complexes trapped in the glomerular filter. The glomeruli become edematous and are infiltrated with polymorphonuclear leukocytes, which occlude the capillary lumen. This condition results in decreased plasma filtration, causing excessive accumulation of water and retention of sodium. The resultant plasma and interstitial fluid volumes lead to circulatory congestion and edema. Hypertension is associated with glomerulonephritis.

INCIDENCE

1. Glomerulonephritis is most common in school-age children.
2. Ages of peak incidence are from 2 to 6 years.
3. There is a male predominance in childhood, but no male or female predilection in adolescents.

4. Sixty percent to 80% of children with acute glomerulo-nephritis have a history of a preceding upper respiratory tract infection or otitis media (typically, the child has been in good health before the infection).

CLINICAL MANIFESTATIONS

1. Nephritis tends to have an average latent period of approximately 10 days, with onset of symptoms 10 days after the initial infection.
2. Initial signs are puffiness of the face, periorbital edema, anorexia, and dark urine.
3. Edema tends to be more prominent in the face in the morning; then it spreads to the abdomen and the extremities during the day (moderate edema may not be recognized by someone who is unfamiliar with the child).
4. Urinary output is decreased.
5. Urine is cloudy, smoky, or described as the color of tea or cola.
6. The child is pale, irritable, and lethargic.
7. Younger children may appear ill but seldom express specific complaints.
8. Older children may complain of headaches, abdominal discomfort, vomiting, and dysuria.
9. Mild to moderate hypertension may be present.

COMPLICATIONS

Once acute glomerulonephritis progresses to the chronic stage, the following complications may be seen.
1. Deteriorating renal function (generally reflected by clinical manifestations and laboratory findings)
2. Proteinuria
3. Edema
4. Hypertension
5. Hematoria
6. Anemia (manifestation of progressive disease)
7. Hypertensive encephalopathy (characterized by headache, vomiting, irritability, convulsions, and coma)—can result from the chronic hypertension

8. Cardiac failure, possibly a result of an increase in blood volume secondary to retention of sodium and water—associated with pulmonary congestion
9. End-stage renal disease

LABORATORY AND DIAGNOSTIC TESTS

No diagnostic tests are specifically indicated for the diagnosis of glomerulonephritis. However, the following are commonly done:

1. Examination of urine—proteinuria (1–4+), hematuria; presence of casts, red blood cells, and white blood cells; decreased creatine clearance rates
2. Blood tests—elevated blood urea nitrogen, serum creatinine, and uric acid; electrolyte alterations (metabolic acidosis; decreased sodium and calcium; increased potassium, phosphorus, serum albumin, and cholesterol); mild anemia and leukocytosis; elevated antibody titers (antistreptolysin, antihyaluronidase, or anti-DNAase B) and erythrocyte sedimentation rate
3. Renal biopsy—may be indicated; if it is performed, possible findings are an increased number of cells in each glomerulus and subepithelial "humps" containing immunoglobulin and complement

MEDICAL MANAGEMENT

Acute glomerulonephritis has no specific treatment; thus therapy is targeted at the symptoms. Marked hypertension may be treated with diuretics and/or antihypertensives. Appropriate antibiotics are used for acute infections. Some medicinal approaches for chronic glomerulonephritis have included glucocorticoids and immunosuppressive agents.

NURSING ASSESSMENT

1. See the section on renal assessment in Appendix A.
2. Assess nutritional intake.
3. Assess fluid status.

NURSING DIAGNOSES

- Fluid volume excess
- Altered nutrition: less than body requirements
- Knowledge deficit

NURSING INTERVENTIONS

1. Maintain bed rest, and keep the child comfortable until diuresis occurs; after diuresis, encourage quiet activity.
2. Closely monitor vital signs (especially blood pressure).
3. When hypertension is present, limit sodium intake and administer ordered medications.
4. Monitor urine for protein and occult blood.
5. Promote adequate nutritional intake: encourage high-carbohydrate meals, serve preferred foods, and try small, frequent feedings.
6. Limit potassium intake if hyperkalemia occurs.
7. Record weight daily, and record accurate intake and output.
8. Monitor for complications—significant changes in vital signs, change in appearance or volume of urine, excessive weight gain, visual disturbances, motor disturbances, seizure activity, severe pain, or any behavioral changes.

♠ Discharge Planning and Home Care

1. Provide the family with education about the child's illness and treatment plan.
2. Instruct about any medications the child will take at home.
3. Instruct parents and child to monitor blood pressure and weight, and to obtain urinalyses for several months; follow-up appointments should be arranged.
4. Instruct parents to contact the physician if there is any change in the child's condition, such as signs of infection, edema, alteration in eating habits, abdominal pain, headaches, change in appearance or amount of urine, or lethargy.
5. Explain any dietary restrictions to the parents.

CLIENT OUTCOMES

1. Child will have a return to normal renal function.
2. Child and family understand home care and follow-up needs.

REFERENCES

Edelmann CM: *Pediatric kidney disease,* ed 2, Boston, 1992, Little, Brown & Company.

Matsell DG, Wyatt RJ, Gaber LW: Terminal complement complexes in acute poststreptococcal glomerulonephritis, *Pediatr Nephrol* 8(6):671, 1994.

Welch TR: Current management of selected childhood renal diseases, *Curr Probl Pediatr* 22(10):432, 1992.

29

Hemolytic-Uremic Syndrome

PATHOPHYSIOLOGY

Hemolytic-uremic syndrome is an intravascular coagulation condition that primarily affects the kidney. It consists of the following symptomatology: (1) renal failure, (2) hemolytic anemia with fragmented red blood cells (RBCs) and platelets, and (3) thrombocytopenia. The exact cause is unknown, although findings suggest the majority of cases of idiopathic hemolytic-uremic syndrome are associated with one or the other of the enteric pathogens *Escherichia coli* and *Shigella dysenteriae.* The clinical manifestations and features result from changes in the capillary endothelium caused by the etiologic agent. The endothelial changes result in the following pathologic responses: (1) mechanical trauma to erythrocytes and platelets, shortening their life span and resulting in anemia and thrombocytopenia; and (2) decreased renal blood flow and glomerular filtration rate, resulting in cortical necrosis, which leads to renal failure and acquired hemolytic anemia in infants and children. The severity of the condition varies. The length of the oliguria phase correlates with the ultimate prognosis for recovery. In addition, the prognosis is related to the efficiency and promptness of treatment.

INCIDENCE

1. A seasonal variation exists, with an increased incidence during spring and fall.

2. Hemolytic-uremic syndrome is most commonly seen in children 6 months to 5 years old.
3. The incidence of hypertension as a long-term complication varies from 10% to 50%.
4. Hemolytic-uremic syndrome affects male and female individuals equally.
5. It is uncommon for a sibling to be affected.
6. Mortality is 10% to 25%.

CLINICAL MANIFESTATIONS
Prodromal Period

1. Hemolytic-uremic syndrome usually follows gastroenteritis or viral illness.
2. Prodromal illness in older children resembles upper respiratory tract illness.
3. Prodromal symptoms may last a week, whereas other symptoms may recur in children who appear to have recovered; severity varies (see the box on p. 175 for four types of clinical manifestations).

Acute Phase

1. Oliguric, amber urine
2. Renal failure (metabolic disturbance or acidosis; hypocalcemia or hyperkalemia)
3. Oligoanuric for more than 1 week, then diuresis
4. Abdominal pain (caused by splenic enlargement or gastrointestinal [GI] involvement)
5. Edema
6. Hypertension
7. Mild icterus
8. Pallor
9. Systemic bleeding manifestations—purpura, petechiae
10. Alteration in neurologic status
11. Anemia associated with uremia
12. Anorexia
13. Seizures
14. Moderate to severe respiratory distress caused by congestive heart failure (CHF) and circulatory overload

Clinical Manifestations

Mild

No anemia
Oliguria*
Hypertension*
Convulsions*

Severe

Anuria for more than 24 hours

Deteriorating Renal Function

Progressive oliguria
Azotemia
Complete renal failure—may not occur
Severe hypertension
Cardiac failure

Recurrent Hemolytic-Uremic Syndrome

First occurrence—mild
Recurrent occurrence—mild to severe

* Child may manifest one or more symptoms but not all three.

COMPLICATIONS

1. Neurologic—mortality rate in children with neurologic symptoms (seizures, coma) is 90%, compared to overall mortality rate of 45%.
2. Disseminated intravascular coagulation (DIC)—primarily affects vasculature of kidney, nervous system, and GI tract.

LABORATORY AND DIAGNOSTIC TESTS

1. Renal scan—to assess renal perfusion
2. Renal biopsy—to assess renal involvement
3. Serum protein—increased
4. Complete blood count—decreased hemoglobin; increased white blood count (WBC); significant reticulocytosis; reticulocyte count greater than 2%
5. Platelet count—less than 140,000; remains low for 7 to 14 days
6. Serum albumin—decreased
7. Arterial blood gas values—decreased pH; acidosis with acute renal failure
8. Electrolytes—consistent with renal failure (hyponatremia, hyperkalemia)
9. Tests for hyperuricemia, hypocalcemia, hyperphosphatemia
10. Urinalysis—gross hematuria, proteinuria, casts
11. Blood urea nitrogen (BUN), creatinine—increased; reflects severity of renal failure

MEDICAL MANAGEMENT

Early diagnosis and aggressive treatment are the goals of therapy. Early intervention with peritoneal dialysis is the most effective treatment for children who have been anuric for 24 hours or who demonstrate oliguria with hypertension and seizures. Supportive care is directed toward vascular support and stabilization.

Drugs such as corticosteroids, anticoagulants, or antiplatelet agents have not been found effective.

NURSING ASSESSMENT

1. See the section on renal assessment in Appendix A.
2. Assess hydration status.
3. Assess cardiovascular status.

NURSING DIAGNOSES

- Fluid volume excess
- Decreased cardiac output
- High risk for infection

- Impaired tissue integrity
- Knowledge deficit
- Anxiety

NURSING INTERVENTIONS

1. Monitor and maintain fluid and electrolyte balance.
   a. Monitor types of fluids and administration rate to avoid fluid overload and cerebral edema.
   b. Record accurate input and output.
   c. Record daily weights (twice a day during acute phase).
   d. Monitor blood pressure and pulse pressure.
   e. Replace fluids from urinary loss with isotonic solution (normal saline or lactated Ringer's).
   f. Assess hydration status every 4 to 6 hours during acute phase.
   g. Perform arterial pressure and central venous pressure (CVP) monitoring.
2. Monitor electrolytes and observe for signs of imbalance.
   a. Hyperkalemia—muscular instability; electrocardiogram (ECG) changes (peaked T waves, wide QRS complex, prolonged PR interval); cardiac arrhythmias
   b. Hypocalcemia—coma, convulsions
   c. Hyponatremia—seizures
   d. Hypoglycemia—seizures
3. Transfuse with blood products as indicated.
   a. Washed packed red blood cells (PRBCs)—for low hemoglobin level; transfuse slowly; do not raise hemoglobin level higher than 7 to 8 g
   b. Platelets—as needed for bleeding
4. Observe and report signs and symptoms of impending complications.
   a. Shock
   b. Infection
   c. Disseminated intravascular coagulation
   d. Heart failure
   e. Potassium intoxication
   f. Overhydration
   g. Seizures

  h. Neurologic disturbance—lethargy, coma, hyperactivity
  i. Pulmonary edema
  j. Hypertension
5. Monitor for nutritional status; nasogastric (NG) feedings or hyperalimentation may be needed.
6. Prepare child and family for peritoneal dialysis or hemodialysis if indicated; indications include the following.
  a. Anuria for 24 to 48 hours
  b. Central nervous system (CNS) disturbance
  c. Congestive heart failure
  d. Bleeding (GI and cutaneous)
  e. BUN greater than 150 mg/100 ml
  f. Uncontrollable hyperkalemia
  g. Hyponatremia less than 130 mEq/L
  h. Change in neurologic status—lethargy to coma or hyperactivity
  i. Hyperphosphatemia greater than 8 mg/100 ml
  j. Uncontrollable acidosis
  k. Hypocalcemia less than 8 mg/100 ml
7. Provide information about procedures before they are performed, and reinforce data provided to parents.

♠ Discharge Planning and Home Care
1. Instruct child and family regarding dietary restrictions.
2. Instruct child and family regarding medications.

CLIENT OUTCOMES
1. Child will have normal or near-normal renal function.
2. Child will have a return to normal or control of blood pressure.
3. Child will have a return to normal neurologic function or control of central nervous system symptoms.

REFERENCES

Grimm PC, Ogborn MR: Hemolytic uremic syndrome: the most common cause of acute renal failure in childhood, *Pediatr Ann* 23(9):505, 1994.

Jernigan SM, Waldo FB: Racial incidence of hemolytic uremic syndrome, *Pediatr Nephrol* 8(5):545, 1994.

Rowe PC et al: Epidemiology of hemolytic-uremic syndrome in Canadian children from 1986-1988, *J Pediatr* 119(2):218, 1991.

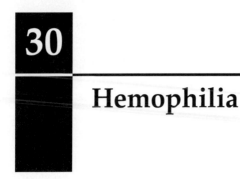

Hemophilia

PATHOPHYSIOLOGY

Hemophilia is a congenital blood coagulation disorder in which the child is deficient in clotting factor VIII (hemophilia A) or factor IX (hemophilia B or Christmas disease). It is an inherited disorder that is transmitted by an X-linked recessive gene from the maternal side. Factor VIII and factor IX are plasma proteins that are necessary components of blood coagulation; they are needed for the formation of fibrin clots at the site of vascular injury. Severe hemophilia results when plasma concentrations of factors VIII and IX are less than 1%. Moderate hemophilia has plasma concentrations between 1% and 5%, and mild hemophilia is between 5% to 25% of the normal level. The clinical manifestations depend on the child's age and the severity of the deficiency of factors VIII and IX. Severe hemophilia is characterized by recurrent hemorrhages, occurring either spontaneously or after relatively minor trauma. The most common sites of hemorrhage are within the joints of the knees, elbows, ankles, shoulders, and hips. The muscles most often affected are the forearm flexor, the gastrocnemius, and the iliopsoas. Because of improvements in treatment, almost all hemophiliac patients are expected to live a normal life span.

INCIDENCE

1. Incidence is 20 per 100,000 male births.
2. Twenty-five thousand male individuals are severely affected.
3. The family histories of two thirds of affected children reveal an X-linked recessive form of inheritance.
4. Central nervous system (CNS) bleeding occurs in 3% of affected children.
5. Spontaneous bleeding and posttraumatic intracranial bleeding are associated with a 34% mortality rate and 50% long-term morbidity.
6. Ten percent of patients with hemophilia A and hemophilia B develop IgG antibodies that inhibit the activity of factors VIII and IX.

CLINICAL MANIFESTATIONS
Infancy (for Diagnosis)

1. Prolonged bleeding after circumcision
2. Subcutaneous ecchymoses over bony prominences (at 3 to 4 months of age)
3. Large hematoma after infections
4. Bleeding from oral mucosa
5. Soft-tissue hemorrhages

Bleeding Episodes (throughout Life Span)

1. Initial symptom—pain
2. After pain—swelling, warmth, and decreased mobility

Long-Term Sequelae

Prolonged bleeding into the muscle causes nerve compression and muscle fibrosis.

COMPLICATIONS

1. Progressive, crippling arthropathy
2. Muscular contracture
3. Paralysis
4. Intracranial bleeding
5. Hypertension

6. Renal impairment
7. Splenomegaly
8. Hepatitis
9. Acquired immunodeficiency syndrome (AIDS) from exposure to contaminated blood products
10. Antibodies formed as antagonists to factors VIII and IX
11. Allergic transfusion reaction to blood products
12. Hemolytic anemia
13. Thrombosis and/or thromboembolism

LABORATORY AND DIAGNOSTIC TESTS

1. Screening tests for blood coagulation
   a. Platelet count (normal)
   b. Prothrombin time (normal)
   c. Partial thromboplastin time (increased; measures adequacy of intrinsic coagulation cascade)
   d. Bleeding time (normal; assesses formation of platelet plugs in capillaries)
   e. Functional assays of factors VIII and IX (confirm diagnosis)
   f. Thrombin clotting time
2. Liver biopsy (sometimes) used to obtain tissue for pathologic examination and culture
3. Liver function tests (sometimes) used to detect presence of liver disease (e.g., serum glutamic-pyruvic transaminase [SGPT], serum glutamic-oxaloacetic transaminase [SGOT], alkaline phosphatase, bilirubin)

MEDICAL MANAGEMENT

The management of hemophilia consists of the administration of factor VIII or IX. The amount depends on the plasma level of the deficient factor needed to treat the specific bleeding episode, and it must be sufficient to allow for the distribution of the factor throughout the body and its clearance from plasma.

Other methods that are used to treat bleeding episodes are the infusion of frozen plasma and that of cryoprecipitate (factor VIII). Desmopressin (DDAVP) is also used to increase plasma levels of factor VIII and can be used for nontransfusional treatment of patients with mild or moderate hemophilia.

NURSING ASSESSMENT

1. See the section on neurologic assessment in Appendix A.
2. Assess child for verbal and nonverbal behaviors indicating pain.
3. Assess site of involvement for extent of bleeding and extent of sensory, nerve, and motor impairment.
4. Assess child's ability to engage in self-care activities (i.e., brushing teeth).
5. Assess child's level of development.
6. Assess child's and family's readiness for discharge and ability to manage home treatment regimen.

NURSING DIAGNOSES

- High risk for fluid volume deficit
- Pain
- High risk for injury
- Knowledge deficit
- High risk for altered growth and development
- High risk for altered family processes
- High risk for ineffective management of treatment regimen
- High risk for impaired physical mobility

NURSING INTERVENTIONS

The following interventions relate to acute episodes.
1. Monitor child's or adolescent's response to administration of plasma products.
2. Monitor child's response to administration of pain medication and to measures to relieve pain.
   a. Acetaminophen (avoid aspirin)
   b. Narcotic analgesics
   c. Application of ice to affected joint
   d. Immobilization of affected limb
3. Monitor child or adolescent for further bleeding episodes; observe for signs and symptoms of bleeding.
4. Protect child or adolescent from further injury.
   a. Pad child's crib or bed.
   b. Apply pressure after venipunctures.
   c. Apply fibrin or gelatin foam to bleeding sites.

5. Instruct and monitor child regarding dental care.
   a. Use of soft-bristle toothbrush
   b. Good nutritional intake
   c. Avoidance of excessive amounts of sweets
   d. Chewing of sugarless gum
   e. Need for regular dental visits
   f. Use of factor replacement before dental work
6. Instruct child about monitoring self for bleeding episodes—an intuitive feeling or "knowing" that bleeding is occurring.
7. Encourage quiet age-appropriate play or diversional activities (see section on growth and development, Appendix B).
8. Provide age-appropriate explanations before treatments and procedures (see Appendix J, section on preparation for procedure/surgery).
9. Provide emotional support to family (see Appendix J, section on supportive care).

♠ Discharge Planning and Home Care

1. Instruct child and parents about administering replacement for deficient factor.
2. Instruct child and parents about signs and symptoms of bleeding episodes.
3. Discuss options and plan life-style activities to support (sedentary) living and to prevent further injuries (avoiding contact sports and physical play).
4. Discuss with parents and child methods to make life-style more normal and to avoid being labeled as having a disability.
5. Encourage parents and child to express feelings about the disease and the limitations it imposes on activities.
6. Link family to appropriate community-based resources (see Appendix K, section on community resources, referral).

CLIENT OUTCOMES

1. Child's bleeding episodes will be controlled.
2. Child and family will adhere to the long-term treatment regimen.
3. Child will attain developmental milestones.

REFERENCES

Colegrove RW Jr, Huntzinger RM: Academic, behavioral, and social adaptation of boys with hemophilia/HIV disease, *J Pediatr Psychol*, 19(4):457, 1994.

Girvan DP et al: Subcutaneous infusion ports in the pediatric patient with hemophilia, *J Pediatr Surg*, 29(9):1220, 1994.

Loveland KA et al: Hemophilia growth and development study: baseline neurodevelopmental findings, *J Pediatr Psychol*, 19(2):223, 1994.

Peterson CW: Treating hemophilia, *Am Pharm* 34(8):57, 1994.

Spitzer A: Children's knowledge of illness treatment experiences in hemophilia, *J Pediatr Nurs* 7(1):42, 1992.

31

Hepatitis

PATHOPHYSIOLOGY

Hepatitis, a liver disease that is typically self-limiting and uncomplicated, is caused by a viral agent. Hepatitis viruses can be classified into five types: hepatitis A (HAV), hepatitis B (HBV), hepatitis C (HCV), hepatitis D (HDV), and hepatitis E (HEV). The hepatocytes (epithelial cells of the liver) are damaged either directly by the virus or by the body's immune response to the virus; in either case, there is altered cellular function that leads to inflammation, necrosis, and autolysis of the liver. Regeneration of cells begins when damaged cells are removed by phagocytosis. Usually recovery is with minimal residual damage, although chronic hepatitis and cirrhosis may develop.

Hepatitis A

Hepatitis A is the most highly contagious form of hepatitis. It is transmitted primarily through the fecal-oral route. It can also be transmitted by unsanitary food handlers, contaminated food supplies, and shellfish from sewage-contaminated waters. It is rarely transmitted through transfusions. Epidemics of hepatitis A have been reported in institutions housing or caring for large numbers of children such as day care centers, schools, and homes for the mentally retarded. The incubation period is approximately 1 month. Jaundice appears 4 to 6 weeks after exposure. The child is contagious 2 weeks prior to the onset of jaundice due to the high concentration of virus in the stool before definitive symptoms are exhibited. The communicable state continues up to 1 week after the onset of jaundice. Hepatitis A manifests a wide spectrum of symptoms; it rarely (10% of cases) leads to chronic hepatitis. Children may have minimal symptoms or be asymptomatic. The child is rarely hospitalized, and there is no known carrier state.

Hepatitis B and Hepatitis C

The viruses are transmitted through blood or blood derivatives and body secretions (semen, saliva, breast milk, urine). Hepatitis B occurs most commonly in the following populations of children: (1) infants whose mothers are chronic carriers of the viral antigen HB_SAg, (2) children receiving frequent transfusions or hemodialysis (may also develop hepatitis C), (3) children involved in intravenous drug abuse (may also develop hepatitis C), (4) institutionalized children, and (5) preschool children in areas where the disease is endemic. The incubation period is 2 to 6 months. Children with hepatitis C are typically asymptomatic. In the United States more than 90% of the cases of hepatitis C are associated with transfusions of blood or blood products. A carrier state and the development of chronic liver disease are possible with hepatitis B and C.

Hepatitis D

The virus can only cause infection and clinical manifestations in association with hepatitis B infection. The virus acts as a parasite of hepatitis B. Coinfection with hepatitis D increases the severity of the hepatitis B infection, creating a more fulminating course and enhancing the potential for chronic liver disease. Hepatitis D is most common in hemophiliac individuals and intravenous drug abusers.

Hepatitis E

Hepatitis E is epidemic or enterally transmitted non-A, non-B hepatitis. Transmission occurs via contaminated water and is often seen after natural disasters in the developing regions of the world. No diagnostic test is available, so other forms of hepatitis must be ruled out.

INCIDENCE

1. Approximately 90% of young children and infants with hepatitis do not exhibit jaundice.
2. Ten percent of children with hepatitis B develop chronic hepatitis.
3. Hepatitis A is the most common type of hepatitis in children.
4. Approximately 30,000 cases of hepatitis A are reported each year; they represent a small proportion of actual cases.
5. Tropical and developing nations have a higher incidence than industrialized and temperate-zone nations.
6. Approximately 200,000 persons, mainly young adults, acquire hepatitis B annually.
7. Incidence of hepatitis D is difficult to measure because it occurs concurrently with hepatitis B and may not be readily diagnosed.

CLINICAL MANIFESTATIONS
Hepatitis A

1. Acute febrile illness
2. Jaundice (develops as fever drops)
3. Anorexia
4. Nausea and vomiting
5. Malaise
6. Dark urine (precedes jaundice)
7. Children under three—often asymptomatic
8. Hepatomegaly
9. Splenomegaly

Hepatitis B, C, D, and E

1. Insidious onset
2. Jaundice
3. Anorexia
4. Malaise
5. Nausea
6. Papular acrodermatitis (Gianotti-Crosti syndrome)
7. Prodromal symptoms—arthralgia, arthritis, erythematous maculopapular rash
8. Polyarteritis nodosa

9. Glomerulonephritis
10. Hepatitis D intensifies the symptoms of hepatitis B and increases the possibility of a chronic condition
11. Hepatitis C is characterized by mild asymptomatic infection with insidious onset of jaundice and malaise

COMPLICATIONS
Hepatitis A

1. Progression to fulminating disease (rare)
2. Encephalopathy
3. Aplastic anemia

Hepatitis B and C

1. Hepatocellular cancer
2. Liver failure
3. Aplastic anemia
4. Cirrhosis
5. Fulminating hepatitis
6. Massive hepatic necrosis
7. Carrier state (persistent viral infection without symptoms)
8. Chronic liver disease (in 50% of patients with hepatitis C)

Hepatitis D

1. Fulminating hepatitis
2. Liver failure
3. Carrier state

LABORATORY AND DIAGNOSTIC TESTS

1. Serum glutamic-oxaloacetic transaminase (SGOT)—increased
2. Serum glutamic-pyruvic transaminase (SGPT)—increased
3. Bilirubin—elevated
4. IgM antibodies (hepatitis A virus antibody and anti-hepatitis A IgM)—diagnostic for hepatitis A
5. IgM antibodies (hepatitis B core antigen; anti-HB$_S$, IgM)

6. IgG antibodies (hepatitis A virus antibody and antihepatitis)—indicates susceptibility or past exposure to hepatitis A
7. Hb$_S$Ag titer—diagnostic for hepatitis B; if persists more than 6 months, indicates acute chronic hepatitis B
8. Anti-Hb$_c$ Ag titer—diagnostic for chronic hepatitis
9. Anti-Hb$_s$—presence indicates recovery and immunity to hepatitis B
10. Anti-Hb$_e$—presence indicates low titers of hepatitis B and insufficient disease transmission
11. Anti-HCV (IgG, IgM)—diagnostic for hepatitis C; approximately two thirds of individuals with HCV will not develop antibodies until 5 to 12 months after the infection
12. Aspartate aminotransferase (AST)—increase indicates acute hepatitis
13. Alanine aminotransferase (ALT)—increased in acute hepatitis

MEDICAL MANAGEMENT

Treatment is mainly supportive and includes rest, hydration, and adequate dietary intake. Hospitalization is indicated with severe vomiting, dehydration, abnormal clotting factors, or signs of fulminating hepatic failure (restlessness, personality changes, lethargy, decreased level of consciousness, and bleeding). Intravenous therapy, frequent laboratory studies, and physical examinations for progression of disease are the mainstay of hospital management.

The following medications may be used:

1. Immune globulin (Ig)—used for prophylaxis before and after exposure to hepatitis A (administered within 2 weeks of exposure)
2. HBIG—given as prophylaxis after exposure (Unvaccinated: give intramuscularly [IM] and initiate HB vaccine series. Vaccinated: give IM plus booster doses of vaccine. Perinatal: 0.5 ml IM within 12 hours of birth.)
3. Hepatitis B vaccine (Heptavax-B)—used to prevent occurrence of hepatitis B (Perinatal: give IM within 12 hours of birth; repeat at 1 and 6 months. Children younger than 10 years: three doses of IM [anterolateral

thigh/deltoid]; first two doses are given 1 month apart, and a booster is given 6 months after the first dose. Children older than 10 years: three doses into the deltoid muscle. Note that children undergoing long-term hemodialysis and children with Down syndrome should be routinely vaccinated because of increased risk for acquisition of hepatitis B infection.)

NURSING ASSESSMENT

1. See section on gastrointestinal assessment in Appendix A.
2. Assess for areas of jaundice—skin and sclera.
3. Assess nutritional status.

NURSING DIAGNOSES

- Fluid volume deficit
- Altered nutrition: less than body requirements
- Pain
- Impaired home maintenance management
- Knowledge deficit

NURSING INTERVENTIONS

1. Provide and maintain adequate fluid and food intake.
   a. Monitor for signs of dehydration.
   b. Monitor and record intake and output.
   c. Provide small, frequent meals; antiemetics may be needed.
   d. Offer child's favorite foods.
2. Prevent secondary infections.
   a. Avoid child's contact with infectious sources.
   b. Use and encourage appropriate hand-washing technique.
   c. Monitor for signs of infection.
   d. Provide for rest periods.
3. Prevent or control spread of hepatitis.
   a. Refer to institutional procedures for isolation techniques.
   b. Inoculate those people exposed to hepatitis during the incubation period.
      (1) Immune globulin
      (2) HBIG vaccine

    c. Vaccinate those individuals at high risk with hepatitis B vaccine.
4. Provide pain relief and comfort measures.
    a. Position of comfort
    b. Avoidance of unnecessary palpation of abdomen (hepatomegaly and splenomegaly)
5. Monitor for bleeding.
    a. Monitor coagulation studies.
    b. Intramuscular vitamin K may be ordered.
6. Monitor child closely for progression into fulminating hepatitis.
    a. Behavioral changes
    b. Lethargy
    c. Coma

♠ Discharge Planning and Home Care

1. Ensure that all family members and others exposed to child receive inoculation of Ig or HBIG.
2. Instruct parents and child about signs and symptoms of hepatitis so they can observe for them in those individuals exposed to child.
3. Provide instruction to parents about sanitary measures to institute in home.
4. Refer to public health nurse or community nurse for assessment of use of preventive measures for hepatitis.

CLIENT OUTCOMES

1. Child will have a return to normal gastrointestinal and hepatic function.
2. Child will return to normal activity levels without recurrence of illness.
3. Child and family understand home care instructions, disease process, instructions for preventing spread or recurrence of disease, and importance of follow-up needs.

REFERENCES

American Academy of Pediatrics: *Report of the Committee of Infectious Diseases*, Elk Grove Village, Ill, 1994, The Academy.

Behrman R, Kliegman R: *Nelson essentials of pediatrics*, ed 2, Philadelphia, 1994, WB Saunders.

Hazinski MF: *Nursing care of the critically ill child,* ed 2, St Louis, 1992, Mosby.
Ingalls A, Salerno M: *Maternal and child health nursing,* ed 7, St Louis, 1991, Mosby.
Lisanti P, Talotta D: An overview of viral hepatitis, *AORN J* 59(5):997, 1994.

32

Hernia (Inguinal) and Hernia Repair

PATHOPHYSIOLOGY

Inguinal hernia is the prolapse of a portion of the intestine into the inguinal ring above the scrotal sac, caused by a congenital weakness or failure of closure. An incarcerated hernia occurs when the prolapsed intestine causes constriction of the blood supply to the scrotal sac. The infant then develops pain and symptoms of intestinal obstruction (abdominal distention, colicky abdominal pain, no flatus, no stool, vomiting). A communicating hydrocele is always associated with hernia. The child is initially seen with an intermittent lump or bulge in the groin, scrotum, or labia. It becomes prominent with intraabdominal pressure such as that resulting from crying or straining. Contents of the hernia sac usually can be reduced with gentle pressure. Surgical repair (herniorrhaphy) is usually performed on an outpatient basis.

INCIDENCE

1. Of all children, 1% to 3% have a hernia, with increased incidence in premature infants.
2. The incidence is greatest during infancy (more than 50%), with the remaining cases generally occurring before age 5.
3. Incidence is greater in male individuals than female individuals (6:1).

CLINICAL MANIFESTATIONS (IF HERNIA IS INCARCERATED)

1. Continuous crying
2. Vomiting
3. Abdominal distention
4. Bloody stools

COMPLICATIONS

1. Recurrence of hernia
2. Incarcerated hernia
3. Atrophy of gonad

LABORATORY AND DIAGNOSTIC TEST

A complete blood count (CBC) is routine preoperative testing.

SURGICAL MANAGEMENT

Children with reducible hernias are scheduled for elective surgery on an outpatient basis. A 2- to 4-cm transverse incision is made in the area overlying the inguinal canal. Children with suspected incarcerated hernias are admitted, with immediate surgical repair performed to avoid bowel necrosis and, in boys, testicular infarction. Postoperatively these children are observed for at least 24 hours to be assessed for adequate return of gastrointestinal function and to receive prophylactic intravenous antibiotics. Analgesic medications are used for pain management. Oral feedings are begun when adequate peristalsis is established.

NURSING ASSESSMENT

1. See the section on gastrointestinal assessment in Appendix A.
2. Assess for presence of lump in area of groin, scrotum, or labia.

NURSING DIAGNOSES

- Impaired tissue integrity
- Fluid volume deficit

- Pain
- Knowledge deficit

NURSING INTERVENTIONS
Preoperative Care

1. Assess child's clinical status before surgery.
   a. Signs of infection
   b. Hemoglobin (Hb) level higher than 10 g
2. Explain anticipated preoperative and postoperative events using age-appropriate measures.

Postoperative Care

1. Monitor child's clinical status.
   a. Vital signs as often as every 2 hours for first 24 hours, then every 4 hours
   b. Signs and symptoms of infection
   c. Temperature, drainage from site, redness, inflammation
2. Monitor for signs and symptoms of complications.
   a. Recurrence of hernia
   b. Development of items
3. Promote nutritional and fluid intake.
   a. Record input and output.
   b. Monitor for signs of dehydration.
   c. Advance diet as tolerated.
4. Promote and maintain respiratory function.
   a. Have child turn, cough, and deep breathe.
   b. Perform postural drainage and percussion.
   c. Change child's position every 2 hours.
   d. Keep head of bed in semi-Fowler's position.
5. Alleviate child's pain as needed.
   a. Maintain position of comfort.
   b. Use recreational and diversional activities and toys.
   c. Administer analgesics.
6. Provide and reinforce information given to parents about child's condition.

🏠 Discharge Planning and Home Care

1. Instruct parents about care of dressing (if present).
   a. Keep incision covered with plastic-coated dressing.
   b. Bathe child with incision covered by a dressing.

     c. Protect incision from fecal and urinary contamination.
2. Instruct parents about short- and long-term management.
     a. Do not restrict activities.
     b. Administer acetaminophen (Tylenol) for pain as needed.
     c. Monitor for complications.

CLIENT OUTCOMES

1. Child will have a return to normal gastrointestinal function.
2. Pain will be eliminated.
3. Child and family will understand home care and follow-up needs.

REFERENCES

Ashby D: Susan's first pregnancy and first surgery, *J Post Anesth Nurs* 4(6):406, 1990.

Behrman R, Kliegman R: *Nelson essentials of pediatrics*, ed 2, Philadelphia, 1994, WB Saunders.

Ingalls J, Salerno C: *Maternal and child health nursing*, ed 7, St Louis, 1991, Mosby.

Nyhans L, Rogers F: Inguinal hernia repairs, *AORN J* 52(1):292, 1994.

33

Hirschsprung's Disease and Surgical Repair

PATHOPHYSIOLOGY

Hirschsprung's disease, or congenital megacolon, is the absence of ganglion cells in the rectum or the rectosigmoid portion of the colon. This absence results in abnormal or absent peristalsis and the total absence of spontaneous bowel evacuation. In addition, the rectal sphincter fails to relax, preventing the normal passage of stool. Intestinal contents are propelled to an aganglionic segment, causing fecal material to accumulate there and causing dilation of the bowel proximal to this area. It is speculated that Hirschsprung's disease is caused by both genetic and environmental factors, but the exact etiology is unknown. Hirschsprung's disease may manifest itself at any age, although it is most commonly observed in neonates.

INCIDENCE

1. Hirschsprung's disease occurs once in 5000 live births.
2. This disease is three to four times more common in male individuals than female individuals.
3. Incidence increases in siblings and offspring of affected children.
4. Among affected infants, 10% to 15% are diagnosed with Down syndrome.
5. This disease accounts for 15% to 20% of neonatal obstructions.

CLINICAL MANIFESTATIONS
Neonatal Period

1. Failure to pass meconium within 48 hours of birth
2. Bile-stained vomitus
3. Reluctance to ingest fluids
4. Abdominal distention

Infancy and Childhood

1. Constipation
2. Recurrent diarrhea
3. Ribbonlike, foul-smelling stool
4. Abdominal distention
5. Failure to thrive

COMPLICATIONS

1. Respiratory distress (acute)
2. Enterocolitis (acute)
3. Anal strictures (postsurgical)
4. Incontinence (long term)

LABORATORY AND DIAGNOSTIC TESTS

1. Abdominal x-ray films (supine, erect, prone, lateral decubitus)—diagnostic
2. Barium enema—diagnostic
3. Rectal biopsy—to detect absence of ganglion cells
4. Anorectal manometry—to record reflux response of internal and external rectal sphincter

SURGICAL MANAGEMENT

Surgical treatment of Hirschsprung's disease is a two-stage process. Initially, a double-barrel or loop colostomy is performed so that the dilated and hypertrophied portion of the bowel can regain normal tone and size (takes approximately 3 to 4 months). When the infant is between 6 and 12 months of age (or when the infant weighs 18 to 20 pounds), one of three procedures is performed as a means of resectioning the aganglionic bowel and of anastomosing the ganglion-containing bowel to the rectum within 1 cm of the anus.

The Duhamel procedure is generally performed on infants less than 1 year old. It consists of pulling down the normal colon and anastomosing it behind the aganglionic bowel, creating a double wall composed of both the aganglionic sheath and the posterior section of the normal pulled-through colon. In the Swenson procedure, the aganglionic portion of colon is resected. An end-to-end anastomosis of the ganglionic colon to the dilated anal canal is performed. A sphincterotomy is performed posteriorly. The Soave procedure is performed on older children and is the most frequently used procedure for treating Hirschsprung's disease. The muscular wall of the rectal segment is left intact. The normally innervated colon is pulled through to the anus, where an anastomosis between the normal colon and the remaining rectosigmoid muscular tissue is performed.

NURSING ASSESSMENT

See the section on gastrointestinal assessment in Appendix A.

Preoperative

1. Assess child's clinical status (vital signs, intake and output).
2. Assess for signs of bowel perforation.
3. Assess for signs of enterocolitis.
4. Assess child's and family's ability to cope with upcoming surgery.
5. Assess child's level of pain.

Postoperative

1. Assess child's postoperative status (vital signs, bowel sounds, abdominal distention).
2. Assess for signs of dehydration or fluid overload.
3. Assess for complications.
4. Assess for signs of infection.
5. Assess child's level of pain.
6. Assess child's and family's ability to cope with the hospital and surgical experience.
7. Assess parents' ability to manage the treatment regimen and ongoing care.

NURSING DIAGNOSES

- Anxiety
- High risk for infection

- High risk for injury
- Pain
- Fluid volume deficit
- High risk for impaired skin integrity
- Knowledge deficit
- High risk for ineffective management of treatment regimen

NURSING INTERVENTIONS
Preoperative Care

1. Monitor nutritional status before surgery.
   a. Offer diet high in calories, protein, and residue.
   b. Use alternative route of intake if patient cannot take oral fluids.
   c. Assess intake and output accurately every 8 hours.
   d. Weigh patient every day.
2. Prepare infant and family emotionally for surgery (see Appendix J).
3. Monitor clinical status preoperatively.
   a. Monitor vital signs every 2 hours as needed.
   b. Monitor intake and output.
   c. Observe for signs and symptoms of bowel perforation.
      (1) Vomiting
      (2) Increased tenderness
      (3) Abdominal distention
      (4) Irritability
      (5) Respiratory distress (dyspnea)
   d. Monitor for signs of enterocolitis.
   e. Measure abdominal girth every 4 hours (to assess for abdominal distention).
4. Monitor infant's reactions to presurgical preparations.
   a. Enemas until clear (to sterilize bowel preoperatively)
   b. Intravenous (IV) tube insertion
   c. Foley catheter insertion
   d. Preoperative medication
   e. Diagnostic testing
   f. Decompression of stomach and bowel (nasogastric [NG] or rectal tube)
   g. Nothing by mouth for 12 hours before surgery

Postoperative Care

1. Monitor and report child's postoperative status.
   a. Auscultate for return of bowel sounds.
   b. Monitor vital signs every 2 hours until stable, then every 4 hours (dependent on hospital protocol).
   c. Monitor for abdominal distention (maintain patency of NG tube).
2. Monitor child's hydration status (dependent on child's status and hospital protocol).
   a. Assess for signs of dehydration or fluid overload.
   b. Measure and record NG drainage.
   c. Measure and record colostomy drainage.
   d. Measure and record Foley catheter drainage.
   e. Monitor IV infusion (amount, rate, infiltration).
   f. Observe for electrolyte imbalances (hyponatremia or hypokalemia).
3. Observe and report signs of complications.
   a. Intestinal obstruction caused by adhesions, volvulus, or intussusception
   b. Leakage from anastomosis
   c. Sepsis
   d. Fistula
   e. Enterocolitis
   f. Frequency of stooling
   g. Constipation
   h. Bleeding
   i. Recurrence of symptoms
4. Promote return of peristalsis.
   a. Maintain patency of NG tube.
   b. Irrigate with normal saline solution every 4 hours and as needed.
5. Promote and maintain fluid and electrolyte balance.
   a. Record intake per route (IV, oral).
   b. Record output per route (urine, stool, emesis, stoma).
   c. Consult with physician about disparities.
6. Alleviate or minimize pain and discomfort (see Appendix I).
   a. Maintain patency of NG tube.
   b. Maintain position of comfort.
   c. Monitor child's response to administration of medications.

7. Prevent infection.
   a. Monitor incision site.
   b. Provide Foley catheter care every shift (protocols vary according to institutions).
   c. Change dressing as needed (perianal and colostomy).
   d. Refer to institutional procedure manual for care related to specific procedure.
   e. Change diaper frequently to avoid fecal contamination.
8. Perform interventions specific to procedure; refer to institutional procedure manual.
9. Provide emotional support to child and family (see Appendix J, section on preparation for procedure/surgery).

♠ Discharge Planning and Home Care

1. Instruct parents to monitor for signs and symptoms of the following long-term complications.
   a. Stenosis and constrictures
   b. Incontinence
   c. Inadequate emptying
2. Provide instructions to parents and child about colostomy care.
   a. Skin preparation
   b. Use of colostomy equipment
   c. Stomal complications (bleeding, failure to pass stool, increased diarrhea, prolapse, ribbonlike stools)
   d. Care and cleaning of colostomy equipment
   e. Irrigation of colostomy (refer to Chapter 41 for further information)
3. Provide and reinforce instructions about dietary management.
   a. Low-residue diet
   b. Unlimited fluid intake
   c. Signs of electrolyte imbalance or dehydration
4. Encourage parents' and child's ventilation of concerns related to colostomy.
   a. Appearance
   b. Odor
   c. Discrepancy between their child and "ideal" child
5. Refer to specific institutional procedures for information distributed to parents about home care.

CLIENT OUTCOMES

1. Infant remains without signs of infection.
2. Infant has adequate hydration.
3. Infant stoma site is without tissue breakdown.

REFERENCES

Ross AJ III: Intestinal obstructions in the newborn, *Pediatr Rev* 15(9):338, 1994.

Sondheimer JR, Silverman A: Gastrointestinal tract. In Hay WW et al, editors: *Current pediatric diagnosis and treatment,* ed 12, East Norwalk, Conn, 1995, Appleton & Lange.

34

Hodgkin's Disease

PATHOPHYSIOLOGY

Hodgkin's disease is a malignancy of the lymphoid system. The cause is unknown. It is characterized by a proliferation of Reed-Sternberg cells that are surrounded by a pleomorphic infiltrate of reactive cells, predominantly composed of helper T cells. Although no tissue is exempt from involvement, Hodgkin's disease primarily affects the nonnodal or extralymphatic sites, particularly the liver, spleen, bone marrow, lungs, and mediastinum. Hodgkin's disease is classified according to the predominating cells and is characterized by four histologic states: (1) lymphocytic predominance, (2) nodular sclerosis, (3) mixed cellularity, and (4) lymphocytic depletion. High survival rates have been achieved in children with Hodgkin's disease as a result of improved staging procedures and various treatment strategies.

INCIDENCE

1. Hodgkin's disease accounts for 5% of malignancies in children in the United States.
2. Hodgkin's disease has been reported in infants and young children, but is rare before the age of 5 years.
3. Hodgkin's disease is more common in male individuals.
4. The survival rate for stages I and II is approximately 90%; for stages III and IV, 65%.
5. If the disease is left untreated, a 5-year survival rate of less than 5% is expected.

CLINICAL MANIFESTATIONS

1. Nontender, firm lymphadenopathy, usually centripetal and axial in nature with cervical, supraclavicular, and mediastinal presentation
2. Painless, movable lymph nodes in tissues surrounding the involved area
3. Elevated leukocyte count
4. Elevated erythrocyte sedimentation rate (ESR)
5. Fever
6. Malaise
7. Weight loss

COMPLICATIONS (RELATED TO TREATMENT)

1. Hypothyroidism
2. Cardiac dysfunction, including pericardial effusion, valvular heart disease, coronary artery disease, and constrictive pericarditis with tamponade
3. Pulmonary dysfunction, including fibrosis or pneumonitis
4. Impaired immunity
5. Soft-tissue and bone growth impairment
6. Ovarian dysfunction in female individuals and sterility in male individuals
7. Secondary malignancy, including thyroid carcinoma, basal cell carcinoma, osteosarcomas, breast and colon carcinomas, and soft-tissue sarcomas

LABORATORY AND DIAGNOSTIC TESTS

1. Complete blood count (CBC)—diagnostic (anemia may indicate advanced disease)
2. ESR—elevated at diagnosis
3. Serum copper and iron levels—elevated at diagnosis
4. Liver and renal function tests—to assess organ involvement
5. Chest x-ray study—to determine mediastinal or hilar node involvement
6. Computed tomography—to evaluate mediastinal, pulmonary, and upper abdominal disease

7. Radionuclide scan—to determine extent of involvement at site
8. Lymphangiogram (LAG)—to evaluate retroperitoneal involvement and to visualize size, architecture, and filling defects of nodes
9. Excisional lymph node biopsy—essential to diagnosis and staging
10. Surgical staging laparotomy—for pathologic staging

MEDICAL MANAGEMENT

Staging is used to determine the anatomic extent of the disease at the time of diagnosis, and to select the most appropriate therapy (Table 2). Staging includes biopsy, history, physical examination, and radiographic data collection. At the time of diagnosis, approximately 60% of children with Hodgkin's disease have pathologic stage I or II disease. Pathologic stage III disease is diagnosed in approximately 30% of children, and 10% have pathologic stage IV disease.

The treatment approach is guided by the stage of the disease at diagnosis. The goal of treatment is cure of the disease with minimal treatment-related toxicities and sequelae. For stage I and IIA Hodgkin's disease, external-beam radiation therapy is used. For stage IIB and IIIB Hodgkin's disease, total nodal irradiation is the treatment approach of choice. Treatment for stage IIIA Hodgkin's disease consists of radiotherapy and combination chemotherapy, and stage IV Hodgkin's disease is treated with combination chemotherapy.

The following medication regimens may be used:
1. MOPP drug regimen
    a. Mechlorethamine (nitrogen mustard)—interferes with deoxyribonucleic acid (DNA) replication and ribonucleic acid (RNA) protein synthesis; causes myelosuppression
    b. Oncovin (vincristine)—antineoplastic agent; inhibits cell division by arresting mitosis at metaphase
    c. Procarbazine (Matulane)—antineoplastic agent; inhibits cell division by suppressing mitosis at interphase

Table 2. System for Hodgkin's Disease: Ann Arbor Staging

Stage*	Description
I	Involvement of a single lymph node region or a single extralymphatic organ or site
II	Involvement of two or more lymph node regions on the same side of the diaphragm or localized involvement of an extralymphatic organ or site and one or more lymph node regions on the same side of the diaphragm
III	Involvement of lymph node regions or extralymphatic organs or sites or spleen on both sides of the diaphragm
IV	Diffuse involvement of one or more extralymphatic organs or tissues with or without associated lymph node involvement

* Subdivision A has no defined symptoms; subdivision B symptoms include unexplained recent weight loss or fever or night sweats.

    d. Prednisone—corticosteroid used for its inflammatory effect; inhibits phagocytosis and suppresses other clinical symptoms of inflammation
2. ABVD drug regimen (for MOPP-resistant therapy)
    a. Adriamycin (doxorubicin)—antitumor antibiotic
    b. Bleomycin—antitumor antibiotic
    c. Vinblastine—causes metaphase arrest and protein synthesis
    d. Dacarbazine—causes myelosuppression

NURSING ASSESSMENT

1. Assess child's physiologic status (see Appendix A).
   a. Signs and symptoms of Hodgkin's disease
   b. Involvement of other body systems (e.g., respiratory, gastrointestinal)
   c. Adverse effects of treatment
2. Assess family's psychosocial needs (see Appendix J).
   a. Knowledge
   b. Body image
   c. Family structure
   d. Family stressors
   e. Coping mechanisms
   f. Support systems
3. Assess child's developmental level (see Appendix B).
4. Assess family's ability to manage home care.

NURSING DIAGNOSES

- High risk for impaired tissue integrity
- Anxiety
- Fluid volume deficit
- Altered nutrition: less than body requirements
- Impaired skin integrity
- Altered oral mucous membranes
- Pain
- Fatigue
- Altered growth and development
- High risk for ineffective management of therapeutic regimen

NURSING INTERVENTIONS
Staging Procedure

1. Provide preprocedural education to the child and family (see Appendix J).
2. Prepare the child for clinical staging procedures with age-appropriate approach (see Appendix J).
3. Assist and support the child in the collection of laboratory specimens.
4. Provide instruction, support, and family crisis intervention.

Radiation and/or Chemotherapy Phase

1. Provide sedation for radiation treatments.
2. Monitor cardiorespiratory status during treatments.
3. Prepare for treatment-induced emergencies.
   a. Metabolic
   b. Hematologic
   c. Space-occupying tumors
4. Assess for signs of extravasation.
   a. Cell lysis
   b. Tissue sloughing
5. Monitor signs and symptoms of infection.
6. Assess skin integrity.
7. Minimize side effects of radiotherapy and/or chemotherapy.
   a. Bone marrow suppression
   b. Nausea and vomiting
   c. Anorexia and weight loss
   d. Oral mucositis
   e. Pain
8. Provide ongoing emotional support to the child and family (see Appendix J).
9. Refer to child life specialist for continued coping strategies.
10. Provide ongoing education about treatment and medications.
11. Refer family to social services for support and resource utilization (see Appendix K).

♠ Discharge Planning and Home Care

Instruct child and parents about home care management.

1. Signs of infection and when to seek medical attention
2. Care of child's central venous access device, including site care, dressing change, flushing, and emergency care
3. Medication administration (provide written information)
4. Adherence to treatment and medical appointments
5. Proper nutrition for optimal weight gain and health maintenance
6. School attendance and/or activity restrictions
7. Potential behavioral changes in the child and/or siblings

CLIENT OUTCOMES

1. Child and family demonstrate ability to cope with life-threatening illness.
2. Child will be free of infection.
3. Child and family understand home care and long-term follow-up care.

REFERENCES

Foley G, Fochtman D, Mooney K, editors: *Nursing care of the child with cancer,* ed 2, Philadelphia, 1993, WB Saunders.

Hockenberry M, Coody J, Bennett B: Childhood cancers: incidence, etiology, diagnosis and treatment, *Pediatric Nursing* 16(3):239, 1990.

Rosenthal J et al: Hodgkin's disease in childhood: treatment modalities, outcomes and epidemiological aspects, *The American Journal of Pediatric Hematology/Oncology* 16(2):138, 1994.

Sullivan M: Hodgkin's disease in children, *Hematol Oncol Clin North Am* 4(1):603, 1987.

Weinshel E, Peterson B: Hodgkin's disease, *CA Cancer J Clin* 43(6):327, 1993.

35

HIV and AIDS

PATHOPHYSIOLOGY

Research findings have demonstrated that the cause of acquired immunodeficiency syndrome (AIDS) is the human immunodeficiency virus (HIV), which attaches and enters T-helper CD4+ lymphocytes. The virus infects CD4+ lymphocytes and other immunologic cells, and the person experiences a gradual destruction of CD4+ cells. These cells, which amplify and replicate immunologic responses, are necessary to maintain good health, and when they are reduced and damaged, other immune functions begin to fail.

HIV can also infect macrophages, cells that the virus uses to cross the blood-brain barrier into the brain. B-lymphocyte function is also affected, with increased total immunoglobulin production associated with decreased specific antibody production. As the immune system progressively deteriorates, the body becomes increasingly vulnerable to opportunistic infections and is also less able to slow the process of HIV replication. HIV infection is manifested as a multisystem disease that may be dormant for years as it produces gradual immunodeficiency. The rate of disease progression and clinical manifestations vary from person to person.

The virus is transmitted only through direct contact with blood or blood products and body fluids, through intravenous drug use, sexual contact, perinatal transmission from mother to infant, and breast-feeding. There is no evidence that HIV infection is acquired through casual contact.

Currently, the majority of reported cases of HIV infection and AIDS in the United States occur in gay and bisexual men. However, the highest rates of new transmission of HIV are among heterosexual individuals. Sixty-five percent of HIV-positive adolescents age 13 to 19 were infected through sexual exposure or intravenous drug use. With recent advances in use of screening of blood products for HIV, the incidence of new infections from blood transfusions has been greatly reduced in developed countries.

Four populations in the pediatric age group have been primarily affected:

1. Infants infected through perinatal transmission from infected mother (also referred to as vertical transmission); this accounts for more than 85% of AIDS cases among children younger than 13 years
2. Children who have received blood products (especially children with hemophilia)
3. Adolescents infected after engaging in high-risk behavior
4. Infants who have been breast-fed (primarily in developing countries)

INCIDENCE

1. Eighty percent of children diagnosed with AIDS are younger than 6 years of age.
2. Ethnic distribution is 59% African American, 26% Hispanic, and 15% white.
3. The majority of children with AIDS (60%) live in New York, New Jersey, Florida, and California.
4. Gender distribution is 61% male and 39% female.

CLINICAL MANIFESTATIONS
Infants and Children

Children with perinatally acquired HIV infection appear normal at birth but develop symptoms during the first 2 years of life. Clinical manifestation include the following:

1. Low birth weight
2. Failure to thrive

3. Generalized lymphadenopathy
4. Hepatosplenomegaly
5. Sinusitis
6. Recurrent upper respiratory tract infections
7. Parotitis
8. Chronic or recurrent diarrhea
9. Recurrent bacterial and viral infections
10. Persistent Epstein-Barr virus infection
11. Oropharyngeal thrush
12. Thrombocytopenia
13. Bacterial infections such as meningitis
14. Chronic interstitial pneumonia

Fifty percent of children with HIV infection have neurologic involvement that primarily manifests itself as a progressive encephalopathy, developmental delay, or loss of motor milestones.

Adolescents

Most adolescents who are infected experience an extended period of asymptomatic illness that may last for years. This may be followed by signs and symptoms that begin weeks to months before the development of opportunistic infections and malignancies (see the box on pp. 215-217, Category C for list of diagnoses that define AIDS in adolescents and adults). The signs and symptoms include the following:
1. Fever
2. Malaise
3. Fatigue
4. Night sweats
5. Insidious onset of weight loss
6. Recurrent or chronic diarrhea
7. Generalized lymphadenopathy
8. Oral candidiasis
9. Arthralgias and myalgias

Descriptions of each clinical category are shown in the box.

LABORATORY AND DIAGNOSTIC TESTS:

1. ELISA: enzyme-linked immunosorbent assay (usual initial test)—detects antibody to HIV antigens (almost

Clinical Categories of HIV

Category N: Not Symptomatic

Children with no signs or symptoms felt to be the result of HIV infection

Category A: Mildly Symptomatic

Children who have two or more of the following:
- Lymphadenopathy
- Hepatomegaly
- Splenomegaly
- Dermatitis
- Parotitis
- Recurrent/persistent upper respiratory tract infection, sinusitis, or otitis media

Category B: Moderately Symptomatic

Children who have symptomatic conditions that are attributed to HIV infection and/or are indicative of immunologic deficits attributable to HIV infection; examples of conditions are the following:
- Anemia, neutropenia, thrombocytopenia persisting >30 days
- Bacterial meningitis, penumonia, or sepsis
- Thrush persistent for more than 2 months in a child over 6 months old
- Cardiomyopathy
- Cytomegalovirus infection with onset *before* 1 month of age
- Diarrhea, recurrent or chronic
- Hepatitis

Continued

- Herpes stomatitis, recurrent
- HSV bronchitis, pneumonitis, or esophagitis with onset *before* 1 month of age
- Herpes zoster (shingles), two or more episodes
- Leiomyosarcoma
- Lymphoid interstitial pneumonia or pulmonary lymphoid hyperplasia complex (LIP/PLH)
- Nephropathy
- Nocardiosis
- Persistent varicella zoster
- Persistent fever >1 month
- Toxoplasmosis, onset *before* 1 month of age
- Varicella, disseminated (complicated chicken pox)

Category C: Severely Symptomatic

Children who have any of the following conditions:
- Multiple or recurrent bacterial infections
- Candidiasis of the trachea, bronchi, lungs, or esophagus
- Coccidioidomycosis, disseminated or extrapulmonary
- Cryptosporidiosis, chronic intestinal
- Cytomegalovirus disease (other than liver, spleen, nodes), onset at age >1 month
- Cytomegalovirus retinitis (with loss of vision)
- HIV encephalopathy
- Chronic herpes symplex ulcer (>1 month duration) or pneumonitis or esophagitis, onset at >1 month of age
- Histoplasmosis, disseminated or extrapulmonary

- Isosporiasis, chronic intestinal (>1 month duration)
- Kaposi's sarcoma
- Lymphoma, primary in brain
- Lymphoma (Burkitt's or immunoblastic sarcoma)
- *Mycobacterium avium* complex or *Mycobacterium kansasii*, disseminated or extrapulmonary
- *Pneumocystis carinii* pneumonia
- Progressive multifocal leukoencephalopathy
- Salmonella septicemia, recurrent
- Toxoplasmosis of brain, onset at age >1 month
- Wasting syndrome caused by HIV

Modified from Centers for Disease Control: 1994 revised classification system for human immunodeficiency virus infection in children less than 13 years of age, *MMWR* 43(12): 1994.

universally used to screen for HIV in persons more than 2 years of age)

2. Western blot (usual confirmatory test)—detects antibody against several specific HIV proteins

3. HIV culture—the gold standard for establishing diagnosis in infants

4. Polymerase chain reaction (PCR)—detects HIV deoxyribonucleic acid (DNA) (this direct test is useful for diagnosis in infants and children)

5. HIV antigen test—detects HIV antigen

6. HIV, IgA, IgM—detect HIV antibody produced by the infant (have been used experimentally to diagnose HIV in infants)

The diagnosis of HIV infection in infants born to HIV-infected mothers has been difficult. By using a combination of these laboratory tests, diagnosis can be made in a majority of infected children before age 6 months.

These laboratory findings are commonly seen in HIV-infected infants and children:

1. Reduced absolute CD4+ lymphocyte count
2. Reduced CD4 percentage
3. Reduced CD4 to CD8 ratio
4. Lymphopenia
5. Anemia, thrombocytopenia
6. Hypergammaglobulinemia (IgG, IgA, IgM)
7. Decreased response to skin tests (*Candida* albicans, tetanus)
8. Poor response to vaccines that have been given (diphtheria, tetanus, measles, *Haemophilus influenzae* type B)

An infant who is born to an HIV-positive mother, who is less than 18 months of age, and who has tested positive on two separate determinations from the HIV culture, HIV polymerase chain reaction, or HIV antigen is "HIV infected." An infant who is born to an HIV-positive mother, who is less than 18 months of age, and who has not tested positive to these three tests is "perinatally exposed." Infants who are born to HIV-infected mothers, who have been determined to be HIV-antibody negative, and who have no other laboratory evidence of infection are "seroreverters."

MEDICAL MANAGEMENT

There is currently no cure for HIV infection and AIDS. Management begins with a staging evaluation to determine disease progression and the appropriate course of treatment. Children are categorized according to Table 3 using three parameters: immune status, infection status, and clinical status. A child with mild signs and symptoms but with no evidence of immune suppression is categorized as A2. The immune status is based on the CD4 count or CD4 percentage , which is dependent on the child's age, according to Table 4.

In addition to controlling disease progression, treatment is directed at preventing and managing opportunistic infections such as candidiasis and interstitial pneumonia.

Azidothymidine (zidovudine), videx, and zalcitabine (ddc) are medicines indicated in HIV infections with a low CD4 count. Videx and ddc have been less beneficial for central nervous system disease. Trimethoprim sulfamethoxazole

Table 3. Categorization of Children with HIV Infection and AIDS

Immune Categories	Clinical Categories			
	(N) No Signs or Symptoms	(A) Mild Signs or Symptoms	(B) Moderate Signs or Symptoms	(C) Severe Signs or Symptoms
(1) No evidence of suppression	N1	A1	B1	C1
(2) Evidence of moderate suppression	N2	A2	B2	C2
(3) Severe suppression	N3	A3	B3	C3

Table 4. Determination of Immune Category Based on Age and CD4 Count

Immune Categories	Age Groups: CD4 Count and Percentage		
	0-11 months	1-5 years	6-12 years
(1) No evidence of suppression	>1500 >25%	>1000 >25%	>500 >25%
(2) Evidence of moderate suppression	750-1499 15-25%	500-999 15-25%	200-499 15-25%
(3) Severe suppression	<750 <15%	<500 <15%	<200 <15%

Modified from Centers for Disease Control: 1994 revised classification system for human immunodeficiency virus infection in children less than 13 years of age, *MMWR* 43(12):1994.

(Septra, Bactrim) and pentamadine are used for treatment and prophylaxis of *Pneumocystis* carinii pneumonia (PCP). Monthly administration of intravenous immunoglobulin has been useful in preventing serious bacterial infections in children, as well as hypogammaglobulinemia.

Immunizations are recommended for children with HIV infection. Instead of the oral poliovirus vaccine (OPV), the inactivated poliovirus vaccine (IPV) is given.

NURSING ASSESSMENT

1. See the section on nursing assessment in Appendix A.
2. Assess nutritional status.
3. Assess for opportunistic infections.
4. Assess for knowledge of transmission—safe sex, sharing needles, etc.

NURSING DIAGNOSES

- High risk for infection
- Altered growth and development
- Altered nutrition: less than body requirements
- Altered family processes
- Anticipatory grieving
- Noncompliance with treatment plan
- Impaired social interactions

NURSING INTERVENTIONS

1. Protect infant, child, or adolescent from infectious contacts (see the box on p. 222); although casual person-to-person contact does not transmit HIV, a number of recommendations have been made for children with HIV and AIDS.
   a. Providers in foster homes should be educated on precautions regarding blood exposure, saliva contamination, and infection protection.
   b. Day care attendance should be evaluated on an individual basis.
   c. The patient should attend school if health, neurologic development, behavior, and immune status are appropriate.
2. Prevent the transmission of HIV infection.
   a. Clean spills of blood or other body fluids with bleach solution (10:1 ratio of water to bleach).
   b. Wear latex gloves when exposure to blood or body fluids is anticipated.
   c. Wear masks with protective eyewear if aerosolization or splashing with blood or body fluids with visible blood is anticipated.
   d. Wash hands after exposure to blood or body fluids and after removing gloves.

Preventive Measures

Preventive efforts are of vital importance in dealing with AIDS. Reducing the number of sexual partners, especially those in high-risk groups, would decrease the incidence of this disease in the adolescent population, as would involvement in drug rehabilitation programs and avoidance of nonsterile needles. Also, sexual abuse of adolescents contributes to AIDS risk.

Prevention of AIDS in the adult population would result in the greatest decrease of this disease in children. In addition, elimination of infected blood and blood products would decrease the likelihood of transmission to children. Blood and blood products are now screened for the antibody HIV, so that 95% of infected blood is eliminated from the market.

Research indicates that hepatitis B vaccine is safe from AIDS virus contamination. An HIV-positive mother should not breast-feed, because transmission via breast milk is supported, if not proven.

e. Place uncapped needles attached to syringes (and other sharps) in a closed, puncture-proof container labeled as biohazardous/infectious waste.
f. Dispose of waste contaminated with visible blood in a biohazardous plastic bag.

3. Protect child from infectious contacts when he or she is immunocompromised.
   a. Screen for infections.
   b. Place child in room with noninfectious children.
   c. Restrict visitors with active illnesses.
4. Assess child's achievement of developmental milestones and nutritional status.
   a. Provide age-appropriate, stimulating activities (see section on growth and development, Appendix B).
   b. Monitor growth pattern (height, weight, head circumference) and refer to dietitian for assistance with nutritional interventions.
5. Involve social services and other health team members to assist child and family with the crisis and stresses of a chronic and fatal illness.
   a. Encourage ventilation of feelings.
   b. Refer to clergy for spiritual support.
   c. Discuss likelihood of child's death with parents and child.
   d. Encourage family members to discuss with each other, relatives, and friends the likelihood of the child's death.
   e. Encourage family to discuss likelihood of parent's death (if applicable).
6. Assist family in identifying factors that impede compliance with treatment plan.
   a. Educate patient and family about the risks of noncompliance.
   b. Assist family in establishing a schedule that optimizes the therapeutic effect of the medication and fits into the family's lifestyle.
7. Encourage child to participate in activities with other children.
   a. Assist child and family in identifying personal strengths.
   b. Educate school or day care personnel and classmates about HIV infection and AIDS.
   c. Educate adolescent about sexual transmission, abstinence, use of condoms with nonoxynol-9, dangers of promiscuity, and other risky behaviors.

d. Educate adolescent about the relationship between substance abuse and practicing risky behaviors.

e. Encourage use of support network of family and friends and refer to AIDS support group as needed.

f. Collaborate with school nurse regarding child's condition.

🏠 Discharge Planning and Home Care

1. Instruct child and family to contact medical team in case of signs or symptoms of infection.
2. Instruct child and family to observe response to medications and notify physician of adverse reactions.
3. Instruct child and family about follow-up appointments.
   a. Name and phone number of physician and appropriate health care team members
   b. Date and time and purpose of follow-up appointments

CLIENT OUTCOMES

1. Child exhibits no signs or symptoms of infection.
2. Child and family demonstrate understanding of home care and follow-up needs.
3. Child participates in activities with family and peers.

REFERENCES

Boland MG: The child with AIDS: special concerns. In Durham JD, Cohen FL, editors: *The person with AIDS: nursing perspectives,* ed 2, New York, 1991, Springer Publishing.

Centers for Disease Control: 1994 revised classification system for human immunodeficiency virus infection in children less than 13 years of age, *MMWR* 43(12):1994.

Clark PJ, Byrne MW: Clinical issues in long term pediatric HIV disease, *MCN* 18(3):164, 1993.

Cohen D: Similarities between the nursing care needs of children with human immunodeficiency virus infection, *J Pediatr Oncol Nurs* 7(4):149, 1990.

Parrott RH, Rathlev M: Access to primary care for children with HIV: a guide for physicians, nurses, and social workers, *Pediatric AIDS and HIV Infection: Fetus to Adolescent* 2(5):243, 1991.

Pizzo PA, Wilfert CM: *Pediatrics AIDS: the challenge of HIV infections in infants, children and adolescents,* ed 2, Baltimore, 1993, Williams & Wilkins.

36

Hydrocephalus and Surgical Repair

PATHOPHYSIOLOGY

Hydrocephalus results from (1) obstruction of cerebrospinal fluid (CSF) flow, (2) interference with absorption of CSF, and (3) overproduction of CSF. Several causative factors account for hydrocephalus. These include tumors, vascular malformations, abscesses, intraventricular cysts, intraventricular hemorrhage, meningitis, aqueductal stenosis, and cerebral trauma. There are two types of hydrocephalus, congenital and acquired.

INCIDENCE

1. Congenital hydrocephalus occurs in 0.5 to 1 out of 1000 live births.
2. Seventy percent of the children with untreated hydrocephalus have a 5-year survival rate, and 75% of these children have an intelligence quotient (IQ) greater than 75.

CLINICAL MANIFESTATIONS

1. Vital sign changes (decreased apical pulse, decreased respiratory rate, increased blood pressure)
2. Vomiting
3. Increased head circumference
4. Irritability
5. Lethargy

6. Change in cry (pitch)
7. Seizure activity

Infants

1. Progressive head enlargement (above 95th percentile)
2. Prominence of frontal portions of the skull
3. Bulging, tense fontanels (especially nonpulsatile)
4. Distention of superficial scalp veins
5. Symmetrically increased transillumination over the skull
6. Downturned eyes ("sunset eyes")

Older Children

1. Frontal headache, nausea, and vomiting
2. Anorexia
3. Ataxia
4. Lower-extremity spasticity
5. Deterioration in child's school performance or cognitive ability

Signs and symptoms are the results of increased intracranial pressure (ICP) and vary with the child's age and the skull's ability to expand.

COMPLICATIONS

1. Increased ICP
2. Infection
3. Shunt malfunction
4. Delays in cognitive, psychosocial, and physical development
5. Decreased IQ

LABORATORY AND DIAGNOSTIC TESTS

1. Computed tomography (CT) scan—most useful method of diagnosis
2. Direct puncture into ventricle through anterior fontanel—to monitor CSF pressure
3. Magnetic resonance imaging (MRI)—may be used for a complex lesion

SURGICAL MANAGEMENT

The main therapeutic management is surgical shunt insertion. A shunt is inserted into the right ventricle as a surgical treatment for hydrocephalus. The shunt removes the excessive cerebrospinal fluid and decreases intracranial pressure. The proximal end is inserted in the lateral ventricle; the distal end is extended to the peritoneal cavity or right atrium as a means of draining excessive fluid into another body cavity. The ventricular peritoneal shunt is used most frequently because the atrioventricular (AV) shunt requires repeated revisions as a result of growth and the risk of bacterial endocarditis. The symptoms of increased ICP are relieved. After surgery, the child is more alert, and vomiting, anorexia, and bulging of the fontanel are decreased. Because seizure activity remains a possibility after the shunt placement, anticonvulsants may be given. Phenobarbital is used for generalized tonic-clonic and partial simple seizures because it limits the seizure activity by increasing the threshold for motor cortex stimuli. Antibiotics, depending on the results of culture and sensitivity, are used for shunt infections.

The following are possible complications of surgery:
1. Shunt malfunction (blockage)
2. Shunt infection
3. Meningitis
4. Progressive mental deterioration
5. Seizures

NURSING ASSESSMENT
1. See the section on neuromuscular assessment in Appendix A.
2. Assess for increased ICP.

NURSING DIAGNOSES
■ Altered tissue perfusion, cerebral
■ High risk for infection
■ High risk for injury
■ Altered family processes
■ Knowledge deficit

NURSING INTERVENTIONS
Preoperative Care

1. Monitor for, prevent, and intervene in case of increased ICP.
   a. Place child in position of comfort; raise head of bed to 30 degrees (to decrease congestion and increase drainage).
   b. Monitor for signs of increased ICP.
      (1) Increased respiratory rate, decreased apical pulse, increased blood pressure, and increased temperature
      (2) Decreased level of consciousness (LOC)
      (3) Seizure activity
      (4) Vomiting
      (5) Alteration in pupil size, symmetry, and reactivity
      (6) Fullness of fontanels—tense to bulging
   c. Decrease external stimuli.
   d. Maintain oxygen and suction at bedside.
2. Prepare child and parents for surgical procedure.
   a. Provide age-appropriate explanations (see Appendix J, section on preparation for procedure/surgery).
   b. Provide and reinforce information given to parents about child's condition and treatment.

Postoperative Care

1. Monitor child's vital signs and neurologic status; report signs of increased ICP (size, fullness, tension of anterior fontanel), decreased LOC, anorexia, vomiting, convulsions, seizures, or sluggishness.
2. Monitor and report signs of site infection (fever, tenderness, inflammation, nausea, and vomiting).
3. Monitor and maintain functioning of shunt.
   a. Report signs of shunt malfunction (irritability, decreased LOC, vomiting).
   b. Check shunt for fullness.
   c. Elevate head of bed 30 degrees (to increase drainage and decrease venous congestion).
   d. Position child on left side (nonoperative side).
   e. Maintain bed rest for 24 to 72 hours.
   f. Monitor for seizure activity.

4. Support child and parents to help them deal with emotional stresses of hospitalization and surgery.
   a. Provide age-appropriate information before procedures.
   b. Encourage participation in recreational and divisional activities.
   c. Incorporate child's home routine into daily activities.

🏠 Discharge Planning and Home Care

1. Instruct parents to monitor for and report signs of shunt complications.
   a. Shunt malfunction
   b. Shunt infection
2. Provide parents with assistance in contacting community resources.
   a. Follow-up by home health nurse (see Appendix K)
   b. Selection of preschool and recreational programs
3. Assess cognitive, linguistic, adaptive, and social behaviors to determine development; use developmental history to assess early milestones, and refer to appropriate specialists as needed.

CLIENT OUTCOMES

1. Child will not have signs or symptoms of increased ICP.
2. Child and parents will understand the surgical procedure.
3. Child and parents will understand how to monitor for and report shunt complications.
4. Child will achieve optimal developmental functioning.

REFERENCES

Bayston R: Hydrocephalus shunt infections, *J Antimicrobial Chemo* 34(suppl A):75, 1994.

Fletcher JM et al: Behavioral adjustment of children with hydrocephalus: relationships with etiology, neurological, and family status, *J Pediatr Psychol* 20(1):109, 1995.

Jackson P: Primary care needs of children with hydrocephalus, *J Pediatr Health Care* 4(2):54, 1990.

Kokkonen J et al: Long-term prognosis for children with shunted hydrocephalus, *Childs Nerv Syst* 10(6):384, 1994.

Scheinblum S, Hammond M: The treatment of children with shunt infections: extraventricular drainage system care, *Pediatr Nurs* 16(2):139, 1990.

Scott R: *Hydrocephalus: concepts in neurosurgery, vol 3,* Baltimore, 1990, Williams & Wilkins.

Shaw N: Common surgical problems in the newborn, *J Perinat Neonat Nurs* 3(3):50, 1990.

Thompson J, Thompson H: Applying the decision-making model: case studies, *Neonat Network: J Neonat Nurs* 9(4):57, 1990.

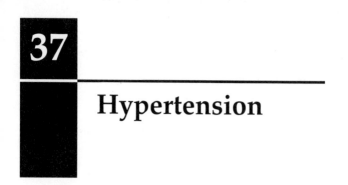

37

Hypertension

PATHOPHYSIOLOGY

Hypertension in the pediatric patient is described as blood pressures that are persistently between the 90th and 95th percentile. The box on p. 232 identifies guidelines (based on age and sex) for suspect blood pressure values. A variety of mechanisms are associated with hypertension. The renin-angiotensin-aldosterone system maintains fluid volume and vascular tone through the production of angiotensin II (a vasoconstrictor) and the stimulation of aldosterone production (for sodium retention). The sympathetic nervous system affects peripheral vascular resistance, cardiac output, and renin release, influencing the regulation of blood pressure.

Hypertension is classified as primary or secondary. Primary hypertension can be attributed to no identifiable cause, whereas secondary hypertension is attributable to a structural abnormality or to an underlying disease (renal, cardiovascular, endocrine, central nervous system [CNS], or collagenous). A variety of factors have been identified as contributing to hypertension, including diet (high in calories, saturated fats, and sodium), contraceptives, positive family history, obesity, and minimal physical exercise. Children generally manifest no overt symptoms. If symptomatic, the disease may be quite severe. Prognosis is variable, depending on the age of onset and response to treatment.

Approximate Guidelines for Suspect Blood Pressures

Blood Pressure Values

Supine position—lowest of three readings

Boys and Girls

Age in years	3-5	6-9	10-14
Blood pressure mm Hg	>110/70	>120/75	>130/80

Seated position—average of second and third readings

	Girls			Boys
Age in years	14-18	14	15	16-18
Blood pressure mm Hg	>125/80	>130/75	>130/80	>135/85

Modified from Gilles S, Kagan B: *Current pediatric therapy,* ed 13, Philadelphia, 1990, WB Saunders.

Problems evident in adults may have originated during the first or second decade of life. The earlier the onset, the more severe the disease will be.

INCIDENCE

1. There is an increased incidence among children in a lower socioeconomic status.
2. There is an increased incidence among black adolescents.
3. Incidence rates vary from 0.6% to 20.5% (depends on methodology used).
4. Noncompliance with treatment occurs among more than 50% of the affected children; compliance improves when child is dependent on parent.
5. Male individuals are affected more often than female individuals.

6. Forty-five percent to 100% of cases of hypertension in individuals 2 to 18 years of age are attributed to primary hypertension.
7. Twenty-five percent of children with primary hypertension have positive family history.
8. One percent to 2% of children and 11% to 12% of adolescents are affected.

CLINICAL MANIFESTATIONS

1. Severe headaches
2. Blurred vision; symptoms of increased intracranial pressure (ICP)
3. Marked irritability
4. Nosebleeds
5. Dizziness
6. Fatigue
7. Nervousness
8. Anorexia, failure to thrive (FTT), weight loss
9. Focal or generalized seizures
10. Severe back and/or abdominal pain
11. Papilledema
12. Retinal hemorrhage or exudate
13. Left-ventricular hypertrophy
14. Altered renal function

COMPLICATIONS

1. Ischemic (coronary) heart disease
2. Side effects associated with use of antihypertensives (e.g., postexercise syncope, depression, and dizziness)
3. Altered renal function

LABORATORY AND DIAGNOSTIC TESTS

1. Urinalysis, urine culture—to assess for renal cause
2. Serum electrolytes—to assess for renal and metabolic status
3. Complete blood count (CBC)—to assess for infection, fluid overload
4. Creatinine, blood urea nitrogen (BUN)—to assess for renal cause

5. Serum cholesterol—greater than 250 mg/100 ml
6. Serum triglyceride level—increased
7. Lipoprotein electrophoresis—elevated lipoprotein
8. Electrocardiogram (ECG)—left-ventricular hypertrophy
9. Chest x-ray film—left-ventricular hypertrophy
10. Rapid-sequence intravenous pyelogram—to assess activation of renin-angiotensin system
11. Plasma renin activity—to assess activation of renin-angiotensin system
12. Excretory venogram—to detect renal and renovascular abnormalities
13. Arteriogram—to detect renal and renovascular abnormalities
14. Radionuclide studies—to detect renal and renovascular abnormalities

MEDICAL MANAGEMENT

The aim of controlling hypertension is to reduce the associated risk of cardiovascular and renal complications. The step approach to treatment for the pediatric patient is to educate the child and family on the importance of prevention. Nonpharmacologic interventions such as diet, exercise, and weight control should be the first approach when possible. The goal of antihypertension therapy is to maintain pressures below the 90th percentile using the least amount and number of drugs. Medications should be started one at a time using a diuretic, beta-blocker, or a calcium antagonist. Keeping the medication schedule as simple as possible helps to promote compliance.

NURSING ASSESSMENT

1. See the section on renal assessment in Appendix A.
2. Assess neurologic status.
3. Assess nutritional history.

NURSING DIAGNOSES

- Altered tissue perfusion
- Decreased cardiac output
- Knowledge deficit

NURSING INTERVENTIONS

1. Monitor child's clinical status and assess for changes.
   a. Blood pressure (see Appendix E)
   b. Neurologic status
   c. Presence of bleeding
   d. Blurred vision
   e. Renal function
2. Monitor the child's therapeutic and untoward response to administered medications.
3. Monitor and encourage child's nutritional intake.
   a. Administer diet restricted in sodium, fats, and calories.
   b. Reinforce dietary information and management plan provided by dietitian.

♠ Discharge Planning and Home Care

Instruct child and family about management of hypertension:
1. Explanation of hypertension
2. Medications
3. Dietary restrictions and weight control
4. Use of oral contraceptives
5. Salt intake
6. Exercise
7. Smoking

CLIENT OUTCOMES

1. Child will remain normotensive.
2. Child and family will understand follow-up needs.
3. Child will remain compliant with medications and diet.

REFERENCES

Hohn AR: *Guidebook for pediatric hypertension*, Armonk, New York, 1994, Futura Publishing.

Kaplan N: *Clinical hypertension*, ed 5, Baltimore, 1990, Williams & Wilkins.

Rocchini AP: *The pediatric clinics of North America: childhood hypertension*, Philadelphia, 1993, WB Saunders.

Schieken RM: Genetic factors that predispose the child to develop hypertension, *Pediatr Clin North Am* 40(1):1, 1993.

38

Hypertrophic Pyloric Stenosis

PATHOPHYSIOLOGY

Hypertrophic pyloric stenosis is one of the more frequently occurring conditions of infancy that cause malnutrition. Hypertrophy and hyperplasia of the circular muscle of the pylorus cause obstruction at the pyloric sphincter. The circular muscle thickens to as much as twice the normal thickness, and the pylorus increases in length, with severe narrowing of the lumen as a result. In addition, the stomach dilates in size and hypertrophy of the antrum occurs. The cause is unknown, although evidence suggests that local innervation is involved. It may be associated with intestinal malrotation, esophageal or duodenal atresias, and anorectal anomalies. In addition, there is a genetic disposition.

INCIDENCE

1. Hypertrophic pyloric stenosis occurs once in 500 live births.
2. Hypertrophic pyloric stenosis is rare in black and Chinese individuals.
3. Gender ratio of male to female is 4:1.

CLINICAL MANIFESTATIONS

1. Projectile vomiting
2. Feeding hungrily; eagerness to be fed after vomiting

3. Not vomiting after each feeding; retained feeding vomited with current feeding
4. Nonbilious vomitus; may be blood streaked
5. Signs of dehydration (decreased tears, poor skin turgor, dark circles under eyes, sunken fontanel)
6. Failure to gain weight
7. Loss of fat pads
8. Pain behaviors—arching back, stretching, screaming
9. Visible right-to-left gastric peristaltic waves
10. Palpable olive-size pyloric tumor during feeding

COMPLICATIONS

1. Jaundice (8% of cases)—caused by deficiency of hepatic glucuronide transferase
2. Metabolic alkalosis (acute)
3. Severe dehydration (acute)
4. Persistant pyloric obstruction
5. Gastroesophageal reflux (GER)

LABORATORY AND DIAGNOSTIC TESTS

1. Complete blood count (CBC)—anemia
2. Serum electrolytes—hypochloremia, hypokalemia
3. Serum glucose and glucose oxidase strips—hypoglycemia
4. Blood urea nitrogen (BUN)—increased level is indicative of dehydration
5. Arterial blood gas values—metabolic alkalosis
6. Upper gastrointestinal (GI) x-ray examination—diagnostic; shows delayed gastric emptying
7. Ultrasound—diagnostic

MEDICAL AND SURGICAL MANAGEMENT

The infant or child is admitted to the hospital and started on intravenous (IV) fluids to correct the metabolic alkalosis (due to the chloride loss in the vomitus and the renal compensation). Fluid and electrolyte imbalances are corrected prior to the pyloromyotomy (incision down to mucosa and fully across pyloric length), the standard surgical treatment for this disorder.

NURSING ASSESSMENT

1. See the section on gastrointestinal assessment in Appendix A.
2. Assess for signs and symptoms of dehydration.
3. Assess for signs and symptoms of electrolyte imbalances.
4. Assess child's response to oral intake.
5. Assess child's response to pain.
6. Assess wound for drainage and infection.
7. Assess child and family coping.

NURSING DIAGNOSES

- Fluid volume deficit
- Altered nutrition: less than body requirements
- Pain
- High risk for infection
- Knowledge deficit

NURSING INTERVENTIONS
Preoperative Care

1. Promote and maintain fluid and electrolyte balance.
   a. Maintain patent IV route for administration of ordered fluids at specified rate.
   b. Replace nasogastric (NG) output with IV fluids as ordered.
   c. Strictly monitor input and output (including number and characteristics of stools and amount of vomiting).
   d. Record urine specific gravity every 8 hours.
   e. Record daily weight.
   f. Monitor for signs and symptoms of dehydration (vital signs [VS], mucous membranes, fontanel status).
   g. Maintain patent nasogastric tube (NGT) if present.
   h. Perform gastric lavage with normal saline through NGT until clear (preoperative preparation).

2. Monitor and report child's response to electrolyte imbalance.
   a. Monitor and report lab results.
   b. Monitor for signs of electrolyte imbalances.
3. Prepare parents preoperatively for child's upcoming surgery (see Appendix J, section on preparation for procedure/surgery).

Postoperative Care

1. Promote and maintain fluid and electrolyte balance.
   a. Maintain patent IV route for administration of ordered fluids at specified rate.
   b. Strictly monitor input and output.
   c. Monitor for signs of dehydration (VS, mucous membranes, fontanel status, urine output).
   d. Maintain patent NGT if present.
2. Monitor child's response to oral intake.
   a. Initiate fluids by mouth 3 to 4 hours postoperatively; assess response.
   b. Provide small, frequent feedings (15 to 20 ml per feeding) as tolerated.
   c. Begin with clear liquids (glucose and electrolytes); increase to full-strength formula as tolerated (progression of fluids: D_5W, one-fourth, one-half, three-fourths, full-strength formula).
   d. Feed infant in upright position.
   e. Monitor blood sugars with strips with glucose oxidase.
   f. Observe for signs of vomiting and hematemesis (may delay feedings by mouth for 48 hours).
   g. Monitor for weight gain.
3. Provide pain relief measures as indicated.
   a. Monitor for signs of pain—crying, irritability, stretching, arching back, increased motor activity.
   b. Assess child's therapeutic and untoward reactions to medications.
4. Monitor and maintain integrity of incisional site.
   a. Assess for signs of infection—redness, drainage, inflammation, warmth to touch.
   b. Perform incision site care per institution protocols.

5. Provide psychosocial support (see Appendix J, section on supportive care).

♠ Discharge Planning and Home Care

1. Instruct parents to observe for child's response to feedings and untoward symptoms.
   a. Persistent vomiting
   b. Signs of infection
   c. Weight gain
2. Instruct parents about care of incisional site.
3. Provide follow-up support and management for parents.
   a. Name and phone number of primary physician
   b. Phone number of clinic
   c. Name and phone number of clinical nurse specialist and primary nurse

CLIENT OUTCOMES

1. Child will be adequately hydrated.
2. Child will have appropriate weight gain.
3. Parents will demonstrate understanding of infant's or child's condition, possible complications, and home care.

REFERENCES

Rollins M et al: Pyloric stenosis: congenital or acquired, *Arch Dis Child* 64:138, 1989.

Ross AJ III: Intestinal obstructions in the newborn, *Pediatr Rev* 15(9):338, 1994.

Sondheimer JM, Silverman A: Gastrointestinal tract. In Hay WW et al, editors: *Current pediatric diagnosis and treatment*, ed 12, East Norwalk, Conn, 1995, Appleton & Lange.

Wong DL: *Essentials of pediatric nursing*, ed 4, St Louis, 1993, Mosby.

39

Idiopathic Thrombocytopenic Purpura

PATHOPHYSIOLOGY

Idiopathic thrombocytopenic purpura (ITP) is one of the most common acquired bleeding disorders. ITP is a syndrome in which there is a reduction in the number of circulating platelets in the presence of normal marrow. The exact cause of this condition is unknown, although it is speculated to be caused by viral agents that damage platelets. Generally, ITP is preceded by a vaguely defined febrile illness 1 to 6 weeks before onset of symptoms. Clinical manifestations vary considerably. ITP can be classified into three types: acute, chronic, and recurrent (see the box on p. 242). Children are initially seen with the following symptoms: (1) fever, (2) bleeding, (3) petechiae, (4) purpura with thrombocytopenia, and (5) anemia. Prognosis is favorable, especially in children with the acute form.

INCIDENCE

1. The age range of peak incidence is 2 to 6 years.
2. ITP affects male and female individuals equally.
3. ITP occurs more commonly in white individuals.
4. Eighty percent of ITP in children is the acute type.
5. Incidence is seasonal—occurrence is more frequent in winter and spring.
6. Fifty percent to 85% of affected children have a viral illness before ITP.

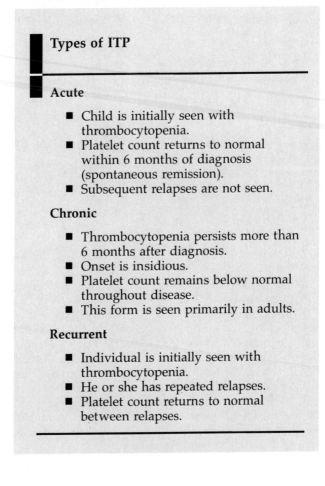

Types of ITP

Acute

- Child is initially seen with thrombocytopenia.
- Platelet count returns to normal within 6 months of diagnosis (spontaneous remission).
- Subsequent relapses are not seen.

Chronic

- Thrombocytopenia persists more than 6 months after diagnosis.
- Onset is insidious.
- Platelet count remains below normal throughout disease.
- This form is seen primarily in adults.

Recurrent

- Individual is initially seen with thrombocytopenia.
- He or she has repeated relapses.
- Platelet count returns to normal between relapses.

7. Ten percent to 25% of affected children develop the chronic form of ITP.

CLINICAL MANIFESTATIONS

1. Prodromal period—fatigue, fever, and abdominal pain
2. Spontaneous appearance on skin of petechiae and ecchymoses
3. Bruising easily

4. Epistaxis (initially seen symptom in one third of children)
5. Menorrhagia
6. Hematuria (infrequent)
7. Bleeding from oral cavity (infrequent)
8. Melena (infrequent)

COMPLICATIONS

1. Transfusion reaction
2. Relapse
3. Central nervous system hemorrhage (less than 1% affected individuals)

LABORATORY AND DIAGNOSTIC TESTS

1. Platelet count—decreased to less than 40,000 mm^3, and often less than 20,000 mm^3
2. Complete blood count (CBC)—anemia results from inability of red blood cells (RBCs) to use iron
3. Bone marrow aspiration—increased megakaryocytes
4. White blood count (WBC)—mild to moderate leukocytosis; mild eosinophilia
5. Platelet antibody tests—done with questionable diagnosis
   a. Tissue biopsy of skin and gingiva—diagnostic
   b. Antinuclear antibody test—to rule out systemic lupus erythematosus (SLE)
   c. Slit lamp examinations—to screen for uvetis
   d. Renal biopsy—to diagnose renal involvement
   e. Chest x-ray examination and pulmonary function test—diagnostic for pulmonary manifestations (effusion, interstitial pulmonary fibrosis)

MEDICAL MANAGEMENT

The goal of treatment in ITP is the reduction of antibody production and platelet destruction, and an elevation and maintenance of the platelet count. Corticosteroids are often used as the initial therapy for ITP. If the child does not respond to the corticosteroid regimens, intravenous immune globulin (IVIG) is administered. IVIG stimulates a rapid rise in platelet count within 24 hours of administration. Immunosuppressants (vincristine and cyclophosphamide) may be used in difficult cases. A splenectomy may be done if ITP lasts more than a year or child is older than 5 years.

NURSING ASSESSMENT

1. See the section on hematologic assessment in Appendix A.
2. Determine location of purpuric areas.
3. Determine sites of bleeding.

NURSING DIAGNOSES

- High risk for injury
- Impaired tissue integrity
- Altered peripheral tissue perfusion
- Fluid volume deficit
- Fatigue
- Diversional activity deficit
- Knowledge deficit

NURSING INTERVENTIONS

1. Monitor child's clinical status.
   a. Vital signs every 2 hours (during acute phase)
   b. Bleeding sites
   c. Level of activity
   d. Purpuric area
   e. Areas susceptible to bruising
2. Monitor for and prevent infection.
   a. Screen contacts with child.
   b. Institute clean techniques when in contact with child.
   c. Monitor for signs of infection (pulmonary, systemic, localized).
   d. Administer medications.
3. Monitor child's response to blood product transfusions (whole blood, packed cells, platelets).
4. Monitor child's therapeutic and untoward response to administration of medications.
   a. Antibiotics
   b. Antipyretics (avoid aspirin)
   c. Iron preparations
   d. Immunosuppressives
5. Promote rest and conservation of the child's energy.
   a. Maintain complete bed rest during acute stages.
   b. Assess child's response to activity as means of assessing tolerance and progression.

6. Provide diversional and age-appropriate activities for child during periods of limited activities (see section on growth and development, Appendix B).
7. Provide age-appropriate explanations before procedures; treatments; and surgery, if splenectomy is indicated (see Appendix J, section on preparation for procedure/ surgery).

♠ Discharge Planning and Home Care

1. Provide parents and child with instructions about administration of medications.
   a. Time and route of administration
   b. Monitoring for untoward effects
2. Instruct parents and child to monitor for signs and symptoms of thrombocytopenia and report immediately (i.e., petechiae, ecchymosis, blood in urine or stool, and headache).
3. Instruct parents to monitor child's activities.
   a. Encourage quiet activities; have child avoid contact sports until platelet level returns to normal.
   b. Balance rest and activity periods; increase activity as tolerated.
4. Instruct parents to avoid child's contact with persons who have infections, especially upper respiratory tract infections.
5. Instruct parents to avoid use of over-the-counter medications that may affect clotting (i.e., aspirin, antihistamines, and nonsteroidal antiinflammatory drugs).

CLIENT OUTCOMES

1. The child will be free of complications of the disease.
2. The child will not demonstrate signs and symptoms of infection.
3. The child and family will verbalize knowledge of the treatment regimen.

REFERENCES

Aronis S et al: Seventeen years of experience with chronic idiopathic thrombocytopenic purpura in childhood: is therapy always better? *Pediatr Hematol Oncol* 11(5):487, 1994.

Burstein Y, Berns L: Immune thrombocytopenic purpura, *Pediatr Ann* 11(3):323, 1982.

Byrnes J: Thrombotic thrombocytopenic purpura: an epidemiologic study, *J Pediatr* 83:31, 1980.

Nazarian LF: Index of suspicion, case 1: idiopathic thrombocytopenic purpura, *Pediatr Rev* 14(6):215, 1993.

Reynolds M: Role of immune globulin in the treatment of idiopathic thrombocytopenic purpura, *J Pediatr Health Care* 3(2):109, 1989.

Thomas G, O'Brien R: Idiopathic thrombocytopenic purpura in children, *Nurs Pract: Am J Prim Health Care* 12(4):24, 1987.

Thomas G et al: Idiopathic thrombocytopenic purpura in children, *Nurs Pract* 12(4):24, 1987.

40

Imperforate Anus

PATHOPHYSIOLOGY

The congenital malformation known as imperforate anus involves the anus, the rectum, or the junction between the two. There are two classifications of imperforate anus, related to the placement of the distal end of the colon (rectum). In high imperforate anus, the rectum ends above the puborectalis sling, the main muscle complex responsible for sphincter control and fecal continence. In low imperforate anus, the rectum has transversed the puborectalis sling, with an abnormal location in the perineum. Affected infants can be expected to have rectal continence after repair.

Along with the imperforate anus, the following may also occur:

1. In female individuals, a fistula may be present between the rectum and the vagina.
2. In male individuals, a fistula may be present between the rectum and the urinary tract at the scrotum.

The appearance of the defect varies, depending on its severity. A less involved imperforate anus appears as a deep anal dimple and exhibits strong muscular reaction to pinprick, indicating innervation of that area. More severe involvement is initially seen as a flat perineum with no dimple and poor muscular response to pinprick, a result of defective perineal innervation and muscle formation. A highly involved defect includes other anomalies as well (Table 5). The infant may initially be seen with poorly developed labia, undescended testicles, and ambiguous genitalia. Outcomes are favorable after definitive surgery is performed.

Table 5. Associated Anomalies	
Type	**Incidence (%)***
Esophageal atresia	13
Intestinal atresia	4
Intestinal malrotation	4
Cardiovascular defects	7
Skeletal deformities (spina bifida, agenesis of sacrum)	6
Genitourinary anomalies (renal agenesis, hypospadias, epispadias)	40

* Approximate percentage.

INCIDENCE

1. Imperforate anus occurs in 1 of every 1500 to 5000 live births.
2. Twenty percent to 75% of affected infants have an associated anomaly.
3. Imperforate anus affects male and female individuals with equal frequency.

CLINICAL MANIFESTATIONS

1. Meconium not passed within first 24 hours after birth
2. Inability to take infant's rectal temperature
3. Meconium passed through a fistula or misplaced anus
4. Gradual distention and signs of bowel obstruction if no fistula present

COMPLICATIONS

1. Hyperchloremic acidosis
2. Continuing urinary tract infection
3. Urethral damage (result of surgical procedure)

4. Long-term complications
   a. Eversion of anal mucosa
   b. Stenosis (result of contraction of scar from anastomosis)
   c. Impactions and constipation (result of sigmoid dilation)
   d. Problems or delays associated with toilet training
   e. Incontinence (result of anal stenosis or impaction)
   f. Prolapse of anorectal mucosa (results in persistent seepage and incontinence)
   g. Recurrent fistulas (result of tension in surgical site and infection)

LABORATORY AND DIAGNOSTIC TESTS

1. Visual and digital rectal examination is generally diagnostic.
2. If fistula is present, urine may be examined for meconium epithelial cells.
3. Inverted lateral x-ray examination (Wangensteen-Rice technique) may demonstrate air collected in the blind-ending rectum at or near the perineum; may be misleading if the rectum is filled with meconium preventing air from reaching the end of the rectal pouch.
4. Ultrasound may be helpful in locating rectal pouch.
5. Needle aspiration for detecting the rectal pouch involves advancing the needle while attempting to aspirate; if no meconium has been obtained by the time the needle has been advanced 1.5 cm, the defect is assumed to be of a high type.

SURGICAL MANAGEMENT

Surgical therapy in the newborn varies with the severity of the defect. The higher the lesion, the more complicated the surgical correction procedure. For high anomalies, a colostomy is performed a few days after birth. The definitive surgery, a perineal anoplasty (an abdominal-perineal pull-through procedure), is generally delayed 9 to 12 months. This delay allows the pelvis to enlarge and the musculature to develop. It also enables the infant to gain weight and attain satisfactory nutritional status. Low lesions are corrected by pulling the rectal pouch through the sphincter to the opening on the anal skin. Fistulas, if present, are closed.

Membranous defects require only minimal surgical treatment. The membrane is punctured with a hemostat or scalpel.

In most instances, correction of the imperforate anus requires a two-stage surgical approach. For mild to moderate defects, the prognosis is favorable. The defect can be repaired, and normal peristalsis and continence can be obtained. More serious defects are usually associated with other anomalies, compounding the surgical outcomes.

NURSING ASSESSMENT

1. See the section on gastrointestinal assessment in Appendix A.
2. Assess nutritional status.

NURSING DIAGNOSES

- High risk for fluid volume deficit
- Altered nutrition: less than body requirements
- Impaired tissue integrity
- High risk for infection
- Pain
- Impaired home maintenance management

NURSING INTERVENTIONS
Preoperative Care

1. Monitor infant's condition before surgery.
   a. Measure abdominal girth (assess for abdominal distention).
   b. Monitor vital signs every 4 hours.
   c. Monitor for bowel complications (perforation and enterocolitis).
   d. Monitor fluid and electrolyte balance (input and output, nasogastric [NG] drainage).
2. Prepare infant for surgery.
   a. Monitor infant's response to evacuation of bowel.
   b. Using NG tube, decompress stomach.
   c. Using catheter, decompress bladder.
   d. Provide only clear liquids 24 to 48 hours before surgery.
   e. Monitor infant's response to antibiotics (e.g., neomycin) used to sterilize bowel.
3. Prepare infant for procedures and surgeries.

Postoperative Care

1. Monitor infant's response to surgery.
   a. Vital signs
   b. Intake and output—report discrepancies
   c. Surgical site—bleeding, intactness, signs of infection
2. Monitor for signs and symptoms of complications.
   a. Urinary tract infection
   b. Hyperchloremic acidosis
   c. Decreased urinary output
   d. Constipation
   e. Obstruction
   f. Bleeding
3. Promote and maintain fluid and electrolyte balance.
   a. Record intake per route (intravenous, NG, oral).
   b. Record output per route (urine and stool, NG drainage, emesis, Penrose drain).
   c. Assess hydration status (signs of dehydration, electrolyte imbalance).
4. Provide dressing care; maintain integrity of surgical site (depends on type of surgery).
   a. Monitor dilation of anus.
   b. Monitor endorectal pull-through incision (made over anal dimple and colon directly through to muscle cuff).
   c. Do not take rectal temperatures, give rectal medications, or perform rectal examinations.
   d. Keep anus clean and dry.
   e. Apply zinc oxide for skin lesions and irritation surrounding surgical site.
   f. Avoid tension on suture line; position infant on side or abdomen.
5. Promote adequate nutritional intake.
   a. Monitor bowel sounds; begin fluids when bowel sounds are heard.
   b. Advance to full diet as tolerated.
6. Protect infant from infection.
   a. Provide Foley catheter care.
   b. Change dressing and note drainage.
   c. Monitor incisional site for drainage, redness, inflammation.

   d. Clean anal area frequently to prevent fecal contamination.
   e. Perform pulmonary toilet every 2 to 4 hours.
   f. Change infant's position every 2 hours.
   g. Monitor for signs of systemic infection or local abscess.
7. Promote functioning and maintain patency of colostomy.
8. Promote comfort and minimize pain.
   a. Provide sitz bath (initiate 1 week after surgery).
   b. Apply zinc oxide to excoriated and irritated areas of skin.
   c. Provide position of comfort.
   d. Use distractions (play activities).
   e. Monitor child's response to medication.

♠ Discharge Planning and Home Care

1. Encourage parents to ventilate concerns about outcomes of surgery.
2. Refer to specific institutional procedures for information distributed to parents about home care.
3. Instruct parents on the signs of intestinal obstruction, poor tolerance of feedings, and impaired healing processes.
4. Instruct parents about follow-up techniques to promote optimal surgical outcomes.
   a. Colostomy care
   b. Dilation of anus
   c. Sitz bath

CLIENT OUTCOMES

1. Infant will return to normal gastrointestinal function.
2. Infant growth will continue at a steady pace.
3. Parents will verbalize understanding of home care and follow-up needs.

REFERENCES

Bellet P: *The diagnostic approach to common symptoms and signs in infants, children and adolescents,* Philadelphia, 1989, Lea & Febiger.

McCollum L et al: Assessment and management of gastrointestinal dysfunction. In Kenner C et al, editors: *Comprehensive neonatal nursing,* Philadelphia, 1993, WB Saunders.

Seashore J: Disorders of the anus and rectum. In Gellis S, Kagan B, editors: *Current pediatric therapy,* ed 13, Philadelphia, 1990, WB Saunders.

Tarnowski KJ et al: Congenital gastrointestinal anomalies: psychosocial functioning of children with imperforate anus, gastroschisis, and omphalocele, *J Consult Clin Psychol* 59(4):587, 1991.

41

Inflammatory Bowel Disease

PATHOPHYSIOLOGY

Inflammatory bowel disease refers to two gastrointestinal conditions: ulcerative colitis and Crohn's disease. Differentiating ulcerative colitis from Crohn's disease may be difficult; in 10% of the cases, a differential diagnosis is not made. The causes of both diseases are unknown, although recent research has focused on genetic, immunologic, dietary, and infectious causes.

An association between ankylosing spondylitis and the histocompatibility of human leukocyte antigen (HLA-B27) and inflammatory bowel disease is a possibility. Ulcerative colitis and Crohn's disease have similar initial signs, including diarrhea, rectal bleeding, abdominal pain, fever, malaise, anorexia, weight loss, and anemia. Children may initially be seen with vague symptoms such as growth failure, anorexia, fever, and joint pains with or without gastrointestinal symptoms. Both conditions are characterized by remissions and exacerbations. Extracolonic manifestations such as joint problems, skin rashes, and eye irritation can occur. Although the peak incidence of inflammatory bowel disease occurs between 15 and 25 years of age, 15% of all cases occur at age 15 years and younger. Prognosis is dependent on the following factors: (1) age at onset and rapidity of onset; (2) response to medical treatment; and (3) extent of involvement.

Ulcerative colitis is a recurrent inflammatory and ulcerative disease affecting primarily the large intestine. Lesions are continuous and involve the superficial mucosa, causing vascular congestion, capillary dilation, edema, hemorrhage, and ulceration. Muscular hypertrophy and deposition of fibrous tissue and fat result, giving the bowel a "lead pipe" appearance because of narrowing of the bowel itself.

Crohn's disease is an inflammatory and ulcerative disease affecting any part of the alimentary tract from the mouth to the anus. The disease affects the deep walls of the bowel. The lesions are discontinuous, resulting in a "skipping" effect, with the diseased portions of the bowel separated by normal tissue. Fissures, fistulas, and thickened intestinal walls result. Granulomas occur in approximately 50% of cases.

INCIDENCE

1. Annual incidence of ulcerative colitis and Crohn's disease is four to seven cases per 100,000 children.
2. Ulcerative colitis represents more than half of the 20,000 to 25,000 newly diagnosed cases of inflammatory bowel disease each year.
3. Age range of peak incidence is 15 to 20 years.
4. White individuals are affected more often than black individuals.
5. There is a high preponderance among American Jews.
6. Twenty-nine percent of those with ulcerative colitis have a family history of the disease.
7. Thirty-five percent of those with Crohn's disease have a family history of the disease.

CLINICAL MANIFESTATIONS
Ulcerative Colitis

1. Frequent, bloody stools (number of stools varies from 4 to 24)—major symptom
2. Pain relief after defecation
3. Rectal bleeding
4. Anorexia, pallor, and fatigue
5. Fever
6. Tachycardia
7. Peritoneal irritation
8. Electrolyte imbalance
9. Ten- to 20-pound weight loss over 2 months
10. Anemia, leukocytosis, increased sedimentation rate

11. Extraintestinal symptoms—skin rashes, arthritis
12. Flatulence
13. Severe pain, abdominal rigidity, distention
14. Growth retardation

Crohn's Disease

1. Diarrhea, occult blood
2. Cramping abdominal pain aggravated by eating
3. Pain in the right lower quadrant of abdomen with or without palpable mass
4. Growth retardation
5. Weight loss
6. Abscess formation
7. Spiking fever
8. Leukocytosis
9. Perianal disease—fistula and fissures
10. Nutritional deficiencies—malnutrition, electrolyte imbalances
11. Amenorrhea, delay in sexual maturation
12. Cachexia
13. Finger clubbing
14. Arthritis

COMPLICATIONS
Ulcerative Colitis

1. Predisposition to cancer—20% risk is associated with each decade after the first 10 years
2. Toxic megacolon
3. Hemorrhage
4. Sepsis

Crohn's Disease

1. Perforation
2. Toxic megacolon
3. Hemorrhage
4. Liver abscess and liver disease
5. Ureteral obstruction
6. Retroperitonitis
7. Erythema nodosum
8. Strictures
9. Fistulas

LABORATORY AND DIAGNOSTIC TESTS

1. Complete blood count (CBC)—anemia
2. White blood count (WBC)—increased with inflammation
3. Sedimentation rate—increased with inflammation
4. Hematocrit—decreased because of blood loss
5. Serum electrolytes—decreased potassium
6. Serum protein—decreased proteins
7. Stool culture—for presence of infectious organisms
8. Hematest of stool—for presence of blood in stool
9. D-Xylulose absorption blood and urine test—to measure intestinal absorption when there are fatty stools
10. Sigmoidoscopy—to evaluate mucosa, rectum, sigmoid colon directly
11. Colonoscopy—to evaluate colon directly
12. Upper gastrointestinal tract x-ray series with small bowel follow-through—differential diagnosis
13. Barium enema—differential diagnosis
14. Biopsy—to determine type of inflammatory bowel disease; tissue specimens are taken from several sites

MEDICAL MANAGEMENT
Ulcerative Colitis

Medical management is the primary treatment of ulcerative colitis and centers around drug therapy and nutritional support. Antidiarrheal preparations may be used along with antiinflammatory agents to control or suppress the inflammatory process. Analgesics and narcotics may also be given for pain. Dietary modifications may be needed to control diarrhea, in the presence of fistulas, or for lactose intolerance. Therapy depends on the severity of the illness. If the illness is severe, the child may require intravenous (IV) hyperalimentation, corticosteroids, and close observation for electrolyte imbalances, acidosis, anemia, and intestinal perforation. Surgical intervention is eventually needed in 25% of cases and provides a cure.

Crohn's Disease

Pharmacologic interventions for Crohn's disease are similar to those for ulcerative colitis. Because there is no known cure for this disease, the treatment goals are to reduce bowel inflammation, correct nutritional deficiencies, and provide relief of symptoms. Nutritional support may include dietary modifications, vitamins, oral supplements, or hyperalimentation. Up to 70% of children with Crohn's disease require surgery because of failure of medical management, intestinal fistulas or obstruction, and growth failure.

SURGICAL TREATMENT
Ileostomy

Ileostomy is performed to treat inflammatory bowel disease after medical therapeutic procedures have been unsuccessful. Ileostomy involves removal of the diseased portion of the bowel (small intestine), with the ileum used to form a stoma on the abdominal wall for bowel evacuation. A variety of surgical procedures may be used, depending on the extent and location of the affected portion of the bowel. An ileostomy with subtotal or total colectomy is performed on children who are malnourished and have moderate to severe rectal disease. The Koch ileostomy provides continence without the use of appliances. Use of the Koch pouch procedure is contraindicated in many cases because of the length of the bowel that is lost with recurrence of disease in the pouch (Crohn's disease).

Colostomy

Permanent or temporary colostomies are performed for a variety of conditions. Permanent colostomies are performed for children with severe cases of Crohn's disease. The sigmoid colostomy is most frequently performed. Temporary colostomies (e.g., transverse loop and double-barrel colostomies) are performed in children most often. In all types of colostomies, an intact portion of the colon is brought through an abdominal incision and is sutured to the abdominal wall to form a stoma.

Clinical Manifestations

The response to the surgery should result in amelioration of symptoms associated with the primary disease. The child is left with an abdominal stoma through which bowel contents are emptied into an attached appliance or into an abdominal pouch (Koch pouch). Although the child does not live with a normally functioning bowel after surgery, most children do well. If the child, adolescent, or parent learns to care properly for the colostomy or ileostomy, a life filled with educational, social, and athletic activities can be expected.

Complications

1. Necrosis of colostomy (caused by inadequate blood supply)
2. Stricture formation
3. Retraction of the stoma
4. Prolapsed stoma
5. Herniation
6. Bleeding
7. Intestinal obstruction
8. Wound infection
9. Peritonitis
10. Spillover of stool
11. Constipation bordering on obstruction
12. Nephrolithiasis
13. Fistula (if multiple fistulas or extensive undermining of subcutaneous tissue occurs, stoma must be excised and located elsewhere)

NURSING ASSESSMENT

1. See section on gastrointestinal assessment in Appendix A.
2. Assess for abdominal distention, bowel sounds, tenderness and pain, and abdominal girth.

NURSING DIAGNOSES

- Diarrhea
- Pain
- Impaired tissue integrity
- Altered nutrition: less than body requirements
- High risk for infection
- Potential for fluid volume deficit
- Body image disturbance
- Knowledge deficit
- Impaired home management maintenance
- Potential for injury

NURSING INTERVENTIONS

1. Promote and maintain proper hydration status.
   a. Record input and output.
   b. Record daily weights.
   c. Assess for signs of dehydration.
   d. Promote oral intake when appropriate.
   e. Monitor administration of elemental feedings or hyperalimentation.
2. Provide comfort and pain relief measures as indicated.
   a. Maintain bed rest during acute episode (decreased activity results in decreased peristalsis, diarrhea, pain).
   b. Provide diversional activities.
   c. Provide heating pad.
   d. Change child's position.
   e. Assess intensity, type, time, and pattern of occurrence of pain, and child's response to pain relief measures.
   f. Monitor child's response to analgesics and narcotics.
   g. Provide uninterrupted rest periods.
3. Promote skin integrity.
   a. For perineal care, apply A&D ointment or petroleum jelly to perineal area to prevent skin irritation or breakdown.
   b. Apply body moisturizers liberally.
   c. Provide sitz bath three times a day (for perianal or rectal fistulas or fissures).
   d. Provide foam mattress to prevent pressure sores.
   e. Change child's position every 2 hours.
4. Promote and support optimal nutritional status.
   a. Compile dietary history, including food allergies.
   b. Monitor tolerance to food, noting type and amount.
   c. Monitor response to elemental feedings.
   d. Monitor response to low-residue, bland, high-protein, high-calorie diet.
   e. Monitor for signs of electrolyte imbalances (hypotension, tachycardia, oliguria, atonic muscles, general sense of confusion).
   f. Restrict intake of greasy, spicy, and lactose-containing foods.
   g. Monitor administration of hyperalimentation; observe child's or adolescent's response.
      (1) Maintain sterility of central line.

    (2) Record accurate input and output.
    (3) Obtain daily weights.
    (4) Monitor urinary specific gravity.
    (5) Check urinary glucose and acetone.
    (6) Monitor electrolyte balance (especially blood glucose).

5. Monitor child's or adolescent's response to and untoward side effects of medications.
6. Monitor for, prevent, or report signs of potential or actual complications.
    a. Fistulas or fissures
    b. Hemorrhage
    c. Intestinal obstruction
    d. Liver abscess
    e. Ureteral obstruction
    f. Retroperitonitis
    g. Perforations
    h. Enterocolitis

Preoperative Care

Prepare infant, child, or adolescent physically for surgery.

1. Monitor infant's or child's response to enemas, laxatives, stool softeners (to evacuate bowel preoperatively).
2. Monitor infant's or child's response to decompression of stomach and bowel (nasogastric [NG] tube and rectal tube).
3. Provide nothing by mouth 12 hours before surgery.
4. Insert Foley catheter to decompress bladder.
5. Administer antibiotics to sterilize bowel.
6. Monitor vital signs every 4 hours.
7. Monitor for bowel complications (perforation, toxic megacolon, or enterocolitis).
8. Demonstrate use of appliances.

Postoperative Care

1. Monitor child's response to surgery.
    a. Vital signs
    b. Intake and output (report any discrepancy)
    c. Dressing (amount of drainage, intactness)

2. Monitor for signs and symptoms of complications.
   a. Stoma complications (prolapse, bleeding, excessive diarrhea, ribbonlike stools, failure to pass stool, and flatus)
   b. Intestinal obstruction or constipation
   c. Prolapse of proximal segment
   d. Bleeding
   e. Increased stooling
   f. Infection
3. Promote return of peristalsis.
   a. Maintain patency of NG tube.
   b. Check functioning of suction machine.
   c. Irrigate with normal saline solution every 4 hours and as needed.
   d. Check for placement of NG tube; auscultate and aspirate contents.
4. Promote and maintain fluid and electrolyte balance.
   a. Record intake per route (IV, NG, oral).
   b. Record output per route (urine, stool, NG drainage, emesis, stoma).
   c. Monitor for signs and symptoms of electrolyte imbalances.
   d. Consult with physician about disparities.
5. Alleviate or minimize pain and discomfort.
   a. Maintain patency of NG tube.
   b. Maintain position of comfort.
   c. Monitor child's response to administration of medications.
   d. Provide oral care (mouth can become dry with NG tube in place).
6. Provide stoma and skin care to promote healing and to prevent complications.
   a. Inspect stoma every 4 hours for retraction, prolapse, or protrusion greater than 2 cm.
   b. Check for bleeding at stoma site.
   c. Check for obstruction (enlarged, pale, and edematous stoma).
7. Provide ostomy care (refer to institutional manual for specific technical and institutional procedure).
   a. Care of appliance
   b. Skin care
   c. Prevention of complications

(1) Skin can become irritated by digestive enzymes.
(2) Match adhesive to stoma size.
(3) Apply protective cream to exposed area.

8. Protect child from infection.
   a. Provide Foley catheter care per hospital protocol.
   b. Change dressing as needed (perianal and colostomy).
   c. Monitor incision site.
   d. Refer to institutional procedure manual for care related to specific procedure.
   e. Perform pulmonary toilet every 2 to 4 hours.
   f. Change child's position every 2 hours (prevents atelectasis).
   g. Monitor for signs of systemic infection and local abscess.

9. Facilitate development of realistic adaptive body image.
   a. Encourage ventilation of feelings regarding stoma, outcome of surgery.
   b. Encourage socialization through peer support groups.
   c. Refer to community organizations.
   d. Provide active problem solving for concerns such as dress apparel and sexual activity.

10. Encourage socialization with peers as a means to cope with impact of disease.

11. Modify chronic sick role behavior by promoting socialization and normal daily activities.

12. Encourage ventilation of fears of body mutilation.

♠ Discharge Planning and Home Care

1. Instruct child, parents, and family about ostomy or Koch pouch care.

2. Instruct child or adolescent and parents to monitor for and report signs of complications.
   a. Mechanical obstruction
   b. Peritonitis or wound infection

3. Instruct child or adolescent and parents about administration of total parenteral nutrition or NG feedings.

4. Initiate referral to school nurse and teacher to promote continuity of care.
   a. Observations of child's response to condition
   b. Observations of untoward effects of medications and complications

   c. Observation of social interactions with peers and conduct in school
5. Refer to community organizations.
   a. Ostomy Association of Los Angeles, Inc.
      5015 Eagle Rock Blvd.
      Suite 215
      Los Angeles, CA 90041
      (213) 255-1681
   b. United Ostomy Association, Inc.
      36 Executive Park
      Suite 120
      Irvine, CA 92714-6744
      (714) 660-8624

CLIENT OUTCOMES

1. Child will have stable gastrointestinal function.
2. Child will have positive adaptation to psychosocial aspects of disease and/or surgery.
3. Child and family will understand home care and follow-up needs.

REFERENCES

Behrman R, Kliegman R: *Nelson essentials of pediatrics,* ed 2, Philadelphia, 1994, WB Saunders.

Hampton B, Bryant R: *Ostomies and continent diversions: nursing management,* St Louis, 1994, Mosby.

Hurd L: Presenting a patient's guide to ileoanal reservoir surgery, *Ostomy/Wound Management* 38(5):52, 1992.

Meissner J: Ulcerative colitis, *Nurs 94* 24(7):54, 1994.

42

Iron Deficiency Anemia

PATHOPHYSIOLOGY

Iron deficiency anemia is the most common anemia affecting children in North America. The full-term infant born of a well-nourished, nonanemic mother has sufficient iron stores until the birth weight is doubled, generally at 4 to 6 months. After that period, iron must be available from the diet to meet the child's nutritional needs. If dietary iron intake is insufficient, iron deficiency anemia results. Most often, insufficient dietary iron intake results from inappropriately early introduction of solid foods (before age 4 to 6 months), discontinuation of iron-fortified infant formula or breast milk before age 1 year, and excessive consumption of cow's milk to the exclusion of iron-rich solids in the toddler. Also, the preterm infant, the infant with significant perinatal blood loss, or the infant born to a poorly nourished, iron-deficient mother may have inadequate iron stores. This infant would be at a significantly higher risk for iron deficiency anemia before age 6 months.

Iron deficiency anemia may also result from chronic blood loss. In the infant, this may be due to chronic intestinal bleeding caused by the heat-labile protein in cow's milk. In children of all ages, the loss of as little as 1 to 7 ml of blood through the gastrointestinal tract daily may lead to iron deficiency anemia. In female teenagers, iron deficiency anemia may also be due to excessive menstrual flow.

INCIDENCE

1. Three percent to 24% of infants 6 to 24 months of age have iron deficiency anemia.
2. Twenty-nine percent to 68% of infants 6 to 24 months of age are iron deficient.
3. Incidence of iron deficiency and iron deficiency anemia among adolescent girls is 11% to 17%.
4. The age range of peak incidence for iron deficiency anemia is 12 to 18 months.

CLINICAL MANIFESTATIONS

1. Conjunctival pallor (hemoglobin [Hb] 6 to 10 g/dl)
2. Palmar crease pallor (Hb below 8 g/dl)
3. Irritability and anorexia (Hb 5 g or below)
4. Tachycardia, systolic murmur
5. Pica
6. Lethargy, increased need for sleep
7. Lack of interest in toys or play activities

COMPLICATIONS

1. Poor muscular development (long term)
2. Decreased attention span
3. Decreased performance on developmental tests
4. Decreased ability to process information obtained through hearing

LABORATORY AND DIAGNOSTIC TESTS

1. Free erythrocyte porphyrin level—increased
2. Serum iron concentration—decreased
3. Transferrin saturation—decreased
4. Serum ferritin concentration—decreased
5. Hemoglobin—decreased
6. Erythrocyte porphyrin-hemoglobin ratio—greater than 2.8 μg/g is diagnostic for iron deficiency
7. Mean corpuscle volume (MCV) and mean corpuscle hemoglobin concentration (MCHC)—decreased, yielding a microcytic, hypochromic anemia or small, pale red blood cells (RBCs)

8. During treatment, reticulocyte count—increase within 3 to 5 days of initiating iron therapy indicates a positive therapeutic response
9. With treatment, hemoglobin—return to normal within 4 to 8 weeks indicates adequate iron and nutritional support

MEDICAL MANAGEMENT

Treatment efforts are directed toward prevention and intervention. Prevention includes encouraging mothers to breast-feed, to eat foods that are iron rich, and to take iron-fortified prenatal vitamins. Therapy to treat iron deficiency anemia consists of a medication regimen. Iron is administered by mouth (po) in doses of 2 to 3 mg/kg of elemental iron. All iron forms are equally effective (ferrous sulfate, ferrous fumarate, ferrous succinate, ferrous gluconate). Vitamin C must be administered simultaneously with iron (ascorbic acid increases iron absorption). Iron is best absorbed when taken 1 hour before a meal. Iron therapy should continue for a minimum of 6 weeks after the anemia is corrected to replenish iron stores. Injectable iron is seldom used unless small bowel malabsorption disease is present.

NURSING ASSESSMENT

1. See the section on cardiovascular assessment in Appendix A.
2. Assess child's reaction to iron therapy.
3. Assess child's activity level.
4. Assess child's developmental level.

NURSING DIAGNOSES

- Activity intolerance
- Altered nutrition: less than body requirements
- Fatigue
- High risk for altered growth and development

NURSING INTERVENTIONS

1. Monitor child's therapeutic and untoward effects from iron therapy.
   a. Side effects (e.g., tooth discoloration) of oral therapy are infrequent.

b. Instruct about measures to prevent tooth discoloration.
   (1) Take iron with fluids, preferably orange juice.
   (2) Rinse mouth after taking medication.
c. Encourage increased fiber and water intake to minimize constipating effects of iron.
d. For severe, iron-induced constipation, consider lowering iron dose, but extending length of treatment.

2. Instruct parents about appropriate nutritional intake.
   a. Reduce child's milk intake.
   b. Increase intake of meat and appropriate protein substitutes.
   c. Encourage inclusion of whole grains and green leafy vegetables in diet.

3. Gather information about dietary history and eating behaviors.
   a. Assess for factors contributing to nutritional deficiency—psychosocial, behavioral, and nutritional.
   b. Plan with parents an acceptable approach toward dietary habits.
   c. Refer to nutritionist for intensive evaluation and treatment.

4. Encourage breast-feeding, since breast milk iron is well absorbed.

♠ Discharge Planning and Home Care

1. Instruct about administering iron therapy (see nursing intervention number 1).
2. Instruct about meal planning and nutritional intake (see nursing intervention number 2).

CLIENT OUTCOMES

1. Child's skin color improves.
2. Child's pattern of growth improves (as indicated on growth chart).
3. Child's activity level is appropriate for age.
4. Parents demonstrate understanding of home treatment regimen (i.e., medication administration, appropriate iron-rich foods).

REFERENCES

Belkengren R, Sapala S: Pediatric management problems: iron deficiency anemia, *Pediatr Nurs* 19(4):378, 1993.

Dallman P, Yip R: Changing characteristics of childhood anemia, *J Pediatr* 114(1):161, 1989.

Looker A et al: Iron status: prevalence of impairment in three Hispanic groups in the United States, *Am J Clin Nutr* 49:553, 1989.

Walter T et al: Effectiveness of iron-fortified infant cereal in prevention of iron deficiency anemia, *Pediatrics* 91(5):976, 1993.

43

Juvenile Rheumatoid Arthritis

PATHOPHYSIOLOGY

Juvenile rheumatoid arthritis (JRA) is a chronic inflammatory disease that begins before the affected child is 16 years of age. It is the most common rheumatic disease in children and a leading cause of disability. Although its cause is unknown, a genetic predisposition is thought to exist. JRA causes chronic inflammation of the synovium with joint effusion that can result in eventual erosion and destruction of the articular cartilage. If the process persists long enough, adhesions between the joint surfaces and ankylosis of joints develop. The diagnosis is based on the following criteria:

1. There must be objective evidence of arthritis (defined as joint swelling or joint limitation of motion with tenderness). Pain or tenderness alone is not sufficient for a diagnosis of arthritis.
2. The arthritis must persist for at least 6 weeks in a given joint.
3. Other specific diseases that may cause or be associated with arthritis must be excluded.

   Common characteristics include morning stiffness, joint pain, sluggishness with movement, malaise, fatigue, anorexia, and weight loss.

   Children diagnosed with JRA are classified into one of the following categories that reflect etiology and prognosis:

1. Systemic JRA
2. Polyarticular JRA: rheumatoid factor positive

3. Polyarticular JRA: rheumatoid factor negative
4. Pauciarticular JRA
5. Pauciarticular extended JRA
6. Psoriatic JRA
7. Enthesopathy-related JRA

    For classification purposes, joints are counted individually, with certain exceptions. The cervical region of the spine is considered one joint. The carpal joints of each hand are counted as one joint, as are the tarsal joints of each foot. The metacarpophalangeal, metatarsophalangeal, proximal, distal, and interphalangeal joints are counted individually.

INCIDENCE

1. JRA is twice as common in female individuals.
2. JRA affects 0.1% of children (1 in 1000 children).
3. Age ranges of peak incidence are 1 to 3 years and 8 to 11 years.
4. JRA is the most common pediatric rheumatic disease.
5. Rates of incidence are acute systemic, 10%; polyarticular, 25%; and pauciarticular, 65%.

CLINICAL MANIFESTATIONS
Systemic JRA

1. This type of JRA is characterized by persistent, intermittent fever: daily or twice-daily, "hectic" temperature elevations to 102.2° F (39° C) or higher, with rapid return to normal temperature between fever spikes. This may occur with or without rheumatoid rash or other organ involvement.
2. There is a salmon-colored macular rash on trunk and extremities; the rash is migratory and, in 20% of cases, reported to be pruritic.
3. Arthritis may not occur for weeks or months after the onset of the symptoms.
4. Both large and small joints may be affected.
5. Before a definite diagnosis can be made, objective symptoms must be present.
6. The arthritis pattern may be pauciarticular (1 to 4 joints) or polyarticular (5 or more joints).
7. There are extraarticular symptoms, including pericarditis, lymphadenopathy, hepatosplenomegaly, anemia,

thrombocytosis, leukocytosis (as high as 45,000 to 60,000), and pleuritis.

Polyarticular JRA: Rheumatoid Factor Positive

1. Presence of arthritis in five or more joints
2. Intermittent low-grade fever
3. Possible malaise and fatigue
4. Possible anorexia, weight loss
5. Possible morning stiffness, joint pain, and sluggishness with movement
6. Highest incidence among female individuals, with onset in late childhood or adolescence
7. Similarity to adult rheumatoid arthritis
8. Rheumatoid nodules
9. Early onset of erosive synovitis
10. Symmetric joint involvement
11. Involvement of small joints of hands or feet
12. Frequent involvement of large joints of knees, wrists, elbows, and ankles
13. Possible involvement of cervical region of spine
14. Possible involvement of temporomandibular joint, leading to impaired biting and shortness of mandible

Polyarticular JRA: Rheumatoid Factor Negative

1. Presence of arthritis in five or more joints
2. Intermittent low-grade fever
3. Possible malaise and fatigue
4. Possible anorexia, weight loss
5. Possible morning stiffness, joint pain, and sluggishness with movement
6. Asymmetric joint involvement
7. Less tendency for involvement of large number of joints
8. Rare involvement of joints of hands or feet
9. Frequent involvement of large joints of knees, wrists, elbows, and ankles
10. Possible involvement of cervical region of spine
11. Possible involvement of temporomandibular joint, leading to impaired biting and shortness of mandible

Pauciarticular JRA (Presence of Arthritis in One to Four Joints)

1. The disease primarily affects female individuals, ages 1 to 4 years.
2. The joints affected are knees, ankles, and elbows.
3. Painless swelling of joints is common.
4. Iridocyclitis (20% of cases) is insidious and subacute.

Pauciarticular Extended JRA

1. During the first 6 months of disease, affected children have fewer than five joints involved; but later, more joints develop arthritis.
2. At least one third of children with pauciarticular arthritis fall into this category.
3. Outcome is more typical of rheumatoid factor–positive polyarticular disease.
4. Incidence of iridocyclitis is similar to that seen in pauciarticular JRA.

Psoriatic JRA

1. Arthritis with typical psoriatic rash or with the following accompanying characteristics
   a. Dactylitis (sausagelike swelling of a toe or fingers)
   b. Nail pitting
   c. Family history of psoriasis in close relatives (parents, siblings)
2. Slightly higher incidence among female individuals
3. Often, arthritis that is asymmetric, involving large and small joints

Enthesopathy-Related JRA

1. The disease primarily affects boys 8 years and older.
2. The disease affects large joints of lower extremities.
3. Heel pain and Achilles tendinitis are common.
4. Sacroiliitis occurs in 90% of cases.
5. Iritis occurs in 20% of cases (generally an acute process).
6. Low-grade fevers are characteristic.
7. There is decreased appetite, poor weight gain.

COMPLICATIONS

Uveitis (iritis or iridocyclitis) is a complication found in 20% of children with pauciarticular onset JRA, in 5% of those with polyarticular onset JRA, and rarely in children with systemic onset JRA. At increased risk for development of uveitis are young female individuals with pauciarticular onset disease. Those with a positive antinuclear antibody (ANA) test are at even higher risk. The onset is usually insidious and asymptomatic; however, approximately half of the children have some symptoms (pain, redness, headache, photophobia, change in vision) later in the course of the disease. If not diagnosed early, the disease can result in cataracts, glaucoma, visual loss, and blindness. If the disease is detected early, the prognosis is improved.

Other possible complications of JRA are the following:
1. Flexion contractures, with tendency toward a fetal position
2. Bilateral weakness of grip
3. Limitation of movement
4. Leg length discrepancy and other growth disturbances
5. Cardiopulmonary complications and other systemic complications
6. Severe anemia and malnutrition
7. Renal, bone marrow, gastrointestinal, and liver toxicity to drugs.

LABORATORY AND DIAGNOSTIC TESTS

1. Erythrocyte sedimentation rate (ESR) and C-reactive protein—increased with inflammation (these are useful in measuring disease activity and monitoring response to antiinflammatory medications; however, they are often normal in pauciarticular disease)
2. Rheumatoid factor—positive in only 15% of children with JRA (primarily those with polyarticular disease)
3. Positive ANA—primarily seen in pauciarticular JRA (in 40% of cases)
4. Complete blood count (CBC)—systemic leukocytosis; 45,000 to 60,000 white blood count (WBC) with acute systemic juvenile rheumatoid arthritis; thrombocytosis with normochromic or hypochromic anemia (thrombocytopenia is not seen in JRA)
5. Complement levels—increased
6. Alpha globulins—increased

7. Synovial fluid analysis (cell count and culture)—to rule out other conditions
8. Urinalysis—mild proteinuria accompanying increased fever
9. Radiologic studies (x-ray; nuclear scan; magnetic resonance imaging [MRI]; computed tomography [CT]; ultrasound)—to monitor disease progression and to rule out other conditions

MEDICAL MANAGEMENT

Treatment goals for JRA are to reduce the inflammatory process, to maintain joint function and strength, to decrease pain, and to maintain the patient's self-esteem and self-image in the face of a chronic illness. Drug therapy is used to reduce inflammation. Physical and occupational therapy and a regular daily program of exercise are essential to promote mobility and function. Heat is used to relieve joint pain and stiffness.

The treatment plan also includes frequent slit lamp examinations by an ophthalmologist according to specified guidelines (Table 6).

Nonsteroidal antiinflammatory drugs (NSAIDs) are used to control inflammation.
1. Aspirin and salicilates are no longer used as the first-choice NSAIDs, because of the association with Reye's syndrome during influenza or varicella infection, and the availability of other NSAIDs.
2. Naproxen (Naprosyn), ibuprofen, tolmetin (Tolectin), and indomethacin (Indocin) are common NSAIDs used for control of inflammation.

To be effective as an antiinflammatory medication, NSAIDs must be taken on a routine basis. If adequate effectiveness is not achieved after 2 to 3 months, an alternative NSAID can be tried. Many children require a second-line medication in addition to an NSAID to control disease activity. The following second-line medications may be used:
1. Slower-acting antirheumatic drugs (SAARDs) or disease-modifying antirheumatic drugs (DMARDs)
    a. Methotrexate given orally once a week in small doses has been markedly effective in the treatment of JRA;

Table 6. Slit Lamp Examination Guidelines

Type of JRA	ANA	When Diagnosed	Recommended Frequency of Slit Lamp Examination
Pauciarticular or polyarticular	Positive	Age 7 years or younger	Every 3-4 months for 7 years; then yearly
Pauciarticular or polyarticular	Negative	Age 7 years or younger	Every 6 months for 7 years; then yearly
Pauciarticular or polyarticular	—	Older than 7 years	Every 6 months for 4 years; then yearly
Systemic	—	—	Yearly

Modified from American Academy of Pediatrics, Section on Rheumatology and Section on Ophthalmology: Guidelines for ophthalmologic examinations in children with juvenile rheumatoid arthritis, *Pediatrics* 92(2):295, 1993.

it is also given subcutaneously or intramuscularly once a week for higher doses or in children with poor absorption.

b. Hydroxychloroquine (Plaquenil), sulfasalazine, gold salts, and penicillamine (D-Penicillamine) have been used in the treatment of JRA; however, none of these drugs have been shown to be effective in double-blinded placebo-controlled trials of JRA (parenteral gold and sulfasalazine have not been studied in JRA).

2. Cytotoxic agents (azathioprine, cyclophosphamide, and cyclosporine) are used occasionally in children with JRA that is unresponsive.

3. Glucocorticosteroids are used for life-threatening complication of JRA; oral steroid use should be limited as much as possible because of the potential side effects (intravenous pulse steroids and intraarticular steroid injections offer other methods of administration).

NURSING ASSESSMENT

1. See the section on musculoskeletal assessment in Appendix A.
2. Assess for pain.
3. Assess activities of daily living.
4. Assess growth and development.

NURSING DIAGNOSES

- Pain
- Impaired physical mobility
- Self-care deficit (bathing/hygiene, dressing/grooming, feeding, toileting)
- Altered growth and development
- Impaired social interaction
- Altered family processes

NURSING INTERVENTIONS

1. Provide pain relief measures as necessary.
   a. Tub bath or shower for joint stiffness
   b. Heating pad applied to affected areas
   c. Whirlpool bath, paraffin bath, or hot packs for pain and stiffness
   d. Footed pajamas or a sleeping bag
   e. Heated water bed or electric blanket

    f. Crutches, walker, or other device to avoid full weight bearing

2. Promote joint mobility, maintain strength, and prevent deformity of joints.
   a. Encourage compliance with physical therapy exercises (range of motion [ROM]/passive range of motion [PROM]).
   b. Encourage patient to participate in physical activity exercise.
      (1) Avoid excessive strain on affected joints.
      (2) Participate in creative dance, bicycle riding, swimming, or walking.
      (3) Avoid activities that place total body weight on affected, non–weight-bearing joints (cartwheels, chin-ups, handstands, aerobics, contact sports, roller skating).
   c. Encourage use of splints to prevent flexion contractures.
   d. Encourage compliance with prone and active gluteal exercise with hip involvement.
   e. Provide cast with knee in severe flexion.
   f. Provide cervical collar for neck pain.

3. Collaborate with physical therapist and/or occupational therapist to devise methods that will promote independent functioning.
   a. Use splints as needed.
   b. Make modifications to utensils for easier grasp.
   c. Select clothes that are convenient to put on (Velcro fasteners).
   d. Elevate toilet seat.

4. Monitor growth and development pattern.
   a. Educate family about side effects of corticosteroid therapy and refer to dietitian as needed.
   b. Encourage age-appropriate activities that will conserve energy and promote development of perceptual skills and coordination.

5. Assist child with intervention strategies for common school problems.
   a. Instruct family to meet with school personnel to discuss child's diagnosis and make classroom modifications.
   b. Instruct child to change position every 20 minutes to prevent stiffness.

    c. Have child use "fat" pens or pencils, or felt-tip pens, for writing.

    d. Suggest obtaining extra set of schoolbooks to keep at home.

    e. Suggest use of computer for reports and tape recorder for note taking.

    f. Encourage rest period after lunch.

    g. Plan schedule with less demanding subjects in the morning.

    h. Encourage participation in activities with other children.

    i. Assist family and school personnel in developing individualized education plan (IEP).

6. Provide education and support to child and family to maximize coping with a chronic and often disabling disease.

    a. Encourage participation in support groups with other JRA-affected children and their families (American Juvenile Arthritis Organization).

    b. Monitor child's therapeutic response and adverse reactions to medications.

    c. Prepare child preoperatively for procedures and surgeries as indicated for treatment of condition; they may include the following:
- Arthrocentesis
- Diagnostic biopsy
- Synovectomy
- Capsulotomy
- Soft-tissue release
- Osteotomy
- Arthrodesis
- Epiphysiodesis
- Arthroplasty
- Total joint or hip replacement

7. Provide emotional support to child and family as indicated during hospitalization.

🏠 Discharge Planning and Home Care

1. Instruct child and family about follow-up appointments.

    a. Name and phone number of physician and appropriate health care team members

    b. Date, time, and purpose of follow-up appointments

2. Instruct child and family to observe response to medications and notify physician of adverse reactions.
3. Reinforce information given about JRA and encourage compliance with the treatment plan.
4. Perform evaluation at clinic.
5. Monitor compliance with consultation referrals.

CLIENT OUTCOMES

1. Child will exhibit no signs or symptoms of discomfort and will be able to move with minimal discomfort.
2. Child is able to perform activities of daily living and to participate in age-appropriate activities with minimal fatigue.
3. Child and family understand home treatment plan and follow-up medications.

REFERENCES

American Academy of Pediatrics, Section on Rheumatology and Section on Ophthalmology: Guidelines for ophthalmologic examinations in children with juvenile rheumatoid arthritis, *Pediatrics* 92(2):295, 1993.

Cassidy JT, Petty RE: *Textbook of pediatric rheumatology,* ed 3, Philadelphia, 1995, WB Saunders.

Hughes RB, D'Ambrosia K: Nursing management of a child with juvenile rheumatoid arthritis, *Orthop Nurs* 12(5):17, 1993.

Pediatric Rheumatology Patient Education Task Force: *Understanding juvenile rheumatoid arthritis: a health professional's guide to teaching children and parents,* Atlanta, 1987, Arthritis Foundation.

44

Kawasaki Disease

PATHOPHYSIOLOGY

Kawasaki disease is an acute febrile illness of young children that causes widespread vasculitis. It is distinguished by marked immune system activation that contributes to the injury of small- and medium-size blood vessels. Also known as mucocutaneous lymph node syndrome, Kawasaki disease affects multiple body systems and can have life-threatening cardiovascular consequences. Although researchers speculate that Kawasaki disease has a viral or bacterial cause, the specific etiology is unknown. Typically, the disease occurs in three phases (acute, subacute, and convalescent) and is self-limiting. Diagnosis, which is sometimes confusing, is based on strict adherence to clinical criteria. Initial treatment focuses on reducing the vascular inflammatory process, and prognosis is excellent with early recognition and treatment. The long-term prognosis for children with coronary artery abnormalities who survive the disease is not known.

INCIDENCE

1. Of all children with diagnosed Kawasaki disease, 80% are 4 years of age or younger.
2. Kawasaki outbreaks are more common in the winter and spring.
3. The incidence is higher in boys than in girls.

4. The disease occurs in all races, with a predominance in Japanese and Asian children.
5. Kawasaki disease occurs in siblings of affected children more frequently than in the general population.
6. There is no evidence to suggest that Kawasaki disease is contagious.
7. Mortality is 20% and usually occurs during the subacute phase.
8. Of untreated children with Kawasaki disease, 20% develop coronary artery abnormalities.

CLINICAL MANIFESTATIONS
Acute Phase (10 to 14 Days)

For the diagnosis of Kawasaki disease, the child must meet five of the first six principal criteria.

1. Fever—abrupt onset of high fever that lasts more than 5 days and is unresponsive to antibiotic and antipyretic therapy
2. Conjunctival infection lasting 1 to 2 weeks with no exudate or corneal scarring
3. Oropharyngeal manifestations, with red, dry, cracked lips; red, dry, "strawberry" tongue; and pharyngitis
4. Induration and edema of the extremities, with erythema of the palms and soles, and swelling of digits
5. Erythematous body rash that is typically macular; it begins on the extremities, spreads to the trunk, and is often pruritic (no vesicles or petechiae)
6. Cervical lymphadenopathy, which is usually unilateral, is greater than 1.5 cm in size, and "melts away" as the fever subsides
7. Associated features—pyuria and urethritis, diarrhea, aseptic meningitis, irritability and lability of mood, severe lethargy, and hepatic dysfunction lasting from 7 to 10 days
8. Acute pericarditis and acute perivascularitis of coronary arteries and aorta

Subacute Phase (10 to 25 Days)

1. Anorexia
2. Irritability

3. Arthritis—most commonly in large joints (knees, hips, elbows)
4. Arthralgia caused by joint fluid
5. Desquamation of the extremities, beginning at the digits and then peeling off in sheets from the palms and soles
6. Panvasculitis of coronary arteries and formation of aneurysms; inflammation and thrombosis formation may lead to stenosis or obstruction

Convalescent Phase (26 to 70 Days)

1. Signs of illness subsided
2. Deep transverse groove across the fingers and toenails (Beau's lines)
3. Abnormal lab values
4. Personality, appetite, and energy level returned to normal

COMPLICATIONS

1. Congestive heart failure (CHF)
2. Coronary artery aneurysms
3. Coronary thromboses
4. Myocardial infarction

LABORATORY AND DIAGNOSTIC TESTS

There are no specific diagnostic tests for Kawasaki disease; however, several abnormalities have been identified.
1. Electrocardiogram (ECG) changes
   a. Flat, depressed ST segment
   b. Flat, inverted T wave
   c. Conduction disturbances
2. Echocardiogram—used to assess cardiac enlargement, contractility of the ventricles, and coronary aneurysms
3. Complete blood count (CBC)—mild to moderate anemia, elevated white blood cell (WBC) count (first phase) with a predominance of neutrophils
4. Platelet count—elevated
5. Erythrocyte sedimentation rate (ESR)—elevated
6. C-reactive protein—elevated
7. Serum glutamic-oxaloacetic transaminase (SGOT)—elevated
8. Serum glutamic-pyruvic transaminase (SGPT)—elevated
9. Serum albumin—decreased

MEDICAL MANAGEMENT

Initial therapy is aimed at reducing the vascular inflammatory process and preventing thrombosis by inhibiting platelet aggregation. Surgical interventions may be required if obstructive cardiovascular disease results. Common medical therapy includes the following:

1. Aspirin therapy
   a. Dosage of 80 to 100 mg/kg/day (first 14 days or until fever controlled)
   b. Dosage of 30 mg/kg/day given 14 to 35 days and 10 mg/kg/day for at least 3 months and up to 1 year after onset
2. Intravenous gamma globulin (IVGG)—400 mg to 2 g; dosage and frequency vary based on severity of conditions; decreases inflammation of blood vessels
3. Persantine—4 mg/kg/day three times a day for treatment of coronary aneurysms

NURSING ASSESSMENT

1. See the section on cardiovascular assessment in Appendix A.
2. Assess for clinical criteria of Kawasaki disease.
3. Assess for febrile seizures.
4. Assess adequacy of hydration.

NURSING DIAGNOSES

- Fluid volume deficit
- Hyperthermia
- Decreased cardiac output
- High risk for injury
- Altered oral mucous membranes
- Altered nutrition: less than body requirements
- Pain
- Impaired physical mobility
- Fear

NURSING INTERVENTIONS

1. Monitor child's clinical status.
   a. Rectal temperature
   b. Skin turgor, mucous membranes, and anterior fontanel
   c. Strict record of intake and output

    d. Specific gravity

    e. Measurement of stools

    f. Oral mucous membranes

    g. Erythematous body rash

    h. Blood pressure

2. Institute measures to lower fever.

    a. Medicate with antipyretics; monitor child's response to medications.

    b. Provide tepid sponge baths for temperatures greater than 102.2° F (39° C).

    c. Offer cool fluids.

    d. Assess which fluids (such as Popsicles and gelatin) child prefers.

    e. Maintain seizure precautions, because 3% to 5% of children between 6 months and 3 years of age may develop seizures when they have temperatures as low as 101.8° F (38.8° C).

    f. Explain unusual nature of temperature to parents in terms of its intermittent pattern, duration, and resistance to antipyretics; anticipatory guidance will prevent parental anxiety about the unusual nature of the fever.

3. Monitor child for cardiac complications.

    a. Use cardiac monitor as ordered during acute and subacute phases; report any arrhythmias to physician.

    b. Explain the purpose of the ECG and echocardiogram and the aberrations caused by child's movement to the parents and the child.

    c. Allow child to change his or her own electrodes during daily bath.

4. Monitor for untoward signs and symptoms (hypotension, diaphoresis, nausea and vomiting, chills) during IVGG administrations, and stop infusion until symptoms have subsided. Keep epinephrine available to treat anaphylaxis.

5. Monitor for signs of bleeding due to aspirin therapy.

6. Provide comfort measures for the child.

    a. Perform oral hygiene frequently.

    b. Apply petroleum jelly to lips.

    c. Avoid soaps, ointments, and lotions on skin; keep skin clean, dry, and exposed to air.

    d. Cool, moist compresses may be applied to itching areas.

    e. Provide a sheepskin for child to lie on.

    f. Discourage scratching through diversional activities; for young children, soft, loose mittens may be helpful.

    g. Encourage bed rest and elevation of extremities until swelling has subsided.

    h. Teach parents how to hold and comfort the child who has an IV and electrodes in place.

    i. Keep stimulation to a minimum.

    j. Explain to parents that tactile stimulation may be irritating but a soothing voice may provide security.

    k. Provide dim lights.

    l. Provide quiet music.

7. Provide for and promote the child's nutritional status.

    a. Provide comfort measures for mouth (see number 6).

    b. Begin with bland foods in small amounts.

    c. Encourage parents to bring in favorite foods from home, and assess for favorite foods in hospital.

    d. Avoid hot, spicy foods.

    e. Offer high-calorie liquids.

8. Prevent contractions related to imposed restrictions and range of motion (ROM) limitations.

    a. Perform passive range of motion (exercises on edematous extremities during child's bed rest; teach parents how to do the exercises, and explain their importance to them.

    b. When child is able, use active ROM, making it a game for the child.

    c. Place IVs in a position that allows maximal movement.

9. Alleviate anxiety caused by all of the invasive procedures for diagnostic tests and by pain, a new environment, strange people, knowledge deficit, therapeutic play, and age-related fears.

    a. Provide play therapy during all phases of illness and for each new procedure (i.e., ECGs, needle play); base therapy on child's developmental level.

    b. Explain each procedure at child's and parents' cognitive levels.

   c. Suggest ways for parents to support their child during hospitalization and procedures (e.g., holding the child after the procedure).

   d. Consult parents and child about preferences among "quiet" toys and activities during acute phase of illness; encourage parents and volunteers to play with child, allowing for rest periods and then passive participation.

   e. Explain the meaning of the presence of swollen lymph nodes to parents.

♠ Discharge Planning and Home Care

Instruct about long-term management.

1. Instruct parents and child, in a developmentally appropriate manner, about the importance of follow-up care, including ECGs, echocardiograms, and chest x-ray examinations (two thirds of coronary thromboses and aneurysms regress after 1 year).

2. Instruct parents verbally and with written reinforcement about the signs and symptoms of cardiac complications (i.e., aneurysms and coronary thromboses); tell them to contact the physician immediately if the child has any of these signs and symptoms.

3. Instruct the parents about the importance of anticoagulant therapy such as aspirin and about side effects to watch for; explain to parents why some children with Kawasaki disease may need to have a coronary artery bypass graft performed.

4. Instruct parents about the importance of good nutrition and adequate fluids.

5. Stress the importance of adequate rest.

CLIENT OUTCOMES

1. Temperature will return to normal.
2. Changes in skin will resolve.
3. Child will walk without joint pain.

REFERENCES

Levin M, Tizard E, Dillon M: Kawasaki disease: recent advances, *Arch Dis Child* 66:1369, 1991.

Lux K: New hope for children with Kawasaki disease, *J Pediatr Nurs* 6(3):159, 1991.

Rogers ME: *Textbook of pediatric intensive care,* ed 2, Baltimore, 1992, Williams & Wilkins.

Rowley A, Gonzalez-Crussi F, Shulman S: Kawasaki syndrome, *Adv Pediatr* 38:51, 1991.

Shreve B: Kawasaki disease: early treatment/positive results—one family's story, *Pediatr Nurs* 19(6):607, 1993.

45

Lead Poisoning

PATHOPHYSIOLOGY

Lead poisoning is the excessive accumulation of lead in the blood. The majority of children with lead poisoning are asymptomatic. The 1991 Centers for Disease Control (CDC) guideline indicates levels of intervention based on the blood lead level. A lead level of less than 10 μg/dl indicates no lead poisoning; lead levels of 10 to 14 μg/dl are considered borderline; and lead levels equal to or greater than 15 μg/dl require some degree of intervention. Acute symptoms of lead poisoning are generally not evident until the lead levels reach 50 μg/dl or higher.

Younger children absorb a greater proportion of lead because of their greater intake of dietary fat and their decreased intake of calcium and iron. Excessive amounts of absorbed lead accumulate in the bones, soft tissue, and blood. Soft-tissue absorption is of great concern because it can result in central nervous system (CNS) toxicity and reversible renal failure. Late signs of lead toxicity include coma, stupor, and seizures. Lead poisoning is considered chronic if the lead has been accumulated over a period of time greater than 3 months. Lead interferes with heme synthesis and has a toxic effect on the red blood cells, resulting in a decrease in the number of red blood cells and the amount of hemoglobin in cells, leading to an anemic state.

Lead is absorbed primarily through the gastrointestinal (GI) tract after ingestion of lead-contaminated substances. Lead-based paint is the most "high-dose" source of lead and is the most common and serious cause of lead poisoning. Children are exposed to lead-based paint when they ingest paint chips and paint dust from the walls of old homes. Other sources of lead include soil, ceramics and pottery, printed materials, and auto emissions. Lead is a component of several folk remedies used in Mexico (azarcon and greta for digestive problems), the Middle East (farouk rubbed on gums to help teething, bint al zahib used for colic), and Southeast Asia (pay-loo-ah for fever and rashes). Lead is no longer used in soldering cans for food and beverages in the United States; however, soldering may still be a source of lead in imported containers of food and juices. A high incidence of lead poisoning is associated with pica eaters.

INCIDENCE

1. Age range of peak incidence is 1 to 3 years.
2. Children between ages 6 months and 6 years who live in poorly maintained housing are at a high risk.
3. It is estimated that up to 17% of preschool children in the United States have serum lead levels of greater than 15 μg/dl.

CLINICAL MANIFESTATIONS

Most children are asymptomatic and lead poisoning is detected during routine screening. Symptoms that may be seen as the lead levels rise include the following:

1. Anorexia
2. Constipation or diarrhea
3. Irritability
4. Nausea, vomiting
5. Abdominal pain or colic
6. Malaise
   Symptoms of chronic lead poisoning are the following:
1. Increased incidence of learning disorders
2. Behavioral disorders
3. Perceptual deficits
4. Hyperactivity, decreased attention span

COMPLICATIONS

1. Renal toxicity
2. Cerebral edema
3. CNS toxicity—persistent vomiting, irritability, clumsiness, ataxia, loss of developmental skills
4. Severe and permanent brain damage—occurs in 80% of children who develop severe and acute encephalopathy
5. Late signs—stupor, coma, seizures, hypertension, and death

LABORATORY AND DIAGNOSTIC TESTS

1. Blood lead levels—equal to or greater than 10 μg/dl (venous specimen is preferred; if a fingerstick specimen is obtained, careful cleansing of site is necessary to decrease contamination of the specimen)
2. Erythrocyte protoporphyrin (EP)—although commonly used in the past, no longer recommended because of a poor sensitivity to lead levels less than 25 μg/dl (blood lead levels have replaced the EP level as the primary screening test; in some areas, EP level is still used to assess higher lead levels and effectiveness of treatment)
3. Complete blood count (CBC)—anemia and basophilic stippling
4. Serum iron, total nonbinding capacity, and serum ferritin—to assess for iron deficiency
5. Blood, urea nitrogen, creatinine, and urinalysis—to assess for renal damage
6. Flat plate x-ray examination of abdomen—indicates ingestion of lead if positive
7. Edetate disodium calcium (CaEDTA) mobilization test—provides an indication of the potentially mobile amount of lead in the body; indicates whether chelation therapy will be useful
8. δ-Aminolevulinic acid (ALA) in urine—increased excretion in urine is abnormal
9. Coproporphyrin (coproporphyrin III) in urine—increased excretion associated with increased serum lead levels

MEDICAL MANAGEMENT

The primary focus of medical care is screening and decreasing primary exposure by removing lead sources from the child's environment. Screening includes assessing risk for lead poisoning at each physician's appointment. If the infant or child is at low risk, initial blood lead screening is recommended at 12 months. Infants and children at high risk may require earlier, more frequent blood lead screening. See Table 7 for screening, environmental evaluation, education, and medical management based on blood lead levels.

When blood lead levels rise above 45 μg/dl, chelation therapy is indicated to reduce lead burden in the body. All drugs used for chelation bind to the lead, which facilitates removal of the lead via urine (and with some drugs, also via stool) and depletes the amount of lead in the tissues. Before outpatient therapy is begun, the lead must be removed from the child's environment to prevent possible increased absorption of lead by the chelating drug. Children hospitalized for chelation are not discharged until environmental lead is removed or alternative housing is available. The major chelating agents used for children include succimer, edetate disodium calcium, dimercaprol, and D-Penicillamine. Chelation therapy is also administered to children who are symptomatic with blood lead levels less than 45 μg/dl.

The child admitted with symptoms of encephalopathy receives immediate intravenous (IV) chelation therapy. Lumbar punctures are to be avoided in these children whenever possible. Fluids and electrolytes are closely monitored. Fluids may be restricted to basal requirements plus adjustments for fluid losses such as vomiting. Mannitol is used to decrease cerebral edema and intracranial pressure. Seizures are managed initially with diazepam, followed with long-term anticonvulsant therapy. Iron deficiency anemia needs to be treated in all affected children. Prognosis and residual effects are related to how high and how long the lead levels were elevated. Learning disorders and behavioral problems may result from even low levels of lead.

Table 7. Lead Poisoning Screening and Intervention Guidelines

CDC Classification	Blood Lead Level	Screening Frequency	Education	Environmental Inspection	Chelation Therapy
I	<10 µg/dl	Not lead poisoned; routine screening at 12 and 24 months	—	—	—
IIA	10-14 µg/dl	Borderline; rescreen every 3-4 months	Importance of follow-up lead levels	—	—

Continued

Table 7. Lead Poisoning Screening and Intervention Guidelines—cont'd

CDC Classification	Blood Lead Level	Screening Frequency	Education	Environmental Inspection	Chelation Therapy
IIB	15-19 $\mu g/dl$	Rescreen every 3-4 months	Sources of lead exposure, symptoms of poisoning, and nutritional counseling	If levels do not decrease, environmental evaluation and appropriate intervention are indicated	—

III	20-44 μg/dl	Repeat test for confirmation; rescreen at least every 3-4 months or more often	Sources of lead exposure, symptoms of poisoning, and nutritional counseling	Environment is evaluated; lead sources are identified and removed	Only if symptomatic
IV	45-69 μg/dl	Repeat test for confirmation; closely monitor levels with response to chelation therapy	Sources of lead exposure, symptoms of poisoning, nutritional counseling, and chelation therapy	Environment is evaluated; lead sources are identified and removed	Initiated for both symptomatic and asymptomatic cases
V	$\geq$70 μg/dl	Repeat test for confirmation but do not wait for results to implement therapy	Sources of lead exposure, symptoms of poisoning, nutritional counseling, and chelation therapy	Environment is evaluated; child is not returned to the environment until sources of lead are removed	Considered a medical emergency—hospitalize for immediate IV chelation therapy

NURSING ASSESSMENT

1. See the sections on neurologic and musculoskeletal assessment in Appendix A.
2. Assess hydration status.
3. Assess nutritional status.
4. Assess home environment for lead source.

NURSING DIAGNOSES

- High risk for poisoning
- Impaired home maintenance management
- Knowledge deficit
- Fluid volume deficit
- Altered nutrition: less than body requirements

NURSING INTERVENTIONS

1. Monitor child's neurologic status, and report the following.
   a. Changes in level of consciousness (LOC)
   b. Twitching or seizure activity
   c. Complaint of headaches
   d. Projectile vomiting
   e. Pupillary response
   f. Bulging fontanels
2. Monitor child's vital signs, and report the following.
   a. Increased apical pulse
   b. Decreased or increased blood pressure
3. Refer to community agencies for environmental evaluation and lead removal, if appropriate.
4. Provide education about lead poisoning.
   a. Symptoms of lead poisoning
   b. Sources of lead in the environment
   c. Need to remove sources of lead to protect the child
5. Encourage parent to take precautionary measures.
   a. Make sure child does not have access to peeling paint.
   b. Wash the child's hands and face before he or she eats.
   c. Wash toys and pacifiers frequently.
6. Monitor intake and output.
   a. Record urinary and stool output.
   b. Monitor fluid restrictions.

7. Monitor child's reaction to chelation therapy.
   a. Succimer
      (1) Nausea, vomiting, diarrhea
      (2) Anorexia
      (3) Hypertension
      (4) Infection
   b. Edetate disodium calcium
      (1) Decreased urine output
      (2) Decreased blood pressure (20 to 30 minutes after infusion)
      (3) Pain, erythema at infusion site
      (4) Symptoms of hypercalcemia
      (5) Nausea, vomiting, anorexia
      (6) Numbness, tingling, myalgia, arthralgia
      (7) Maintain fluid restrictions if lead encephalopathy is present
   c. Dimercaprol
      (1) Fever (occurs in 30% of children)
      (2) Local pain, sterile abscess (if not given deep into the muscle)
      (3) Increased blood pressure, tachycardia (may occur within minutes of administration and last for hours)
      (4) Decreased urinary output
      (5) Garliclike odor to breath
      (6) Nausea, vomiting
      (7) Headache
      (8) Burning sensation of lips, mouth, and throat
   d. D-Penicillamine
      (1) Sensitivity reactions—rash, pruritis (common)
      (2) Anorexia, nausea, vomiting (infrequent)
8. Provide diet with regular meals rich in iron and calcium.

♠ Discharge Planning and Home Care

1. Instruct parents to identify and remove lead hazards from environment(s) in which child spends considerable time before discharge.
   a. Scrape off and remove all readily accessible lead-based paint.
   b. Regularly sweep and mop.
   c. Remove toys with lead-based paint and earthenware.

2. Instruct parents about supervising more closely the child who is a pica eater.
3. Instruct and counsel parents about recommended follow-up services (Table 7).
   a. Blood lead level is rechecked 7 to 21 days after chelation therapy to determine the need to retreat.
   b. Children who have had chelation will be closely followed for a year or more.
      (1) Those undergoing chelation will be seen every other week for 6 to 8 weeks, then monthly for 4 to 6 months.
      (2) Those who have had courses of edetate disodium calcium or dimercaprol will be seen weekly for 4 to 6 weeks, then monthly for 12 months.

CLIENT OUTCOMES

1. The child will return to a lead-free environment.
2. Child and family understand home care and the importance of follow-up.

REFERENCES

Centers for Disease Control: *Preventing lead poisoning in young children: a statement by the Centers for Disease Control,* Atlanta, 1991, Centers for Disease Control.

Chao J, Kikano GE: Lead poisoning in children, *Am Fam Physician* 47(1):113, 1993.

DeRienzo-DeVivio S: Childhood lead poisoning: shifting to primary prevention, *Pediatr Nurs* 18(6):565, 1992.

Schonfeld DJ, Needham D: Lead: a practical perspective, *Contemp Pediatr* 11(5):64, 1994.

Sweeney DM: Primary prevention of childhood lead poisoning: a goal for the 1990s, *Pediatr Nurs* 18(3):314, 1992.

46

Leukemia, Childhood

PATHOPHYSIOLOGY

Acute lymphoid, or lymphocytic, leukemia (ALL) is a cancer of the tissues that produce white blood cells (leukocytes). Excessive amounts of immature or abnormal leukocytes are manufactured, and they invade various organs of the body. The leukemic cells invade the bone marrow, displacing the normal cellular elements. As a result, anemia develops, and insufficient numbers of red blood cells are produced. Bleeding occurs as a result of decreased numbers of circulating platelets. Infections occur more frequently because of the decreased number of leukocytes. Invasion of leukemic cells in the vital organs causes hepatomegaly, splenomegaly, and lymphadenopathy.

Acute nonlymphoid leukemia (ANLL) includes the following types of leukemia: acute myeloblastic leukemia, acute monoblastic leukemia, and acute myelocytic leukemia. Bone marrow dysfunction occurs, resulting in decreased numbers of red blood cells, neutrophils, and platelets. Leukemic cells infiltrate lymph nodes, spleen, liver, bones, and the central nervous system (CNS), as well as the reproductive organs. Chloromas or granulocytic sarcomas are found in some affected children.

INCIDENCE
ALL

1. Leukemia is the most common type of childhood cancer; ALL accounts for about 80% of all cases of childhood leukemia.
2. Highest incidence is in children between the ages of 3 and 5 years.
3. Female individuals have a better prognosis overall than male individuals.
4. Black individuals have less frequent remissions and a lower median survival rate.

ANLL

1. There is no peak age of incidence.
2. ANLL accounts for 15% to 25% of all cases of childhood leukemia.
3. Risk of the disorder increases for children with congenital chromosome disorders such as Down syndrome.
4. It is more difficult to induce remission than in children with ALL (70% remission rate).
5. Remission is briefer than in children with ALL.
6. Fifty percent of children undergoing bone marrow transplant have a prolonged remission.

CLINICAL MANIFESTATIONS
ALL

1. Evidence of anemia, bleeding, and/or infections
   a. Fever
   b. Fatigue
   c. Pallor
   d. Anorexia
   e. Petechiae and/or hemorrhage
   f. Bone and joint pain
   g. Vague abdominal pain
   h. Weight loss
   i. Enlargement and fibrosis of organs of the reticuloendothelial system—liver, spleen, and lymph glands
2. Increased intracranial pressure resulting from infiltration of the meninges
   a. Pain and stiffness of the neck
   b. Headache

    c. Irritability
    d. Lethargy
    e. Vomiting
    f. Papilledema
    g. Coma
3. Central nervous system symptoms related to site of involvement in the system
    a. Lower-extremity weakness
    b. Difficulty voiding
    c. Learning difficulties, especially with math and memorization (late side effect of therapy)

ANLL

1. Gingival hypertrophy
2. Chloroma of spine (mass lesion)
3. Perirectal necrotic or ulcerous lesions
4. Hepatomegaly and splenomegaly (in less than 50% of children)
5. Same clinical manifestations as in patient with ALL (see section on ALL)

COMPLICATIONS
ALL

1. Bone marrow failure
2. Infections
3. Hepatomegaly
4. Splenomegaly
5. Lymphadenopathy

ANLL

1. Bone marrow failure
2. Infections
3. Disseminated intravascular coagulation (DIC)
4. Splenomegaly
5. Hepatomegaly

LABORATORY AND DIAGNOSTIC TESTS

1. Complete blood count (CBC)—children with CBC of less than $10,000/mm^3$ at time of diagnosis have the best prognosis; a white blood count of more than $50,000/mm^3$ is an unfavorable prognostic sign in a child of any age

2. Lumbar puncture—to assess CNS involvement
3. Chest x-ray examination—detects mediastinal involvement
4. Bone marrow aspiration—a finding of 25% blast cells confirms the diagnosis
5. Bone scan or skeletal survey—assesses bone involvement
6. Renal, liver, and spleen scans—assess leukemic infiltrates
7. Platelet count—indicates clotting capacity

MEDICAL MANAGEMENT

Drug protocols vary according to the type of leukemia and the type of drug regimen to which the child is assigned. The process of inducing remission in the child consists of three phases: induction, consolidation, and maintenance. During the induction phase (for approximately 3 to 6 weeks) the child receives a variety of chemotherapeutic agents to induce remission. The intensive period is extended for 2 to 3 weeks during the phase of consolidation to combat involvement of the central nervous system and other vital organs. Maintenance therapy is administered for several years after diagnosis to sustain remission. Some medications used to treat childhood leukemias are prednisone, vincristine, asparaginase, methotrexate, mercaptopurine, cytarabine, allopurinol, cyclophosphamide, and daunorubicin.

Prednisone

Prednisone is primarily used for its potent antiinflammatory effects in disorders involving many organ systems. It is used for treatment of acute childhood leukemias. Possible side effects are the following:

1. Fluid and electrolyte disturbances—sodium retention, fluid retention, congestive heart failure in susceptible patients, potassium loss, hypertension
2. Musculoskeletal effects—muscle weakness, osteoporosis, pathologic fracture of long bones
3. Gastrointestinal effects—peptic ulcer with possible hemorrhage, pancreatitis, abdominal distention, increased appetite, weight gain

4. Dermatologic effects—impaired wound healing, pete-chiae and ecchymoses, facial erythema, hirsutism, hypo/hyperpigmentation
5. Neurologic effects—increased intracranial pressure with papilledema, convulsions, vertigo, and headache, irrita-bility, mood swings
6. Endocrine effects—development of cushingoid state, manifestations of latent diabetes mellitus
7. Ophthalmic effects—posterior subcapsular cataracts
8. Metabolic effects—negative nitrogen balance resulting from protein catabolism

Dosage should be individualized according to the severity of the disease and the response of the patient, rather than being determined by strict adherence to the ratio indicated by age or body weight. It is administered by mouth (po).

Vincristine (Oncovin)

Vincristine is an antineoplastic that inhibits cell division during metaphase. It is used with cyclophosphamide (Cytoxan) in treatment of ALL. Possible side effects are the following:

1. Neuromuscular effects—peripheral neuropathy, nerve pain, paresthesias of hands and feet, loss of deep tendon reflexes, jaw pain, foot drop
2. Hematologic effects—thrombocytopenia, anemia, leuko-penia
3. Gastrointestinal effects—stomatitis, anorexia, nausea, vomiting, diarrhea, constipation, paralytic illeus
4. Other—convulsions, hyperkalemia, hyperuricemia

Refer to treatment protocol for dosage. Administered by IV push. Avoid extravasation.

Asparaginase

Asparaginase decreases the level of asparagine (an amino acid necessary for tumor growth). It is used in the treatment of ALL. Possible side effects are the following:

1. Allergic manifestations—most serious side effects of as-paraginase; are lessened by the addition of mercaptopu-rine, cytosine arabinoside, and other immunosuppres-sants
   a. Chills and fever within 1 minute of administration
   b. Skin reactions
   c. Respiratory distress

   d. Hypotension
   e. Substernal pain
   f. Nausea and vomiting
   g. Anaphylaxis
2. Liver toxicity with attendant jaundice, hypoalbuminemia, and occasional depression of clotting factor
3. Pancreatitis
4. Diabetes mellitus
5. Disturbances of calcium metabolism

The dosage of asparaginase is highly individualized. It is administered intramuscularly (IM).

Methotrexate (Amethopterin)

Methotrexate is classified as an antimetabolite. It interferes with folic acid metabolism. Folic acid is essential to the synthesis of the nucleoproteins required by rapidly multiplying cells. Methotrexate is used in the treatment of ALL.

In the presence of infection, methotrexate should be used with caution. Therapy with other bone marrow depressants should also be avoided unless the condition of the patient warrants its use. It can be given orally, intramuscularly (IM), intravenously (IV), or intrathecally. Avoid vitamins with folic acid when the child is receiving methotrexate. Possible sid effects are the following:

1. Skin reactions—generalized erythematous rash, urticaria, acne, pruritus
2. Occasional alopecia
3. Oral and gastrointestinal (GI) tract ulcerations
4. Chills
5. Fever
6. Vomiting
7. Diarrhea
8. Cystitis
9. Bone marrow depression (with occasional hemorrhage or septicemia)
10. Liver toxicity
11. Pneumonitis

Mercaptopurine (Purinethol)

Mercaptopurine interferes with the synthesis of nucleic acid, which is especially needed when the cells are growing and multiplying rapidly.

The primary effects of mercaptopurine occur in tissues in which there are rapid cellular growth and a high rate of nucleic metabolism (e.g., bone marrow and gastric epithelium). There is a reduction in leukocyte, thrombocyte, and reticulocyte formation. It is used in the treatment of ALL. Possible side effects are the following:

1. Anorexia
2. Nausea and vomiting
3. Diarrhea (sometimes bloody) caused by injury to GI epithelium
4. Degenerative liver changes with jaundice with very large doses
5. Bone marrow depression

Mercaptopurine is administered by mouth (po) only. Refer to treatment protocol for dosage.

Cytarabine (Cytosar; Cytosine Arabinoside)

Cytarabine is currently indicated for induction of remission in patients with acute granulocytic leukemia. Cytarabine is a potent bone marrow suppressant. Patients receiving this drug must be under close medical supervision and, during induction therapy, should have leukocyte and platelet counts performed frequently. The treatment is modified or suspended when the drug-induced depression has resulted in a platelet count less than $50,000/mm^3$ or a polymorphonuclear granulocyte count less than $1000/mm^3$. Possible side effects are the following:

1. Nausea and vomiting
2. Leukopenia, thrombocytopenia, bone marrow suppression
3. Anemia
4. Rash
5. Anorexia
6. Bleeding (all sites)
7. Diarrhea
8. Oral inflammation or ulceration
9. Megaloblastosis
10. Hepatic dysfunction
11. Anaphylaxis
12. Headaches

Cytarabine is not active orally. It may be given by IV infusion or injection. It must be stored in a refrigerator until reconstituted.

Allopurinol (Zyloprim)

Allopurinol inhibits the production of uric acid by blocking the biochemical reactions that immediately precede uric acid formation. The result is a lowering of blood and urinary uric acid levels. It is given prophylactically to prevent tissue urate deposits or renal calculi in patients with leukemia who are receiving chemotherapy with a resultant elevation of serum uric acid. Allopurinol also inhibits the oxidation of mercaptopurine, therefore necessitating the use of smaller doses of mercaptopurine (one fourth to one third of the regular dose). Possible side effects are the following:

1. Occasional liver toxicity
2. Asymptomatic increase in serum glutamic-oxaloacetic transaminase (SGOT) and serum glutamic-pyruvic transaminase (SGPT)

Allopurinol is administered po. Increase hydration to at least twice maintenance. Refer to treatment protocol for dosage.

Cyclophosphamide (Cytoxan)

A potent antitumor agent of the nitrogen mustard group and an alkylating agent, the exact mechanism of action of cyclophosphamide has not been determined. In contrast to other mustard compounds, it is inert when placed in direct contact with bacteria, leukocytes, and most tumor cells in culture. Cyclophosphamide is used in the treatment of ALL and acute monocytic leukemia. Possible side effects are the following:

1. Nausea and vomiting
2. Anorexia
3. Alopecia (occurs in at least 50% of patients)
4. Leukopenia (decreased white blood count [WBC])
   a. An expected effect
   b. Ordinarily a guide to therapy
   c. Leaving child susceptible to bacterial infection
5. Sterile hemorrhagic cystitis (bladder mucosa may be injured by some active mustard derivatives that are excreted in the urine)

6. Liver dysfunction
7. Cardiotoxicity

Cyclophosphamide is administered IV, by intravenous fast drip (IVFD), po, or IM.

Daunorubicin (Daunomycin)

Daunorubicin binds to deoxyribonucleic acid (DNA). It is used to inhibit cell division during the treatment of acute leukemia. Possible side effects are the following:

1. Sclerosing of vein (use two-needle technique: mix with one needle and dispose of that needle; administer with new needle)
2. Nausea and vomiting (soon after administration)
3. Bone marrow depression
4. Cardiac dysrhythmia and death (rare; occurs at total dose greater than 650 mg/m^2)
5. Elevated liver enzymes (↑ SGPT, ↑ SGOT)
6. Changes urine color to red

Administer IV push. Refer to treatment protocol

NURSING ASSESSMENT

1. See the sections on cardiovascular, respiratory, and neurologic assessment in Appendix A.
2. Assess child's reaction to chemotherapy.
3. Assess for signs and symptoms of infection.
4. Assess for signs and symptoms of hemorrhaging.
5. Assess for signs and symptoms of complications: radiation somnolence, CNS symptoms, cell lysis.
6. Assess child and family coping.

NURSING DIAGNOSES

- Activity intolerance
- High risk for infection
- Fluid volume excess
- Impaired tissue integrity
- High risk for altered nutrition
- High risk for injury
- Body image disturbance
- Anxiety
- High risk for decreased cardiac output

- High risk for fatigue
- High risk for altered growth and development
- High risk for altered family processes
- High risk for ineffective management of treatment regimen

Table 8. Nursing Interventions Related to the Child Undergoing Chemotherapy and Radiotherapy

Responses	Nursing Interventions
Diarrhea	Offer fluids po.
	Perform skin care to buttocks and perineal area.
	Monitor effectiveness of antidiarrheal medications.
	Avoid high-cellulose foods and fruit.
	Offer small, frequent feedings; include child's favorites if possible.
	Decrease or eliminate meat.
	Observe for signs of dehydration.
	Monitor IV infusions.
Anorexia	Monitor intake and output.
Nausea and vomiting	Offer small, frequent feedings of *any bland foods* high in nutrients and calories.
	Consult with child and parents to develop meal plan that incorporates child's likes and dislikes.

Table 8. Nursing Interventions Related to the Child Undergoing Chemotherapy and Radiotherapy—cont'd

Responses	Nursing Interventions
	Maintain adequate fluid intake, using Popsicles, ice cream, gelatin, and noncarbonated beverages.
	Obtain daily weights.
	Observe for dehydration.
	Monitor side effects of antiemetics (e.g., chlorpromazine [Thorazine], promethazine [Phenergan], hydroxyzine pamoate [Vistaril], diphenhydramine [Benadryl]).
Fluid retention	Monitor input and output.
	Obtain daily weights.
	Evaluate for respiratory distress and edema.
	Provide frequent changes of position.
	Monitor side effects of diuretics.
Hyperuremia	Monitor input and output.
	Encourage fluid intake.
	Provide skin care to decrease itching.
	Monitor serum creatinine and uric acid levels.
	Monitor side effects of allopurinol.
Chills and fever	Monitor vital signs and frequency of symptoms.

Continued

Table 8. Nursing Interventions Related to the Child Undergoing Chemotherapy and Radiotherapy—cont'd

Responses	Nursing Interventions
	Evaluate source of symptoms (e.g., tumor or infection).
	Monitor side effects of antipyretics.
	Provide comfort measures such as blankets and tepid sponge baths.
Stomatitis and mouth ulcers	Provide comfort measures such as frequent mouth rinses, use of mouth swabs, and hard candy.
	Avoid hard-bristle toothbrush.
	Avoid glycerine swabs.
	Avoid hard foods that require excessive chewing and foods that are acid or spicy.
	Avoid hot foods.
Cardiotoxicity (doxorubicin and daunorubicin)	Monitor changes in electrocardiogram (ECG) and vital signs.
	Observe for signs and symptoms of congestive heart failure.
Hemorrhagic cystitis (cyclophosphamide)	Encourage frequent voiding after drug administration.
	Offer oral fluids in *large amounts*.
	Monitor IV fluids.
	Encourage voiding before sleep.

Table 8. Nursing Interventions Related to the Child Undergoing Chemotherapy and Radiotherapy—cont'd

Responses	Nursing Interventions
Alopecia	Prepare child and family for hair loss.
	Reassure child and family that hair loss is temporary.
	Prepare child and family for hair regrowth that differs in color and texture from former hair.
	Arrange for another child in same developmental stage to visit child and talk about the experience.
	Suggest use of scarf, hat, or wig before hair loss as a transition measure.
	Wash scalp frequently to prevent cradle cap.
Pain	Evaluate child's verbal and nonverbal behavior for evidence of pain.
	Note cultural aspects affecting pain behavior.
	Use age-appropriate terminology when asking child about pain experience.
	Monitor vital signs.
	Evaluate sleep patterns that may be altered by pain.
	Monitor side effects of analgesics and narcotics.

Continued

Table 8. Nursing Interventions Related to the Child Undergoing Chemotherapy and Radiotherapy—cont'd

Responses	Nursing Interventions
	Offer approaches to deal with pain such as hypnosis, biofeedback, relaxation techniques, imagery, distraction, cutaneous stimulation, and desensitization.
Leukopenia	Observe for signs and symptoms of infection and inflammation.
	Monitor vital signs.
	Screen visitors for contagious disease and infections.
	Monitor white blood cell count and differential.
	Ensure that good hygienic measures are maintained.
	Prevent breaks in skin integrity (e.g., keep nails short and prevent injuries).
Thrombocytopenia	Observe for signs and symptoms of bleeding (petechiae and/or hemorrhage).
	Monitor vital signs.
	Monitor platelet count.
	Prevent injury or trauma to body.
	Avoid rectal temperature readings.
	Avoid injections.

Table 8. Nursing Interventions Related to the Child Undergoing Chemotherapy and Radiotherapy—cont'd

Responses	Nursing Interventions
Anemia and/or fatigue	Monitor platelet transfusions.
	Provide pressure on bleeding sites.
	Evaluate signs and symptoms of anemia.
	Monitor CBC and differential.
	Provide for periods of rest and sleep.
	Encourage quiet play activities.
Increased risk of fractures	Avoid weight bearing on affected limb.
	Prevent accidents and injuries.
	Encourage nonambulatory play activities.
Delayed physical and sexual development	Provide anticipatory guidance to parents about child's growth retardation, skeletal deformities, and delayed sexual development.
	Discuss possibility of sterility with child and family.
Chromosomal damage	Provide patient and family teaching about effects of radiation and chemotherapy on cells.
	Provide genetic counseling.

Continued

> **Table 8. Nursing Interventions Related to the Child Undergoing Chemotherapy and Radiotherapy—cont'd**
>
> | Responses | Nursing Intervention |
> | --- | --- |
> | Hypersensitivity to the medication, resulting in anaphylactic shock | Have the following medications available: hydrocortisone, epinephrine, and diphenhydramine (Benadryl). Observe for dyspnea, restlessness, and urticaria. |
> | Phlebitis and necrosis of tissue, resulting from infiltration of IV infusion | Avoid vesicant agents near a joint. Stop IV flow if infiltration is suspected. Tissue may be treated with drug-specific antidote and hydrocortisone. Apply cold compress to site. Continue to observe site for signs of inflammation and necrosis. Grafting and surgical excision may be indicated if necrosis results. |

NURSING INTERVENTIONS

1. Monitor child for reactions to medications (Table 8).
2. Monitor for signs and symptoms of infection.
   a. Be aware that *fever* is the most important sign of infection.
   b. Treat all of the children as if they are neutropenic until results of tests are obtained. Isolate them from

other clinic patients, especially those children with infectious diseases, particularly chicken pox.

   c. Have the child wear a mask if he or she is around other people and is severely neutropenic (WBC less than $1000/mm^3$).

   d. Be aware that if the child is neutropenic, he or she may not receive chemotherapy. The child may receive IV antibiotics if a fever is also present. (More patients die from infection than from their disease.)

3. Monitor for signs and symptoms of hemorrhaging.

   a. Check skin for bruising and petechiae.

   b. Check for nosebleeds and bleeding gums.

   c. If an injection is given, apply pressure to the site for longer than usual (approximately 3 to 5 minutes) to be sure bleeding has stopped. Check again later to be sure bleeding has not restarted.

4. Monitor for signs and symptoms of complications.

   a. Radiation somnolence: Beginning 6 weeks after receiving craniospinal radiation, children exhibit great fatigue and anorexia for approximately 1 to 3 weeks. Parents often worry about relapse at this time and need to be reassured.

   b. CNS symptoms: These symptoms—headache, blurred or double vision, vomiting—can indicate CNS leukemic involvement.

   c. Respiratory symptoms: These symptoms—coughing, lung congestion, dyspnea—may indicate pneumocystitis or other respiratory infection.

   d. Cell lysis: Rapid cell lysis after chemotherapy can affect blood chemistries, causing increased calcium and potassium.

5. Monitor for concerns and anxiety about the diagnosis of cancer and its related treatments; monitor for emotional responses such as anger, denial, and grief (see Appendix J, section on supportive care).

6. Monitor disruptions in family functioning.

   a. Base all interventions on the family's cultural, religious, educational, and socioeconomic background.

   b. Involve siblings as much as possible because they have many concerns and feelings about the changes in the child and the family's functioning.

c. Consider the possibility that siblings feel self-blame and guilt.

d. Encourage family unity by having 24-hour visitation privileges for all family members.

♠ Discharge Planning and Home Care

The interventions identified for acute care management apply for long-term care as well.

CLIENT OUTCOMES

1. The child will achieve remission.
2. The child will be free of disease complications.
3. The child and family will learn to cope effectively with the living with and management of the disease.

REFERENCES

Bossert E, Martinson I: Kinetic family drawings revised: a method of determining the impact of cancer on the family as perceived by the child with cancer, *J Pediatr Nurs* 5(3):204, 1990.

Bosworth T: Leukemia through a teenager's eyes, *MCN Am J Matern Child Nurs* 14(2):93, 1989.

Cohen D: Acute lymphocytic leukemia. In Foley GV, Fochtman D, Mooney KH, editors: *Nursing care of the child with cancer,* ed 2, Philadelphia, 1993, WB Saunders.

Foote A et al: Orem's theory used as a guide for the nursing care of an eight-year-old child with leukemia, *J Pediatric Oncol Nurs* 10(1):26, 1993.

Gallagher J: Acute lymphocytic leukemia treatment: effects on learning, *J Pediatr Health Care* 3(5):257, 1989.

Hockenberry M, Coody D, Bennett B: Childhood cancers: incidence, etiology, diagnosis and treatment, *Pediatr Nurs* 16(3):239, 1990.

Hydzik C: Late effects of chemotherapy: implications for patient management and rehabilitation, *Nurs Clin North Am* 25(2):423, 1990.

Hymovich D: A theory for pediatric oncology nursing practice and research, *J Pediatr Oncol Nurs* 7(4):131, 1990.

Munet-Vilaro F, Vessey J: Children's explanation of leukemia: a Hispanic perspective, *J Pediatr Nurs* 5(4):274, 1990.

Peckham V et al: Educational late effects in long-term survivors of childhood acute lymphocytic leukemia, *Pediatrics* 81(1):127, 1988.

Rhoades A: A minor's refusal of treatment, *MCN Am J Matern Child Nurs* 15(4):261, 1990.

Sabio H: Advances in the diagnosis and treatment of hematologic malignancies, *J Pediatr Oncol Nurs* 7(2):69, 1990.

Suderman J: Pain relief during routine procedures for children with leukemia, *MCN Am J Matern Child Nurs* 15(3):163, 1990.

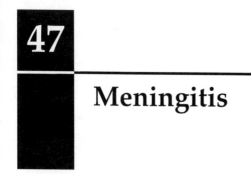

Meningitis

PATHOPHYSIOLOGY

Meningitis is an acute inflammation of the meninges. The organisms responsible for bacterial meningitis invade the area either directly as a result of a traumatic injury or indirectly when they are transported from other sites in the body to the cerebrospinal fluid (CSF). A variety of organisms can produce an inflammation of the meninges. In neonates, the primary organisms responsible are gram-negative enteric bacilli, gram-negative rods, and group B streptococci. In children 3 months to 5 years of age, the primary organism responsible for meningitis is *Haemophilus influenzae* type B. Meningitis in older children is usually the result of a *Neisseria meningitidis* infection or a staphylococcal infection.

Aseptic meningitis is usually caused by a virus and affects young adults more often than children. Older children usually manifest a variety of nonspecific prodromal signs and flulike symptoms that last for 1 to 2 weeks. Although fatigue and weakness may last for a number of weeks, sequelae are uncommon. The child is evaluated and treated until meningitis is ruled out. Viral meningitis usually requires only a brief hospitalization, with supportive care at home the primary intervention.

Otitis media, sinusitis, or respiratory tract infections may be the initial stage of infection. In addition, a predisposition resulting from an immune deficiency increases the likelihood of occurrence of this disorder. Once the meninges are infected, the organisms are spread through the CSF to the brain and adjacent tissues. Prognosis varies, depending on a variety of factors. Neonatal meningitis has a high mortality rate and an increased incidence of neurologic sequelae. Bacterial meningitis results in a large number of patients' having behavioral changes, motor dysfunction, and cognitive changes such as perceptual deficits.

INCIDENCE

1. More male individuals than female individuals have meningitis.
2. Age range of peak incidence is 6 to 12 months.
3. The age range having the highest rate of morbidity is birth to 4 years.

CLINICAL MANIFESTATIONS
Neonates

1. Subnormal temperature
2. Fever
3. Pallor
4. Lethargy
5. Irritability
6. Poor feeding and/or suck
7. Seizures
8. Poor tone
9. Diarrhea and/or vomiting
10. Bulging fontanels
11. Opisthotonus

Infants and Young Children

1. Lethargy
2. Irritability
3. Pallor
4. Anorexia or poor feeding
5. Nausea and vomiting
6. Increased crying
7. Insistence on being held
8. Increased intracranial pressure (ICP)
9. Increased head circumference

10. Bulging fontanel
11. Seizures

Older Children

1. Headache
2. Fever
3. Vomiting
4. Irritability
5. Photophobia
6. Spinal and nuchal rigidity
7. Positive Kernig's sign
8. Positive Brudzinski's sign
9. Opisthotonic posturing
10. Petechiae (*H. influenzae* and meningococcal meningitis)
11. Septicemia
12. Shock
13. Disseminated intravascular coagulation (DIC)
14. Confusion
15. Seizures

COMPLICATIONS

1. Deafness
2. Blindness
3. Subdural effusions
4. Increased secretion of antidiuretic hormone (ADH)
5. Developmental delay
6. Hydrocephalus
7. Cerebral edema
8. Chronic seizure disorder

LABORATORY AND DIAGNOSTIC TESTS

1. Lumbar puncture and culture of CSF with the following results
   a. White blood count (WBC)—increased
   b. Glucose level—decreased (bacterial); normal (viral)
   c. Protein—high (bacterial); slightly elevated (viral)
   d. Pressure—increased
   e. Identification of causative organism—meningococcal, gram-positive (streptococci, staphylococci,

pneumococci, *H. influenzae*), or viral (Coxsackie virus, ECHO virus)
   f. Lactic acid—elevated (bacterial)
   g. Serum glucose—elevated
2. Blood culture—to identify causative organism
3. Urine culture—to identify causative organism
4. Nasopharyngeal culture—to identify causative organism
5. Serum electrolytes—elevated if child dehydrated; increased serum sodium (Na^+); decreased serum potassium (K^+)
6. Urine osmolarity—increased with increased secretion of ADH

MEDICAL MANAGEMENT

Meningitis is considered a medical emergency requiring early recognition and treatment to prevent neurologic damage. The child is placed in respiratory isolation for at least 24 hours after the initiation of intravenous (IV) antibiotics sensitive to the causative organism. Intravenous hydration therapy is instituted to correct electrolyte imbalances, in addition to providing hydration. This fluid administration requires frequent assessment of the infused volume to prevent fluid overload complications such as cerebral edema. Treatment is then directed toward the identification and management of complications of the disease process. The most common complications are subdural effusion, DIC syndrome, and shock.

NURSING ASSESSMENT

1. See the section on neurologic assessment in Appendix A.
2. Assess hydration status.
3. Assess for pain.
4. Assess for sensory deficits.

NURSING DIAGNOSES

- Sensory/perceptual alterations
- Fluid volume deficit
- Pain
- High risk for injury
- Knowledge deficit

NURSING INTERVENTIONS

1. Monitor infant's or child's vital signs and neurologic status as often as every 2 hours.
   a. Temperature, respiratory rate, apical pulse
   b. Level of consciousness (LOC)
   c. Pupils equal, react to light (PERL)
2. Monitor child's hydration status.
   a. Skin turgor
   b. Urinary output
   c. Urinary osmolarity
   d. Signs and symptoms of hyponatremia
   e. Urine specific gravity
   f. Input and output
   g. Daily weights
3. Monitor child for seizure activity (see Chapter 68, Seizure Disorders).
4. Institute isolation procedures with respiratory precautions to protect others from infectious contact; keep child in isolation for 24 hours after antibiotics are started.
5. Monitor the IV infusion and the side effects of medications.
   a. Antibiotics
   b. Anticonvulsants
6. Provide comfort measures in an environment that is quiet and has minimal stressful stimuli.
   a. Avoid bright lights and noise.
   b. Avoid excessive manipulation of the child.
7. Position child with head of bed slightly elevated to decrease cerebral edema; monitor administration of fluids.
8. Reduce temperature through the use of tepid sponge baths or hypothermia mattress.
9. Provide emotional support when the child undergoes a lumbar puncture and other tests.
   a. Provide age-appropriate explanations before procedures.
   b. Restrain child to prevent occurrence of injury.
10. Provide emotional support to family.
    a. Provide and reinforce information about condition and hospitalization.

b. Encourage ventilation of feelings of guilt and self-blame.
c. Encourage use of preexisting support.
d. Provide for physical comforts (e.g., sleeping arrangements, hygiene needs).
11. Provide age-appropriate diversional activities (see section on growth and development, Appendix B).

🏠 Discharge Planning and Home Care

1. Instruct parents about administration of medications and monitoring for side effects.
2. Instruct parents to monitor for long-term complications and their signs and symptoms.

CLIENT OUTCOMES

1. The child will return to normal or control central nervous system symptoms.
2. The child will not experience neck and/or head pain.

REFERENCES

Saez-Llorens X, McCracken GH Jr: Bacterial meningitis in neonates and children, *Infect Dis Clin North Am* 4(4):623, 1990.

Swingler G, Delport S, Hussey G: An audit of the use of antibiotics in presumed viral meningitis in children, *Pediatr Infect Dis J* 13(12):1107, 1994.

Vallejo JG, Kaplan SL, Mason EO Jr: Treatment of meningitis and other infections due to ampicillin-resistant *Haemophilus influenzae* type b in children, *Review Infect Dis* 13(2):197, 1991.

Wilson M, Lilley M: Meningitis in childhood, *Pediatr Nurs* 6(7):23, 1994.

48

Mental Retardation

PATHOPHYSIOLOGY

The term *mental retardation* refers to significant limitations in everyday functioning. This is a cognitive disability manifested during childhood (before age 18) that is characterized by below-normal intellectual functioning (intelligence quotient [IQ] is 70 to 75 or below) with other limitations in at least two adaptive areas of functioning: speech and language, self-care skills, home living, social skills, community use, self-direction, health and safety, functional academics, leisure, and work (American Association on Mental Retardation [AAMR], 1992). This newer definition of mental retardation uses a functional approach rather than the terminology formerly used to describe levels of mental retardation such as mild, moderate, severe, and profound. Refer to the box on p. 324 for diagnostic criteria for mental retardation.

Causes of mental retardation can be classified as prenatal, perinatal, and postnatal. Prenatal causes include chromosomal disorders (trisomy 21 [Down syndrome], Fragile X syndrome), syndrome disorders (Duchenne muscular dystrophy, neurofibromatosis [type 1]), and inborn errors of metabolism (phenylketonuria). Perinatal causes can be classified as those pertaining to intrauterine problems such as abruptio placentia, maternal diabetes, and premature labor; and neonatal conditions including meningitis and intracranial hemmorrhage. Postnatal causes include conditions

Diagnostic Criteria for Mental Retardation

A. Significantly subaverage intellectual functioning: an IQ of approximately 70 or below on an individually administered IQ test (for infants, a clinical judgment of significantly subaverage intellectual functioning).

B. Concurrent deficits or impairments in present adaptive functioning (i.e., the person's effectiveness in meeting the standards expected for his or her age by his or her cultural group) in at least two of the following areas: communication, self-care, home living, social and interpersonal skills, use of community resources, self-direction, functional academic skills, work, leisure, health, and safety.

C. The onset is before age 18 years.

Code based on degree of severity reflecting level of intellectual impairment:

317 Mild mental retardation:
   IQ level 50-55 to approximately 70
318.0 Moderate mental retardation:
   IQ level 35-40 to 50-55
318.1 Severe mental retardation:
   IQ level 20-25 to 35-40
318.2 Profound mental retardation:
   IQ level below 20 or 25
319 Mental retardation, severity unspecified: when there is strong presumption of mental retardation but the person's emintelligence is untestable by standard tests

Modified from American Psychiatric Association: *Diagnostic and statistical manual of mental disorders,* ed 4, Washington, D.C., 1994, The Association.

resulting from head injuries, infections, and demyelinating and degenerative disorders (AAMR, 1992). Fragile X syndrome, Down syndrome, and fetal alcohol syndrome account for one third of the individuals with mental retardation. The occurrence of associated problems such as cerebral palsy, sensory deficits, psychiatric disorders, and seizure disorders is correlated with the more severe levels of mental retardation. Diagnosis is established early in childhood. Long-term prognosis is determined ultimately by the extent to which the individual can function independently in the community (i.e., employment, living independently, social skills).

INCIDENCE

1. More than 85% of persons with mental retardation have an IQ classified within the mild level (IQ is between 50 and 70).
2. Male-female ratio is 1.6:1.
3. Incidence is greater in lower socioeconomic groups.
4. Nearly 18% of very low birth weight (VLBW) infants have severe disabilities.
5. Approximately 500,000 youth have mental retardation.
6. The dropout rate for students with disabilities is 25% to 30%.
7. The unemployment rate for persons with disabilities is 50% to 75%.

CLINICAL MANIFESTATIONS

1. Cognitive impairments
2. Delayed expressive and receptive language skills
3. Failure to achieve major developmental milestones
4. Head circumference above or below normal range
5. Possible delayed growth
6. Possible abnormal muscle tone
7. Possible dysmorphic features
8. Delayed gross and fine motor development

COMPLICATIONS

1. Cerebral palsy
2. Seizure disorder
3. Psychiatric disorders

4. Attention-deficit/hyperactivity disorder (ADHD)
5. Communication deficits
6. Constipation (caused by decreased intestinal motility secondary to anticonvulsant medications, insufficient intake of fiber and fluids)

LABORATORY AND DIAGNOSTIC TESTS

1. Standardized intelligence tests (Stanford-Binet, Weschler, Bayley Scales of Infant Development)
2. Developmental testing such as Denver II
3. Measurement of adaptive functioning (Vineland Adaptive Behavior Scales, Woodcock-Johnson Scales of Independent Behavior, School Edition of the Adaptive Behavior Scales)

MEDICAL MANAGEMENT

The following medications may be used:
1. Psychotrophic medications (thioridazine [Mellaril]) for youth with self-injurious behaviors
2. Psychostimulants for youth who demonstrate attention-deficit/hyperactivity disorder
3. Antidepressants (imipramine [Tofranil])
4. Carbamazepine (Tegretol) and propranolol (Inderal)

NURSING ASSESSMENT

Assessment consists of comprehensive evaluation of deficits and strengths related to these adaptive skills: communication, self-care, social interactions, use of community resources, self-direction, maintenance of health and safety, functional academics, development of leisure and recreational skills, and work.

NURSING DIAGNOSES

- Self-care deficit
- High risk for ineffective management of therapeutic regimen
- Impaired communication
- Altered nutrition: less than body requirements
- Anticipatory grieving
- Altered family processes
- Altered bowel elimination

NURSING INTERVENTIONS

1. Refer to early intervention program for individualized family support plan and interdisciplinary treatment plan.
2. Collaborate with other professionals to formulate an interdisciplinary plan of care.
3. See the section on discharge planning and home care, this chapter, for long-term care.

♠ Discharge Planning and Home Care

1. Refer child and family to agencies and professionals who can provide specialized services related to well child care and dental care and hygiene.
2. Refer family to community resources for genetic counseling, financial assistance, adaptive equipment, and support services.
3. Collaborate with families in forming and implementing a behavior treatment plan.
4. Facilitate learning of appropriate social, community, communication, community safety, and stranger avoidance skills; and development of peer relationships and leisure and recreational interests.
5. Facilitate the child's inclusion into school programs, recreational programs, and community settings.

CLIENT OUTCOMES

1. The child will function at his or her optimal level of functioning.
2. The family and child will cope with the challenges of living with a disability.
3. The family will be adept in accessing community resources.

REFERENCES

American Association on Mental Retardation: *Mental retardation: definition, classification and systems of supports,* ed 9, Washington, DC, 1992, The Association.

American Psychiatric Association: *Diagnostic and statistical manual of mental disorders,* ed 4, Washington, DC, 1994, The Association.

Batshaw M: Mental retardation, *Pediatr Clin North Am* 40(3):507, 1993.

Rauth J: Mentally retarded youth. In McArnarney E et al, editors: *Textbook of adolescent medicine,* Philadelphia, 1992, WB Saunders.

Roth S, Morse J: *A life-span approach to nursing care for individuals with developmental disabilities,* Baltimore, 1994, Paul H Brookes Publishing.

49

Muscular Dystrophy

PATHOPHYSIOLOGY

Muscular dystrophy is a disorder that results in bilateral and symmetric wasting of the voluntary muscles. The muscles pseudohypertrophy, and the muscle tissue is replaced with both connective tissue and fatty deposits. Types of muscular dystrophy include Duchenne, Becker's, limb-girdle, congenital, ocular, and facioscapulohumeral. The onset of sex-linked recessive types (Duchenne, Becker's, limb-girdle, congenital) is earlier than that of dominant types (facioscapulohumeral, ocular). Initially seen symptoms include gait abnormality and clumsiness. Muscles of hands, feet, tongue, palate, and mastication are rarely affected. Mild to moderate retardation is not unusual. Children affected with Duchenne muscular dystrophy rarely live beyond 20 years of age unless they have long-term mechanical ventilatory support. Other characteristics of Duchenne muscular dystrophy are the following:

1. It is transmitted as a sex-linked recessive gene.
2. It is characterized by progressive involvement of voluntary muscles.
3. It runs a rapid course.
4. Onset of symptoms occurs between 3 and 10 years of age.
5. Death occurs approximately 10 to 15 years after onset.

INCIDENCE

1. Duchenne muscular dystrophy affects 1 of every 3000 male children (X-linked recessive).
2. Duchenne muscular dystrophy accounts for approximately 50% of all cases.
3. Becker's muscular dystrophy affects male individuals.
4. Facioscapulohumeral muscular dystrophy affects both sexes equally.
5. Limb-girdle and ocular muscular dystrophies affect either sex (autosomal recessive).
6. Approximately 50% of the sisters of boys with muscular dystrophy will be carriers, and one half of their male offspring will inherit the disease.
7. Approximately 50% of children with muscular dystrophy can be characterized as having normal personalities.

CLINICAL MANIFESTATIONS

Symptoms are related to the voluntary muscles that are affected. The most frequently occurring symptoms are the following:

1. Poor balance
2. Difficulty climbing stairs.
3. Waddling gait or toe walking
4. Gowers' sign indicates hip girdle weakness
5. Difficulty running
6. Difficulty lifting arms above head due to involvement of shoulder girdle muscles
7. Often, loss of ambulation by 10 years of age
8. Pseudohypertrophy of calf muscles, quadriceps, shoulder, and hip girdle
9. Occurrence of scoliosis 2 years after child is wheelchair dependent

COMPLICATIONS

1. Cardiac decompensation
2. Pulmonary infections
3. Osteoporosis
4. Obesity
5. Contractures
6. Scoliosis

LABORATORY AND DIAGNOSTIC TESTS

1. Electromyogram (EMG)—demonstrates less electric activity in affected muscles
2. Muscle biopsy—diagnostic; indicates presence of fat
3. Creatine phosphokinase (CPK)—increase in early stages of disease

MEDICAL MANAGEMENT

A comprehensive, interdisciplinary team approach is used in the long-term management of children with muscular dystrophy. Generally, an interdisciplinary approach including neurology, orthopedics, physical and occupational therapy, and nursing is used. Young adults with Duchenne muscular dystrophy may choose to use long-term mechanical support to survive to their late 20s.

NURSING ASSESSMENT

1. See the section on musculoskeletal assessment in Appendix A.
2. Assess child's adherence to physical therapy regimen.
3. Assess child's level of self-care functioning.
4. Assess child's and family's level of coping.
5. Assess child's and family's management of home treatment regimen.
6. Assess child's and family's need for information.

NURSING DIAGNOSES

- Impaired physical mobility
- Altered growth and development
- Impaired home maintenance management
- Altered family processes
- Diversional activity deficit
- Self-care deficit: bathing/hygiene, dressing/grooming, feeding, toileting
- High risk for dysfunctional grieving
- Knowledge deficit
- High risk for ineffective management of treatment regimen

NURSING INTERVENTIONS

1. Assist parents in expressing and working through feelings of guilt, resentment, and anger.
2. Encourage and support parents' seeking genetic counseling.
3. Encourage parents and siblings to mourn (loss of the "perfect child") and to learn to cope.

♠ Discharge Planning and Home Care

1. Promote optimal muscular functioning.
   a. Reinforce physical therapy exercise regimen.
   b. Discourage inactivity and promote rest (inactivity promotes progression of disease).
2. Promote self-care activities as a means of enhancing child's sense of independence and self-sufficiency.
   a. Investigate and recommend use of adaptive devices as appropriate.
   b. Provide recommendations for home adaptations (e.g., grab bars, overhead slings, raised toilets).
   c. Recommend use of adaptive equipment as necessary (e.g., braces to prevent slumping and to facilitate standing).
3. Encourage parents, in collaboration with the child, to select realistic goals for achievement and living.
4. Provide support for child and family as they cope with disease.
   a. Refer to social worker or psychologist.
   b. Refer to Muscular Dystrophy Association.
   c. Refer to parent support group.
   d. Refer to peer support group.
5. Provide information about and make referrals to available educational resources.
   a. Refer parents to educational specialist.
   b. Promote child's full inclusion in school.
6. Provide information, and assess long-term care needs, pertaining to the following.
   a. Scoliosis
   b. Pulmonary and cardiac problems
   c. Genetic transmission

CLIENT OUTCOMES

1. Child will maintain optimal physical mobility.
2. The child and family will make informed decisions about treatment and management of the disease.
3. The child and family will ventilate feelings as the disease progresses.

REFERENCES

Ahlstrom G, Sjoden PO: Assessment of coping with muscular dystrophy: a methodological evaluation, *J Adv Nurs* 20(2):314, 1994.

Bach JR, Campagnolo DI, Hoeman S: Life satisfaction of individuals with Duchenne muscular dystrophy using long-term mechanical ventilatory support, *Am J Phys Med Rehabil* 70(3):129, 1991.

Cole C et al: Parental testing for Duchenne and Becker muscular dystrophy, *Lancet* 1(8580): 262, 1988.

Fenichel GM et al: A comparison of daily and alternate-day prednisone therapy in the treatment of Duchenne muscular dystrophy, *Arch Neurol* 48(6):575, 1991.

Fenton-May J et al: Screening for Duchenne muscular dystrophy, *Arch Dis Child* 70(6):551, 1994.

Greenberg CR et al: Three years' experience with neonatal screening for Duchenne/Becker muscular dystrophy: gene analysis, gene expression, and phenotype prediction, *Am J Med Genet* 39(1):68, 1991.

Smith RA et al: Assessment of locomotor function in young boys with Duchenne muscular dystrophy, *Muscle Nerve* 14(5):462, 1991.

Willig TN et al: Nutritional assessment in Duchenne muscular dystrophy, *Dev Med Child Neurol* 35(12):1074, 1993.

50

Nephrotic Syndrome

PATHOPHYSIOLOGY

Nephrotic syndrome is the clinical state caused by increased glomerular permeability to plasma proteins, resulting in (1) proteinuria, (2) hypoalbuminemia, (3) hyperlipidemia, and (4) edema. The loss of protein causes decreased plasma osmotic pressure and increased hydrostatic pressure, resulting in the accumulation of fluids in interstitial spaces and abdominal cavities. The decrease in vascular fluid volume stimulates the renin-angiotensin system, resulting in secretion of antidiuretic hormone (ADH) and aldosterone. Tubular reabsorption of sodium (Na^+) and water is increased, expanding the intravascular volume.

Nephrotic syndrome is the pathologic outcome of various factors that alter glomerular permeability. These causes of nephrotic syndrome can be categorized into primary and secondary types (see the box on p. 335). Nephrotic syndrome is classified according to the clinical findings and the microscopic examination of renal tissue. Based on clinical classification, the syndrome types differ according to the course of the disease, treatment, and prognosis. Symptoms may become chronic. Some children experience relapses that gradually decrease with age. Prognosis is poor in children who do not respond to treatment.

Types of Nephrotic Syndrome

Primary

- Congenital disease
  Finnish-type nephrotic syndrome
  (inherited)
- Minimal change nephrotic syndrome
  (most common type)

Secondary

- Postinfectious disease
  Glomerulonephritis
  Systemic bacterial infection
  Hepatitis B
  Human immunodeficiency virus
  (HIV)
  Subacute bacterial endocarditis
- Vascular disease
  Hemolytic-uremic syndrome
  Renal vein thrombosis
  Systemic lupus erythematosis
  Henoch-Schoenlein purpura
  Goodpasture syndrome
- Familial disease
  Alport syndrome
  Diabetes
- Drugs and heavy metals
- Allergic nephrosis

INCIDENCE

1. Incidence is greater in male individuals than in female individuals.

2. The mortality and prognosis of children with nephrotic syndrome vary with the etiology, severity, extent of renal damage, child's age, underlying condition, and response to treatment.
3. Nephrotic syndrome rarely affects children under 1 year of age.
4. Minimal change nephrotic syndrome (MCNS) accounts for 60% to 90% of all cases of nephrotic syndrome in children.
5. The mortality rate from MCNS has declined from 50% to 5% with the advancement of therapy and the introduction of steroids.
6. Infants with Finnish-type nephrotic syndrome are candidates for bilateral nephrectomy and renal transplantation.

CLINICAL MANIFESTATIONS

1. Proteinuria
2. Fluid retention and edema-weight gain, periorbital edema, dependent edema, external genitalia swelling, facial edema, ascites, increased prominence of inguinal and abdominal hernias, pleural effusions
3. Decreased urine output—dark, frothy urine
4. Hematuria
5. Anorexia
6. Diarrhea
7. Pallor
8. Growth failure and muscle wasting (long term)

COMPLICATIONS

1. Intravascular volume depletion (hypovolemic shock)
2. Hypercoagulability (venous thrombosis)
3. Respiratory compromise (related to fluid retention)
4. Skin breakdown
5. Infection
6. Peritonitis (related to ascites)
7. Untoward side effects of steroids

LABORATORY AND DIAGNOSTIC TESTS

Urine Tests

1. Urine protein—increased
2. Urinalysis—hyaline and granular casts, hematuria
3. Urine dipstick—positive for protein and blood
4. Urine specific gravity—elevated

Blood Tests

1. Serum albumen—decreased
2. Serum cholesterol—increased
3. Hemoglobin and hematocrit—increased (hemoconcentration)
4. Erythrocyte sedimentation rate (ESR)—increased
5. Serum electrolytes—varied with individual disease states

Diagnostic Tests

Renal biopsy is diagnostic, but is not routinely done.

MEDICAL MANAGEMENT

Medical management includes the following components of care:

1. Corticosteroid administration (prednisone)
2. Protein replacement (dietary or 25% albumen)
3. Reduction of edema—diuretics and sodium restriction (diuretics should be used with caution to prevent intravascular volume depletion, thrombus formation, and/or electrolyte imbalances)
4. Maintenance of electrolyte balance
5. Angiotensin-converting enzyme inhibitors (decrease the magnitude of proteinuria in membranous glomerulonephritis)
6. Alkylating agents—chlorambucil and cyclophosphamide (for steroid-dependent nephrotic syndrome and patients with frequent relapses)

7. Pain medication (for discomfort related to edema and invasive therapy)

NURSING ASSESSMENT

1. See the section on genitourinary assessment in Appendix A.
2. Assess child's hydration status.
3. Assess for signs and symptoms of electrolyte imbalances.
4. Assess for signs and symptoms of impending complications.
5. Assess child's and family's coping responses.
6. Assess child's developmental level.

NURSING DIAGNOSES

- Fluid volume excess
- Altered nutrition: less than body requirements
- Impaired skin integrity
- High risk for infection
- High risk for injury
- Altered tissue perfusion
- Pain
- Ineffective management of therapeutic regimen

NURSING INTERVENTIONS

1. Monitor child's clinical status.
   a. Report changes to physician.
   b. Monitor urine for proteinuria and hematuria (indicates progression of disease).
2. Monitor and control edema; prevent complications.
   a. Assess edematous areas for changes in condition.
   b. Promote bed rest during periods of severe edema and periods of rapid weight loss during diuresis.
3. Monitor child's response to and untoward effects of therapy.
   a. Record accurate intake and output.
   b. Record daily weights.
   c. Monitor for signs of electrolyte imbalance—hypokalemia, hyponatremia (diuretics), hypernatremia.
   d. Monitor for side effects of medications.

4. Encourage and support nutritional intake and proper nutritional status.
   a. Provide diet high in calories and protein.
   b. Decrease sodium intake (avoid high-sodium foods).
   c. Allow the child as many dietary choices as possible.
   d. Avoid extreme salt restrictions or extremely high protein foods as these may be undesirable to children and/or lead to paradoxical problems.
   e. Consider intravenous (IV) or gastric feedings if patient is unable to maintain proper nutritional status.
5. Provide skin care to maintain integrity and suppleness.
   a. Bathe child frequently.
   b. Dry the moist areas of skin (e.g., folds of skin, male genitalia).
   c. Turn child frequently and position him or her to prevent skin breakdown.
   d. Use pillows, sheepskins, and other padding to protect bony prominences.
6. Monitor for and prevent complications
   a. Monitor for circulatory disturbance (e.g., hypovolemia resulting from protein and fluid loss).
   b. Assess for signs of infection (may be masked by steroids).
   c. Monitor for complications from steroids—gastrointestinal (GI) tract bleeding, decreased resistance to infection, hypertension, increased intracranial pressure (ICP).
   d. Assess for respiratory compromise (caused by compression of lung by pleural effusion and diaphragm).
   e. Monitor for hypercoagulability (from femoral vein or arterial puncture).
   f. Monitor for peritonitis (may result when ascites is present).
7. Monitor for pain and provide pain relief measures as needed.
   a. Administer analgesics as needed.
   b. Use nonpharmacologic pain relief methods as appropriate.
   c. Continually reevaluate the effectiveness of pain relief measures.

8. Provide emotional support to child and family (see Appendix J, section on supportive care).

♠ Discharge Planning and Home Care

Provide child and parents with developmentally appropriate verbal and written instruction regarding home management of the following (see Appendix K):

1. Disease process (include expected clinical progress and signs of relapse)
2. Medications (dose, route, schedule, side effects, and complications)
3. Skin care
4. Nutrition
5. Prevention of infection
6. Pain management
7. Activity limitations
8. Follow-up

CLIENT OUTCOMES

1. The child's renal function will improve as evidenced by absence of clinical signs and symptoms.
2. The child's activity level will be appropriate for age.
3. The child will demonstrate no signs of infection.

REFERENCES

Kelsch R, Sedman A: Nephrotic syndrome, *Pediatr Rev* 14(1):30, 1993.

Kennedy J: Renal disorders. In Hazinski M, editor; *Nursing care of the critically ill child*, ed 2, St Louis, 1992, Mosby.

Melvin T, Bennett W: Management of nephrotic syndrome in childhood, *Drugs* 42(1):30, 1991.

Scipien G et al: *Pediatric nursing care*, St Louis, 1990, Mosby.

Welch T: Current management of selected childhood renal diseases, *Curr Probl Pediatr* 22(10):32, 1992.

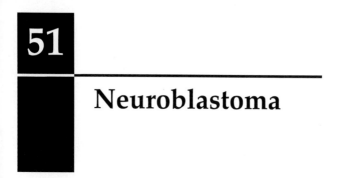

Neuroblastoma

PATHOPHYSIOLOGY

Neuroblastomas are soft, solid tumors that originate from neural crest cells that are precursors of the adrenal medulla and sympathetic nervous system. Neuroblastomas can be present wherever sympathetic nervous tissue is found. Primary tumor sites are usually in the abdomen, either in the adrenal gland or paraspinal ganglia. Less common primary sites include the paraspinal area of the thorax, the neck, and the pelvis. Usually encapsulated, neuroblastomas often impinge on adjacent tissues and organs. The etiology of neuroblastoma is unknown.

INCIDENCE

1. Neuroblastoma is the most common extracranial solid tumor of childhood and the most common neoplasm of infants.
2. Approximately 500 new cases are diagnosed each year in the United States.
3. The estimated incidence is once in 10,000 births.
4. The unique phenomenon of spontaneous tumor regression and maturation into benign forms may allow many cases of neuroblastoma to go undetected.
5. Prognosis is favorable if diagnosis is made before 12 months of age, and if the disease is stage I, II, or IVS (see section on medical management, this chapter).

CLINICAL MANIFESTATIONS

1. Symptoms related to retroperitoneal, adrenal gland, or paraspinal mass
   a. Firm, nontender, irregular abdominal mass that crosses the midline
   b. Altered bowel and/or bladder function
   c. Vascular compression with edema of the lower extremities
   d. Back pain, weakness of lower extremities
   e. Sensory loss
   f. Loss of sphincter control
2. Symptoms related to neck or thoracic mass
   a. Cervical and supraclavicular lymphadenopathy
   b. Congestion and edema of the face
   c. Respiratory dysfunction
   d. Headache
   e. Ecchymotic orbital proptosis
   f. Miosis
   g. Ptosis
   h. Exophthalmos
   i. Anhidrosis

LABORATORY AND DIAGNOSTIC TESTS

1. Complete blood count (CBC)—to detect anemia caused by many secondary factors (e.g., hemorrhage, disseminated intravascular coagulation)
2. Urinary catecholamines (vanillylmandelic acid and hemavanitic acid)—elevated due to overproduction by tumor cells or defective storage within tumor cells
3. Neuron-specific enolase (NSE)—elevated due to correlation with the amount of active neuronal tissue
4. G_{D2} level (sugar-containing lipid molecules)—present on the surface of human neuroblastoma cells; detection confirms presence of neuroblastoma
5. Ferritin level—increased levels correlate with poorer prognosis
6. Bone marrow aspiration and biopsies—to reveal marrow involvement and confirm diagnosis

7. Chest x-ray examination—to delineate primary thoracic neuroblastoma and vertebral and paravertebral involvement
8. Abdominal ultrasound—to reveal location of the mass and any impingement on other organs
9. Computed tomography (CT)—to determine if the tumor is operable
10. Magnetic resonance imaging (MRI)—to detect intraspinal involvement

MEDICAL MANAGEMENT

The International Staging System for Neuroblastoma standardizes definitions for diagnosis, staging, and treatment, and it categorizes patients according to radiographic and surgical findings, plus bone marrow status.

Localized tumors are divided into stages I, II, and III, depending on features of the primary tumor and the status of regional lymph nodes. Disseminated disease is divided into stages IV and IVS (S is for special), depending on the presence of distant cortical bone involvement, extent of bone marrow disease, and features of the primary tumor.

Children with favorable prognostic features usually require no treatment, minimal treatment, or surgical resection alone. Complete surgical resection is the only therapy required for patients with stage I tumors. Surgery may also suffice for stage II, but chemotherapy is widely used and sometimes supplemented with local radiotherapy. Stage IVS neuroblastoma has a high rate of spontaneous regression, and management may be limited to low-dose chemotherapy and close observation.

Stage III and IV neuroblastomas require intensive therapy, including chemotherapy, radiation therapy, surgery, autologous or allogeneic bone marrow transplant, bone marrow rescue, metaiodobenzylguanidine (MIBG), and immunotherapy with monoclonal antibodies specific to neuroblastoma.

Medication consists of simultaneous or rotating use of multiagent chemotherapy:

1. Cyclophosphamide—inhibits deoxyribonucleic acid (DNA) replication

2. Doxorubicin—interferes with nucleic acid synthesis and blocks DNA transcription
3. VP-16—causes metaphase arrest and inhibits nucleic acid and protein synthesis

NURSING ASSESSMENT

1. Refer to Appendix A for system-specific assessment.
2. Be aware that physical assessment is dependent on the tumor site and related system.
3. Be aware that assessment of the child with neuroblastoma should encompass all aspects of medical treatment, including chemotherapy, surgery, radiation, and bone marrow transplantation.
4. Assess child for verbal and nonverbal expressions of pain.
5. Assess child's and family's coping responses.
6. Assess child's level of development.

NURSING DIAGNOSES

- High risk for infection
- Pain
- Fluid volume excess
- High risk for impaired physical mobility
- High risk for ineffective management of therapeutic regimen
- High risk for altered growth and development
- Altered family processes

NURSING INTERVENTIONS
Surgical Phase

1. Prepare the child for clinical staging procedures with age-appropriate approach (see Appendix J, section on preparation for procedure/surgery).
2. Monitor for signs of infection.
3. Monitor respiratory function.
4. Provide fluid support.

Chemotherapy and/or Radiation Phase

1. Assess tumor site using observation and inspection; palpation is contraindicated.
2. Minimize side effects of multiagent chemotherapy.

    a. Bone marrow suppression
    b. Nausea and vomiting
    c. Anorexia and weight loss
    d. Oral mucositis
    e. Pain
3. Observe for medication or transfusion reactions.
4. Assess skin integrity.
5. Monitor for signs of infection.
6. Monitor physical and emotional growth and development of the child (see Appendix B).
7. Teach parents about the medications their child is receiving.
8. Refer child and/or siblings to child life specialist.
9. Refer family to social services for support and resource utilization (see Appendix K).
10. Assess for pain using age-appropriate technique (see Appendix I).
11. Provide pain management (see Appendix I).

♠ Discharge Planning and Home Care

Instruct parents about home care management (see Appendix K).
1. Signs of infection and when to seek medical attention
2. Instructions for wound care
3. Home care of child's central venous access device, including site care, dressing change, flushing, and emergency care
4. Medication administration (provide written information)
5. Compliance with treatment and medical appointments
6. Special nutritional needs
7. Potential behavioral changes in the child and/or siblings

CLIENT OUTCOMES

1. Child and family demonstrate ability to cope with life-threatening illness.
2. Child will be free of infection.
3. Child and family understand home care and long-term follow-up needs.

REFERENCES

Ball J, Bindler R, editors: *Pediatric nursing: caring for children*, East Norwalk, Conn, 1995, Appleton & Lange.

Foley G, Fochtman D, Mooney K, editors: *Nursing care of the child with cancer,* ed 2, Philadelphia, 1993, WB Saunders.

Hockenberry M, Coody D, Bennett B: Childhood cancers: incidence, etiology, diagnosis, and treatment, *Pediatr Nurs* 16(3):239, 1990.

Kushner B, Cheung N: Neuroblastoma: an overview, *Hematol Oncol Ann* 1(3):189, 1993.

Thierry P: Overview of current treatment of neuroblastoma, *Am J Pediatr Hematol/Oncol* 14(2):97, 1992.

52

Nonaccidental Trauma

OVERVIEW OF THE PROBLEM

The lives of youth in America's major cities are being devastated by violence. Health care professionals and professional organizations (such as the American Medical Association [AMA]) have acknowledged violence affecting children in the United States as a public health emergency. Examples of crimes committed by and against youth are rape, robbery, homicide, and aggravated assault. Many fights on school grounds are ending in death, and there are an alarming number of students carrying guns and weapons. Since 1990 there has been a decrease in the childhood mortality rate; however, violence is increasing. Nurses in a variety of settings must be prepared to care for affected children.

INCIDENCE

1. During the period from 1986 to 1991, violent crime arrest rate for children ages 10 to 17 increased by 48%.
2. Juvenile violent crime has increased in 44 states during the period from 1986 to 1991.
3. Male individuals are seven times more likely to be arrested for a violent crime than female individuals.
4. The leading cause of death in African American and white teenagers in America is gunshot wounds.
5. Youths living in disadvantaged, urban areas are more at risk for becoming victims of violent crime and committing them.

6. Incidence is increased in African American individuals versus white individuals.

CLINICAL MANIFESTATIONS

1. Injury-specific manifestations
2. Admitting to "gang" involvement
3. Involvement in high-risk behaviors (substance abuse, criminal activity)

COMPLICATIONS

1. Bleeding from wounds such as gunshot wounds and stab injuries
2. Organ damage
3. Permanent disabilities
4. Death

LABORATORY AND DIAGNOSTIC TESTS

1. Complete blood count
2. X-ray studies
3. Varying diagnostic tests, depending on the site of injury

MEDICAL MANAGEMENT

Management is specific to the injuries, such as surgery, casting, and wound care. Medications may include pain medications and antibiotics as indicated.

NURSING ASSESSMENT

1. Assess risk factors and high-risk behaviors.
2. Assess verbal and nonverbal pain behaviors.
3. Assess presence of injuries.
4. Assess psychosocial factors impacting on the youth and family.

NURSING DIAGNOSES

- Impaired tissue integrity
- Knowledge deficit
- High risk for injury
- High risk for trauma
- High risk for infection
- Impaired skin integrity

- Pain
- Self-esteem disturbance
- Altered family processes
- High risk for violence

NURSING INTERVENTIONS

1. Education of children and parents—distribute information packets, discuss preventive and intervention strategies
2. Prevention, especially of risk-taking behaviors such as violence and substance abuse
3. Steps to decrease gang activity and violence in schools through collaboration with school officials in developing programs
4. Pain management
5. Wound or surgical site care
6. Prevention of infection
7. Encouragement of positive social activities
8. Promotion of self-esteem through referral to community programs, peer support groups, mental health counseling
9. Promotion of use of conflict-resolution skills to deal with confrontational situations

♠ Discharge Planning and Home Care

1. Refer family and youth to prevention and education programs in the community (see the box on p. 350).
2. Refer family and youth to support groups and counseling.
3. Perform wound or surgical site care.
4. Stress the importance of follow-up care.

CLIENT OUTCOMES

1. Youth expresses relief from pain.
2. Youth demonstrates decrease or absence of risk-taking behaviors.
3. Youth and family attend community prevention and education programs.

REFERENCES

Castilia PT: Gangs, *J Pediatr Health Care* 7(1):39, 1993.

Giuliano JD: A peer education program to promote the use of conflict resolution skills among at risk school age males, *Public Health Rep* 109(2):158, 1994.

Resources

Center to Prevent Handgun Violence
1125 Eye Street NW, Suite 1100
Washington, DC 20005
Phone (202) 289-7319

Children's Safety Network
National Center for Education in
Maternal and Child Health
2000 15th Street N, Suite 701
Arlington, VA 22201-2617
Phone (703) 524-7802
Fax (703) 524-9335
E-mail:
rcsnceol@gumedlib.dml.georgetown.edu

Council for Safe Families
210 W 90th Street, Suite 2B
New York, NY 10024
Hotline (212) 914-5800

National SAFEKIDS Campaign
11 Michigan Avenue NW
Washington, DC 20010-2970
Phone (202) 939-4993

Hausman AJ et al: Patterns of teen exposure to a community-based violence prevention project, *J Adolesc Health* 13:668, 1992.

Minall GL: Wounded by violence, can a KISS make it better? *JEMS* 19(1):61, 1994.

Ropp L et al: Death in the city: an American childhood tragedy, *JAMA* 267(14):2905, 1992.

Schinke S et al: Reducing at risk behavior among vulnerable youth: an intervention outcome study, *Fam Community Health* 16(4):49, 1994.

53

Non-Hodgkin's Lymphoma

PATHOPHYSIOLOGY

Non-Hodgkin's lymphoma (NHL) is a highly malignant neoplasm of the lymphatic system and lymphoid tissue. As is the case with most childhood neoplasms, the cause of NHL has not been identified. Several factors, including viral infections, immunodeficiency, chromosomal aberration, chronic immunostimulation, and environmental exposure, have been implicated in precipitating malignant lymphomas.

Childhood NHL tends to have a rapid onset and is characterized by aggressive, widespread involvement that generally has a quick response to treatment. Common sites of the disease include the intraabdominal, mediastinal, peripheral nodal, and nasopharyngeal areas. Common extralymphoid sites include bone, skin, bone marrow, testes, and the central nervous system. With aggressive therapy, the survival rate for children with localized NHL is 90%, and for those with advanced disease, it is 60% to 70%.

Because several classification systems for NHL have been proposed, classification remains complex. NHL can be divided into three groups: (1) lymphoblastic, (2) small noncleaved cell, and (3) large cell. Favorable prognosis is defined by the following:
1. Lymph node involvement
2. An extranodal site in the nasopharynx or oropharynx, or other isolated extranodal site, with or without lymphadenopathy

3. Gastrointestinal involvement, with or without regional lymphadenopathy, limited to the mesentery

INCIDENCE

1. NHL is the third most common malignancy in children.
2. NHL occurs from infancy through adolescence, with a peak incidence between ages 7 and 11 years.
3. Male individuals are affected more than female individuals, with a 3:1 occurrence ratio.
4. Incidence of NHL is approximately 1.5 times that of Hodgkin's disease.
5. The 3-year survival rate for all children with NHL is 50% to 80%.

CLINICAL MANIFESTATIONS
Intraabdominal Involvement

1. Possible symptoms mimicking appendicitis (pain, right lower quadrant tenderness)
2. Intussusception
3. Ovarian, pelvic, retroperitoneal masses
4. Ascites

Mediastinal Involvement

1. Pleural effusion
2. Tracheal compression
3. Superior vena cava syndrome
4. Coughing, wheezing, dyspnea, respiratory distress
5. Edema of the upper extremities
6. Mental status changes

Primary Nasal, Paranasal, Oral, and Pharyngeal Involvement

1. Nasal congestion
2. Rhinorrhea
3. Epistaxis
4. Headache
5. Proptosis
6. Irritability
7. Weight loss

COMPLICATIONS

The major complication is tumor lysis syndrome (as a result of treatment).

1. Hyperuricemia
2. Hyperkalemia
3. Hyperphosphatemia
4. Hypocalcemia

LABORATORY AND DIAGNOSTIC TESTS

1. Bone marrow biopsy—to assess bone marrow involvement
2. Lumbar puncture—to determine presence of malignant cells in the central nervous system (CNS)
3. Complete blood count (CBC)—diagnostic for bone marrow dysfunction
4. Liver and kidney function tests—to assess functional involvement
5. Lactate dehydrogenase (LDH)—elevated due to tumor lysis
6. Serum uric acid—elevated due to cellular tumor load
7. Epstein-Barr virus (EBV)—has been linked to NHL
8. Bone scan—diagnostic

MEDICAL MANAGEMENT

Current therapy for treatment of NHL is based on the stage of the disease, immunophenotype, and histopathology. Treatment for NHL is multiagent chemotherapy to eradicate the disease and to prevent further dissemination.

The following medication regimens may be used:

1. For stage I and II (localized lymphomas)
   a. Induction therapy
      (1) Vincristine—inhibits cell division at metaphase
      (2) Prednisone—used in conjunction with antineoplastic agents
      (3) Doxorubicin—interferes with nucleic acid synthesis
      (4) Cyclophosphamide—blocks deoxyribonucleic acid (DNA), ribonucleic acid (RNA), and protein synthesis

b. Continuation therapy
   (1) Mercaptopurine—interferes with normal cellular metabolism
   (2) Methotrexate—interferes with mitotic process by inhibiting uptake of folinic acid
2. For stage III and IV (advanced lymphomas)—COMP drug regimen
   a. Cyclophosphamide (Cytoxan)
   b. Oncovin (vincristine)
   c. Methotrexate
   d. Prednisone
3. CNS protective medications
   a. Methotrexate
   b. Cytosine arabinoside—interferes with normal cellular metabolism
   c. Hydrocortisone—decreases edema caused by tumor necrosis

NURSING ASSESSMENT

1. Assess child's physiologic status (see Appendix A).
   a. Signs and symptoms of NHL
   b. Involvement of other body systems (e.g., gastrointestinal, respiratory)
   c. Adverse effects of treatment
2. Assess child and family for psychosocial needs (see Appendix J, section on supportive care).
   a. Knowledge
   b. Body image
   c. Family structure
   d. Family stressors
   e. Coping mechanisms
   f. Support systems
3. Assess child's level of development (see Appendix B).

NURSING DIAGNOSES

- High risk for injury
- Fluid volume excess
- Pain
- Altered nutrition: less than body requirements
- Anxiety
- High risk for activity intolerance

- High risk for ineffective management of therapeutic regimen
- High risk for ineffective individual coping
- High risk for ineffective family coping: compromised

NURSING INTERVENTIONS
Diagnosis and Staging Phase

1. Provide preprocedural education to the child and family (see Appendix J, section on preparation for procedure/surgery).
2. Prepare the child for diagnostic procedures with age-appropriate approach (see Appendix J, section on preparation for procedure/surgery).
3. Observe for signs and symptoms of systems involvement.
   a. Respiratory distress
   b. Superior vena cava syndrome
   c. CNS status
4. Refer to child life specialist for preprocedural preparation.
5. Assist and support the child in the collection of laboratory specimens.
6. Provide anticipatory guidance and family crisis intervention.

Treatment Phase

1. Monitor cardiorespiratory status.
2. Prepare for treatment-induced emergencies.
   a. Metabolic
   b. Hematologic
   c. Space-occupying tumors
3. Administer chemotherapeutic agents (see section on medical management, this chapter).
4. Assess for signs of extravasation.
   a. Cell lysis
   b. Tissue sloughing
5. Minimize side effects of chemotherapy.
   a. Bone marrow suppression
   b. Nausea and vomiting
   c. Anorexia and weight loss
   d. Oral mucositis
   e. Pain

6. Monitor for signs and symptoms of infection.
7. Monitor for signs and symptoms of relapse.
   a. CNS changes
   b. Infection
   c. Tumor recurrence
   d. Leukemic conversion
8. Provide ongoing emotional support to the child and family (see Appendix J, section on preparation for procedure/surgery).
9. Refer to child life specialist for continued coping strategies.
10. Provide ongoing education about treatment and medications.
11. Refer family to social services for support and resource utilization.

♠ Discharge Planning and Home Care

Instruct child and parents about home care management.
1. Signs of infection and when to seek medical attention
2. Care of child's central venous access device, including site care, dressing change, flushing, and emergency care
3. Medication administration (provide written information)
4. Compliance with treatment and medical procedures
5. Proper nutrition for optimal weight gain and health maintenance
6. School attendance and/or activity restrictions
7. Signs and symptoms of relapse
8. Potential behavioral changes in the child and/or siblings
9. Accessing support services, such as parent support groups (see Appendix J, section on supportive care, and Appendix K)

CLIENT OUTCOMES

1. Child and family demonstrate ability to cope with life-threatening illness.
2. Child will be free of infection.
3. Child and family understand home care and long-term follow-up needs.

REFERENCES

Foley G, Fochtman D, Mooney K, editors: *Nursing care of the child with cancer,* ed 2, Philadelphia, 1993, WB Saunders.

Hockenberry M, Coody D: Childhood cancers: incidence, etiology, diagnosis and treatment, *Pediatr Nurs* 16(3):239, 1990.

Kurtzberg J, Graham M: Non-Hodgkin's lymphoma: biologic classification and implication for therapy, *Pediatr Clin North Am* 38(2):443, 1991.

Rahr V, Tucker R: Non-Hodgkin's lymphoma: understanding the disease, *Cancer Nurs* 13(1):56, 1990.

Tucker R, Rahr V: Nursing care of the patient with non-Hodgkin's lymphoma: a case study, *Cancer Nurs* 13(4):229, 1990.

54

Osteogenic Sarcoma and Amputation

PATHOPHYSIOLOGY

Osteogenic sarcoma is a tumor found in the diaphysis of a long bone (femur, radius, ulna, proximal humerus, and ilium). It also can affect the flat bones, which include the head, pelvis, and spine. The most common site of occurrence is the femur, followed in order, by the knee joint, tibia, and humerus. The clinical course occurs in the following sequence: (1) the normal bone is destroyed and is replaced by tumor cells, resulting in osteoid tissue and bone; (2) growth penetrates the cortex and extends beyond it (radiating spindles of bone are characteristic of this process); and (3) the tumor extends through the bone marrow cavity. Metastasis occurs through veins and involves lungs first.

INCIDENCE

1. Osteogenic sarcoma is the most common bone tumor in children.
2. It occurs most commonly during the adolescent growth period.
3. It is uncommon before age 10 years.
4. Age range of peak incidence is 10 to 15 years.
5. The survival rate is 50%.

CLINICAL MANIFESTATIONS

Symptoms are gradual in onset. The child may have symptoms for 6 to 9 months before he or she seeks treatment. The symptoms are as follows:

1. Local pain during activity, and more severe pain with passage of time (most common symptom)
2. Limping or gait variation
3. Limitation of joint motion
4. Joint tenderness
5. Local edema

COMPLICATIONS

Pathologic fractures occur with larger lesions and many times are the initially seen symptoms.

LABORATORY AND DIAGNOSTIC TESTS

1. Serum alkaline phosphates—elevated because of osteoid production
2. Tissue biopsy—to confirm diagnosis
3. Anteroposterior lateral x-ray studies—to detect presence of soft-tissue mass associated with destructive bone lesion, and calcification
4. Skeletal bone scan—to detect presence of metastatic bone lesions
5. Computed tomography (CT) scans and magnetic resonance imaging (MRI)—to determine the extent of disease and metastasis

MEDICAL MANAGEMENT

An important component of treatment of osteogenic sarcoma is surgery. Type of surgery is determined by age of the child and tumor size and location. It may be either an amputation or limb salvage. In selected cases, amputation is no longer the surgery of choice. Both procedures are performed to excise the tumor and obtain a biopsy for diagnosis.

Complications of amputation are the following:

1. Reactive hyperemia—reddened skin, particularly at the pressure points; subsides as keratoma layer forms

2. Contact dermatitis—most often caused by contact with prosthetic materials (e.g., polyester resins, chrome)
3. Infections—including fungal and pyogenic infections (e.g., furuncles)
4. Epidermal cysts—evident at points of friction at or near the brim of the socket; most often caused by an ill-fitted prosthesis
5. Stump edema syndrome—consisting of worsening reactive hyperemia, resulting in oozing and capillary rupture
6. Terminal bone overgrowth
7. Bony spurs—developing at the corners or margins of the amputation as a result of periosteal irritation
8. Neuroma
9. "Phantom limb"—feelings of pain and sensation in the amputated limb
10. Stump scarring—caused by inguinal weight bearing and increased shearing force at stump-socket interface

After surgery, chemotherapy is given. The chemotherapy regimens contain various combinations of the following: methotrexate, doxorubicin, bleomycin, cyclophosphamide, cisplatin, and ifosfamide. When methotrexate is given, leucovorin calcium is given to reverse the action of the methotrexate and decrease its toxicity. Leucovorin calcium is given after the infusion of methotrexate. The dosage of leucovorin calcium is equivalent to the amount of methotrexate administered. Allopurinol is also given with chemotherapy to decrease the level of uric acid, which is a by-product of chemotherapy.

NURSING ASSESSMENT

1. Assess for signs of infection at the stump or surgical site.
2. Assess for swelling at the stump or surgical site.
3. Assess child's and family's emotional response to upcoming surgery and need for information.
4. Postoperatively, assess for impending signs and symptoms of complications.
5. Assess for wound drainage and signs and symptoms of infection.
6. Assess child's response to chemotherapy.
7. Assess continuously child's and family's coping.

8. Assess child's and family's ability to manage home treatment regimen.
9. Assess child's and family's use of community resources.

NURSING DIAGNOSES

- Impaired tissue integrity
- Impaired physical mobility
- High risk for injury
- Pain
- Body image disturbance
- Fluid volume excess
- High risk for ineffective management of treatment regimen
- High risk for ineffective individual coping
- High risk for altered family processes
- High risk for altered growth and development

NURSING INTERVENTIONS
Preoperative Care

1. Prepare operative site according to hospital procedure.
2. Encourage use of exercises to strengthen muscles.
3. Provide emotional support to child and parents.
   a. Provide active listening to concerns.
   b. Encourage expression of feelings of loss.
   c. Provide anticipatory information about emotional responses to surgery.
4. Provide preoperative information to decrease anxiety about unknown aspects (see Appendix J, section on preparation for procedure/surgery).
5. Prepare child before laboratory and diagnostic testing.
   a. Complete blood count (CBC) (see Appendix J, section on preparation for procedure/surgery)
   b. Urinalysis
   c. Bone scan
   d. X-ray studies
   e. Type and cross match for blood

Postoperative Care

1. Monitor for signs of complications and report immediately (see section on complications, this chapter).
2. Observe and monitor for signs of hemorrhage every hour for 24 hours, then every 4 hours.

3. Promote patency and healing of surgical site (after amputation).
   a. Apply pressure dressing (figure eight) to stump.
   b. Institute range of motion exercises according to physical therapist's orders.
   c. Reinforce exercise program with physical therapist.
   d. Cleanse stump and socket every day with soap and water; dry thoroughly.
   e. Avoid use of skin lotions (cause maculation and superficial infection).
   f. Pat stump with wet tea bags (tenniten facilitates development of thickened keratin).
4. Position patient correctly to prevent deformities (after amputation).
   a. Trendelenburg position
   b. Pillow beneath knee for 24 hours to decrease edema
   c. After 24 hours, no pillow beneath knee (causes flexion of knee)
   d. Prone position for several hours every day (to prevent hip flexion and contracture)
   e. No external rotation or abduction of amputated limb
5. Monitor for pain; administer pain medication.
6. Promote use of and adaptation to prosthetic device (after amputation).
   a. Perform prosthetic fitting immediately after surgery because this promotes stump maturation, early ambulation, and resumption of normal activities.
   b. Encourage venting of feelings about being disabled.
   c. Explain restrictions on activities.
7. Monitor administration of chemotherapy.
   a. Provide adequate hydration (hydrate 12 hours before infusion of chemotherapy).
   b. Record intake and output hourly.
   c. Measure specific gravity to assess hydration.
   d. Monitor urine pH and hematest (majority of medication is excreted in urine in first 24 hours); urine needs to be alkaline, or its precipitates in kidney will cause tubular necrosis.
   e. Assist with collection of blood chemistry, CBC, and platelet count.
   f. Assist with collection of urine for urinalysis.

8. Monitor for child's or adolescent's untoward and therapeutic responses to chemotherapy.
   a. Oral and gastrointestinal tract ulcerations
      (1) Diarrhea
      (2) Ulcerative stomatitis (hemorrhagic enteritis and death can occur)
   b. Skin reactions—urticaria, rashes
   c. Cystitis—inflammation of urinary tract
   d. Nausea and vomiting
9. Minimize negative consequences of chemotherapy.
   a. Provide good mouth care.
   b. Urge child or adolescent to stop smoking.
   c. Advise child or adolescent to stay out of the sun (methotrexate can cause skin blotches).
   d. Push fluids.
   e. Administer antiemetics.
   f. Provide bland, soft diet.
   g. Elevate head of bed.
   h. Teach self-hypnosis and relaxation techniques.
10. Monitor for complications.
    a. Pneumothorax (symptoms: shortness of breath, dyspnea, chest pain)
    b. Depression of hematologic values 10 days after methotrexate administration
    c. Renal toxicity—dysuria, oliguria (monitor intake and output)
11. Provide emotional support to parents and child (see Appendix J, section on preparation for procedure/surgery).

🏠 Discharge Planning and Home Care Chemotherapy Regimen

1. Instruct parents and adolescents about home management.
   a. Take leucovorin calcium *on time* (wake up child if necessary).
   b. Take antiemetic for nausea and vomiting.
   c. Drink increased amount of fluids (2 qt per day); milk tends to increase mucous secretions.
   d. Check urine for pH.
   e. Stay out of the sun.

2. Refer to community resources for follow-up (see Appendix K).

Postoperative Care

1. Instruct child and parents about stump care.
2. Provide reinforcement information about physical therapy regimen.
3. Refer to school nurse and clinic and advise them about child's status.
4. Explore adherence potential by asking about the following items.
   a. Means of transportation
   b. Resources for child care
   c. Finances
   d. Level of motivation
   e. Understanding of need for long-term follow-up every 3 to 4 months until growth complete

CLIENT OUTCOMES

1. The child will achieve remission.
2. The side effects of chemotherapy experienced by the child will be minimized.
3. The child and family will adhere to the home treatment regimen.

REFERENCES

Betcher D: New trends in osteogenic sarcoma, *J Pediatr Oncol Nurs* 8(2):70, 1991.

Dubousset J, Missenard G, Kalifa C: Management of osteogenic sarcoma in children and adolescents, *Clin Orthop* 270:52, 1991.

Foley GV, Fochtman D, Mooney KH: *Nursing care of the child with cancer,* Philadelphia, 1993, WB Saunders.

Glasser DB et al: Survival, prognosis, and therapeutic response in osteogenic sarcoma: the high-dose methotrexate for osteogenic sarcoma, *Anticancer Drugs* 5(4):480, 1994.

Kiu MC et al: Transient neurological disturbances induced by the chemotherapy of Memorial Hospital experience, *Cancer* 69(3):698, 1992.

Rosen G et al: The role of thoracic surgery in the management of metastatic osteogenic sarcoma, *Chest Surg Clin North Am* 4(1):75, 1994.

Saeter G et al: Systemic relapse of patients with osteogenic sarcoma: prognostic factors for long term survival, *Cancer* 75(5):1084, 1994.

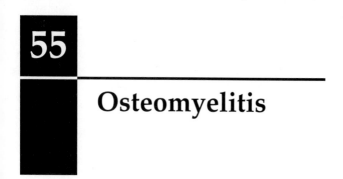

55

Osteomyelitis

PATHOPHYSIOLOGY

Osteomyelitis is an infection of the bone that can occur in any bone in the body. The most common locations are the femur and the tibia. The humerus and the hip are rarely affected. The skull is a common location in infants. Usually a predisposing condition such as poor nutrition or poor hygiene exists.

Bacterial emboli reach the small arteries in the metaphysis, where circulation is sluggish. An abscess forms and replaces bone, causing increased pressure and secondary necrosis. This abscess eventually can rupture into the subperiosteal space. The infection spreads beneath the periosteum, thrombosing vessels and causing increased necrosis. The cycle of impaired circulation is thus established. A sinus can form and extend the infection to the skin. Extension to a joint results in septic arthritis. The condition can become chronic and thus quite resistant to therapy, often requiring involved surgical intervention. The epiphysis is usually spared because it has a separate circulation.

Any organism is capable of causing osteomyelitis, either through the direct (*exogenous*) route or through seeding through the bloodstream from an infection elsewhere (*hematogenous*). Exogenous sources include penetrating wounds, open fractures, contamination during surgery, or secondary extension through an abscess, burn, or wound.

The hematogenous route is more common; sources include furuncles, skin abrasions, upper respiratory tract infections, otitis media, abscessed teeth, and pyelonephritis. The hematogenous form is often subacute because the preceding infection is often treated with antibiotics.

INCIDENCE

1. The greatest incidence of osteomyelitis is found in 5- to 14-year-olds.
2. It is twice as common in male individuals as in female individuals.

CLINICAL MANIFESTATIONS

1. Abrupt pain—point tenderness above the bone, as well as swelling and warmth over the bone
2. Fever
3. Possible dehydration
4. Unwillingness to move the limb or bear weight
5. Holding of extremity in semiflexed position (muscle spasm)
6. Irritability
7. Poor appetite

COMPLICATIONS

Pathologic fractures occur as complications of osteomyelitis.

LABORATORY AND DIAGNOSTIC TESTS

1. Complete blood count (CBC)—marked leukocytosis
2. Sedimentation rate—elevated erythrocyte sedimentation rate (ESR)
3. Blood culture—positive in 50% of cases; common organisms vary with age and other factors
   a. All ages—staphylococci, primarily *Staphylococcus aureus*
   b. Young children—*Haemophilus influenzae*
   c. Neonates—coliforms (*Escherichia coli*)
   d. Sickle cell anemia—*Salmonella* organisms
   e. Foot—*Pseudomonas* organisms
4. X-ray studies—negative first 10 to 12 days until bone destruction occurs (soft-tissue swelling is evident early)
5. Bone scan—often positive early for inflammation

6. Direct needle aspiration—confirms diagnosis and provides culture of site

MEDICAL MANAGEMENT

Intravenous antibiotics are begun after blood cultures have been drawn. Antibiotics are usually administered for 3 to 4 weeks, depending on duration of symptoms, response to treatment, and sensitivity of the organism. The type of antibiotic used to treat osteomyelitis is dependent on the culture and sensitivity. Bed rest may be prescribed, and the affected extremity is usually immobilized with a cast or splint. Surgery may be performed to drain the area and remove necrotic bone. During surgery, polyethylene tubes are placed in the bone—one for instilling an antibiotic solution (usually the upper tube) and the other for drainage.

NURSING ASSESSMENT

1. See the section on musculoskeletal assessment in Appendix A.
2. Assess pain—location, duration, intensity.
3. Assess nutritional status—usually, poor appetite; assess adequacy of caloric intake, as well as intake of protein and fluids.

NURSING DIAGNOSES

- High risk for infection
- Hyperthermia
- Pain
- Altered tissue perfusion: peripheral
- Impaired tissue integrity
- High risk for ineffective management of therapeutic regimen
- Altered nutrition: less than body requirements

NURSING INTERVENTIONS

1. Immobilize extremity to facilitate healing and prevent complications.
   a. Apply splint, bivalved cast, or complete cast with window.
   b. Allow *no weight bearing* (high risk of pathologic fracture).
      (1) Use gurney or wheelchair; elevate extremity slightly.

(2) Use active range of motion (AROM) exercises on unaffected extremity after inflammation subsides.
2. Provide pain relief measures.
    a. Allow comfortable position.
    b. Support affected limb on pillows.
    c. Use care in turning and moving child.
    d. Monitor child's response to analgesia and sedation as necessary.
3. Use wound and skin precautions if any drainage occurs.
    a. Provide diversional activities.
    b. Provide rooming-in for parents of young children.
    c. Refer to procedures manual for institutional isolation techniques.
4. Monitor child's response to antibiotic irrigation of site (up to 6 weeks).
    a. For first 3 days, expect blood, debris, and pus (have tendency to clog tubes).
        (1) Reversing the flow direction of tubes at intervals can prevent blockage; do so with physician consultation only.
        (2) Physician may elect to irrigate with heparin and saline solution if blockage occurs.
        (3) Use prescribed suction (usually low suction).
    b. If tubes are functioning properly, wound and dressing should remain dry.
    c. Maintain records of instillation and output (clarity, color, and volume of drainage); often up to 1000 ml per day is instilled.
    d. When tubes are removed, usually the instillation tube (upper) is removed first, leaving the drainage tube until no further drainage occurs.
    e. Sudden pain at the site of irrigation may indicate blockage of the drainage tube.
5. Monitor child's response to medications.
    a. Antibiotics
    b. Antipyretics
    c. Sedatives
6. Provide cast care.
    a. Monitor skin temperature; casting creates concern for thermoregulation in the young infant and child.
    b. Monitor color, heat, sweating, tenderness, and motion of digital digits.

7. Promote adequate nutritional intake.
   a. Promote high-caloric intake (juices, gelatin, Popsicles).
   b. Appetite usually returns when acute symptoms subside.
8. Monitor for signs of infection and alterations in thermoregulation.
   a. Increased temperature (institute cooling measure)
   b. Signs of inflammation
   c. Drainage or musty odor with cast
9. Provide age-appropriate diversional activities (see section on growth and development, Appendix B).
10. Provide emotional support to parents (see section on supportive care, Appendix J, section on supportive care).

♠ Discharge Planning and Home Care

1. Instruct parents about elements of rehabilitation (see section on home care, Appendix K).
   a. Risks of fractures
   b. Necessity for hospitalization
   c. Necessity for operations
2. Instruct parents about administration of antibiotics.
   a. Therapeutic responses
   b. Side effects—given that many of these antibiotics have negative renal, audiologic, and hepatic effects, these systems must be monitored closely during therapy (intravenous [IV] medication may be prescribed if treatment is longer than 3 weeks)

CLIENT OUTCOMES

1. Child will be free of infection.
2. Child will be free of disease complications.
3. Child and family will learn to cope effectively with the home treatment regimen.

REFERENCES

Faden H, Grossi M: Acute osteomyelitis in children, *Am J Dis child* 145(1):65, 1991.

Morrissy RT, editor: *Lovell and Winter's pediatric orthopaedics* ed 3, Philadelphia, 1990, JB Lippincott.

Pascual A: Index of suspicion: case 3—osteomyelitis, *Pediatr Rev* 15(5):201, 1994.

56

Otitis Media

PATHOPHYSIOLOGY

Otitis media is an inflammation of the middle ear. Children 6 years of age and younger are at particular risk for otitis media because their eustachian tubes lack the cartilaginous support found in older children and adults. This allows the eustachian tube to collapse, causing negative pressure in the middle ear. In turn, there is impaired drainage of middle ear fluid and possible reflux of pharyngeal secretions into this normally sterile area. Otitis media is the most frequently encountered diagnosis in office visits for children under the age of 15. Two types of otitis media are common in clinical pediatrics.

Acute Otitis Media

Acute otitis media is fluid in the middle ear with signs and symptoms of infection, and it can be caused by a variety of pathogens. These include *Streptococcus pneumoniae, Haemophilus influenzae, Streptococcus pyogenes, Moraxella catarrhalis*, viruses, and certain anaerobes. In the neonate, gram-negative enteric organisms or *Staphylococcus aureus* may also be the causative organisms.

Otitis Media with Effusion

Otitis media with effusion is fluid in the middle ear without signs and symptoms of infection. No definitive causative agent has been identified, although otitis media with effusion is seen in children recovering from acute otitis media, as well as those with allergies and viral upper respiratory tract infection.

INCIDENCE

1. The age ranges of peak incidence for otitis media are 5 to 24 months and 4 to 6 years.
2. Seventy percent of affected children have one episode by age 3, with one third having more than three episodes.
3. Children with acute otitis media have a transient conductive hearing loss lasting at least 2 to 4 weeks after the acute infection.
4. Children with otitis media with effusion may have a conductive hearing loss for the duration of the effusion.
5. Fifty percent of children with cleft palate have chronic otitis media before surgical correction.
6. Children exposed to passive cigarette smoke have a significantly higher rate of otitis media.

CLINICAL MANIFESTATIONS
Acute Otitis Media

1. Red tympanic membrane, often bulging with no visible bony landmarks, immobile to pneumatic otoscopy (the application of a positive or negative pressure pulse to the middle ear using a bulb insufflator attachment on the otoscope)
2. Complaint of ear pain (otalgia), or fussiness and ear pulling in the preverbal child
3. Fever (present in about one half of children)
4. Anorexia (common)
5. Anterior cervical lymphadenopathy

Otitis Media with Effusion

1. Dull yellow to gray tympanic membrane, often retracted with poor mobility on pneumatic otoscopy
2. A feeling of fullness or itch deep in the ear
3. Mild to moderate conductive hearing loss

COMPLICATIONS
Common Occurrence

1. Tympanic membrane rupture with otorrhea
2. Short-term conductive hearing loss

Unusual Occurrence

1. Long-term or permanent hearing loss
2. Meningitis
3. Mastoiditis
4. Brain abscess
5. Acquired cholesteatoma (filling of sac in the middle ear with epithelium or keratin)

LABORATORY AND DIAGNOSTIC TESTS

1. Tympanogram is obtained to measure tympanic membrane compliance and stiffness.
2. Culture and sensitivity are only available if tympanocentesis (needle aspiration of the middle ear via the tympanic membrane) is done.

MEDICAL MANAGEMENT

Decongestants and antihistamines have not proven to aid in the resolution of otitis media. Their use should not be encouraged.

Antibiotics may be used for acute otitis media. The first-line medication is amoxicillin; the second-line medication regimen—to be used when an amoxicillin-resistant organism is suspected—is amoxicillin with clavulanate (Augmentin; a second-generation cephalosporin), or trimethoprim sulfamethoxazole. In the penicillin-allergic child, erythromycin with a sulfonamide or trimethoprim-sulfa may be used. Cross allergy to the cephalosporins will occur in about 8% of these children.

For otitis media with effusion, the usual treatment is watchful waiting. This condition will usually spontaneously resolve within 2 months.

For persistent otitis media with effusion, myringotomy may be advised. Myringotomy is the surgical procedure that involves insertion of pressure-equalizer tubes into the tympanic membrane. This allows ventilation of the middle ear, relieves the negative pressure, and permits drainage of fluid. The tubes usually fall out after 6 to 12 months. Complications that may result include atrophy of the tympanic membrane, tympanosclerosis (scarring of the tympanic membrane), chronic perforation, and cholesteatoma.

NURSING ASSESSMENT

1. Assess for verbal and nonverbal pain behaviors.
2. Assess for elevated temperature.
3. Assess for enlarged lymph glands in neck area.
4. Assess nutritional status and adequacy of caloric fluid intake.
5. Assess for hearing loss.

NURSING DIAGNOSES

- Pain
- Altered comfort
- Sensory/perceptual alterations: auditory

NURSING INTERVENTIONS
Acute Otitis Media

1. Treat or teach family to treat the child with analgesics and/or antipyretics as needed for symptoms.
   a. Fever
   b. Ear pain
2. Offer small amounts of liquids frequently with a cup or spoon if breast or bottle is refused (sucking may cause increased ear pain in the younger child).
3. Be aware that increased fluid intake is vital to any child with fever or illness.
4. Teach the family about safe and effective use of prescribed antibiotic.
5. Observe or teach family to observe for signs of complication with acute otitis.
   a. Ear drainage
   b. No improvement of signs and symptoms with treatment, especially after 48 hours of appropriate antibiotic therapy
   c. Stiff neck, severe fussiness and irritability (meningitis)

Otitis Media with Effusion

1. Teach the family about the course of the disease and the lack of definitive etiology and treatment.
2. Support the child and family if conductive hearing loss is present; reassure them that this is likely to spontaneously resolve.

3. If myringotomy is required, supply age-appropriate explanations of the procedure to child and parents.

Postoperative Care

Monitor child's response to surgical intervention (myringotomy with insertion of tympanostomy tubes).

1. Vital signs (increased temperature means infection)
2. Otorrhea from ears (tube insertion)
3. Presence of bleeding
4. Pain (provide pain measures and medications as needed)
5. Hearing

🏠 Discharge Planning and Home Care

1. Instruct child and parents about maintaining patency of tympanostomy tubes (e.g., when child is swimming, plug ears with ear plugs, petroleum jelly).
2. Instruct about limiting child's activities until fully recovered.
   a. Avoid rigorous activities.
   b. Provide frequent rest periods.
   c. Allow return to school after child receives medical approval.
3. Teach the importance of avoiding passive cigarette smoke exposure in children; if household members are unable or unwilling to quit smoking, smoking should be done out-of-doors.

CLIENT OUTCOMES

1. Child is free of pain as demonstrated by verbal and nonverbal behaviors.
2. Child's activity level and appetite return to normal.
3. Child demonstrates no hearing loss.

REFERENCES

Berhman R et al: Disorders of the ear. In *Nelson's textbook of pediatrics*, Philadelphia, 1992, WB Saunders.

Berman S, Schmitt B: The ear: diseases and disorders. In Hay W et al, editors: *Current pediatric diagnosis and treatment*, 1994.

Clark J, Queener S, Karb V: Antiinfective and chemotherapeutic agents. In *Pharmacologic basis of nursing practice*, St Louis, 1993, Mosby.

The Otitis Media Guideline Panel: Managing otitis media with effusion in young children, *Pediatrics* 94(5):766, 1994.

57

Patent Ductus Arteriosus

PATHOPHYSIOLOGY

Patent ductus arteriosus (PDA) is the persistent patency of the ductus arteriosus after birth, resulting in the shunting of blood directly from the aorta (higher pressure) into the pulmonary artery (lower pressure). This left-to-right shunting causes the recirculation of increased amounts of oxygenated blood in the lungs, producing increased demands on the left side of the heart. The additional effort of the left ventricle to meet this increased demand leads to progressive dilation and left-atrial hypertension. The cumulative cardiac effects cause increased pressure in the pulmonary veins and capillaries, resulting in pulmonary edema. The pulmonary edema results in decreased diffusion of oxygen and hypoxia, with progressive constriction of the arterioles in the lungs. Pulmonary hypertension and failure of the right side of the heart ensue if the condition is not corrected through medical or surgical treatment. Closure of the PDA is primarily dependent on the constrictor response of the ductus to the oxygen tension in the blood. Other factors affecting ductus closure include action of prostaglandins, pulmonary and systemic resistances, size of the ductus, and the condition of the infant (premature or full term). PDA occurs more frequently in premature infants and is less well tolerated in these infants because their cardiac compensatory mechanisms are not as well developed and left-to-right shunts tend to be larger.

INCIDENCE

1. Precise incidence varies, depending on gestational age.
2. PDA accounts for 5% to 10% of cardiac defects, excluding those of premature infants.
3. Incidence in full-term infants is 1 in 2500 to 5000 live births.
4. Overall incidence in premature infants is 20% to 75%.
5. PDA is present in 60% to 70% of infants with congenital rubella infection.
6. PDA occurs three times more often in female individuals than in male individuals.

CLINICAL MANIFESTATIONS

Manifestations of PDA in premature infants are often clouded by other problems associated with prematurity (e.g., respiratory distress syndrome). Signs of ventricular overload are not apparent for 4 to 6 hours after birth. Infants with small PDA may be asymptomatic; infants with large PDA may manifest signs of congestive heart failure (CHF).

1. Persistent murmur (systolic, then continuous; heard best at left upper sternal border)
2. Tachycardia (apical pulse greater than 170)
3. Prominent to bounding pulses
4. Hyperactive precordium (result of increased left-ventricular stroke volume)
5. Tachypnea (respiratory rate greater than 70)
6. Wide pulse pressure (greater than 25 mm Hg)
7. Increased ventilator requirement (associated with pulmonary problems)
8. Metabolic acidosis (may not be present)

COMPLICATIONS

1. Hepatomegaly (rare in premature infants)
2. Necrotizing enterocolitis
3. Concurrent pulmonary disorder (e.g., respiratory distress syndrome or bronchopulmonary dysplasia)
4. Gastrointestinal (GI) hemorrhage (decreased platelet count)
5. Hyperkalemia (decreased urinary output)
6. Arrhythmias (digitalis toxicity)
7. Failure to thrive

LABORATORY AND DIAGNOSTIC TESTS

1. Chest x-ray study—prominent or enlarged left atrium and left ventricle (cardiomegaly); increased pulmonary vascular markings
2. Echocardiography—left atrial–to–aortic root ratio greater than 1.3:1 in full-term infants or greater than 1.0 in preterm infants (caused by increased left-atrial volume as a result of left-to-right shunt)
3. Doppler color flow mapping—used to evaluate blood flow and its direction
4. Electrocardiogram (ECG)—varies with degree of severity: no abnormality noted with small PDA; left-ventricular hypertrophy with large PDA
5. Cardiac catheterization—performed only for further evaluation of confusing ECHO or Doppler findings or when there is suspicion that additional defects may be present

MEDICAL MANAGEMENT

Interrupting the left-to-right flow of blood is the goal of management for the uncomplicated patent ductus arteriosus. When the shunt is hemodynamically significant, conservative measures may be tried initially. Conservative management consists of fluid restriction and medications.

Furosemide (Lasix) is used along with fluid restrictions to promote diuresis and minimize the effects of cardiovascular overload.

Indomethacin (Indocin) may be used if fluid management and diuretics fail to significantly decrease the left-to-right ductal shunting. Indomethacin, a prostaglandin inhibitor, promotes closure of the ductus. Its side effects include transitory changes in renal function, increased incidence of occult blood loss via the GI tract, and inhibition of platelet function for 7 to 9 days. Contraindications for the use of indomethacin are as follows:

1. Blood urea nitrogen (BUN) greater than 30 mg/dl
2. Creatinine levels higher than 1.8 mg/dl
3. Urine output of less than 0.6 ml/kg/hr over the preceding 8 hours

4. Platelet count lower than $60,000/mm^3$, because it prolongs platelet activity
5. Stool hematest greater than 3+ (or moderate to large) because GI bleeding has been reported
6. Clinical or x-ray evidence of necrotizing enterocolitis (NEC)
7. Evidence of enlarging central nervous system (CNS) hemorrhage
8. Sepsis, proven or strongly suspected

The ductus reopens in 30% of the patients treated with indomethacin.

Digitalis is controversial and contraindicated in premature infants. It increases the force of contraction of the heart, increases the stroke volume and cardiac output, and decreases cardiac venous pressures. It is used to treat CHF and selected cardiac arrhythmias.

Medical management also includes prophylactic administration of antibiotics to prevent bacterial endocarditis. In older children, there are no exercise restrictions if there is no evidence of pulmonary hypertension.

Surgical management consists of patent ductus arteriosus repair. There are two major categories of children who have been identified as requiring this surgery. The first includes infants with congestive heart failure, usually premature neonates who did not respond to indomethacin therapy. Children more than 1 year of age whose ductus did not close spontaneously (and who are at risk for pulmonary hypertension and subacute endocarditis) make up the second group. Both groups require a left thoracotomy incision, and bypass is unnecessary. Infants are usually at greater risk for complications, so the PDA is doubly ligated in a comparatively quick procedure. For older children, surgery is advised during their preschool years and is performed by dividing the ductus between clamps and suturing the ends closed. A procedure for closing the PDA during cardiac catheterization by depositing a "plug" in the ductus is a recent development being used in the United States.

The hemodynamic results of PDA ligation are truly curative, in contrast to the palliative procedures of many heart surgeries. Closure decreases the pulmonary flow while increasing the systemic flow, creating normal hemodynamics. Unfortunately, if severe pulmonary hypertension existed before surgery, closure will not reverse this process.

NURSING ASSESSMENT

1. See the section on cardiovascular and respiratory assessment in Appendix A.
2. Assess hydration status.
3. Assess child's temperature.
4. Assess postoperative pain.
5. Assess child and family coping strategies.

NURSING DIAGNOSES

- Decreased cardiac output
- Altered tissue perfusion
- Fluid volume excess
- Ineffective thermoregulation
- High risk for infection
- High risk for injury
- Altered family processes

NURSING INTERVENTIONS

1. Monitor cardiac and respiratory status (may need to monitor as often as every hour during acute phase).
2. Observe and report signs of changes in cardiac status (color, vital signs, peripheral perfusion, level of consciousness [LOC], activity level, signs of CHF).
3. Observe and report signs of respiratory distress and changes in respiratory status.
4. Monitor and report responses to ventilator assistance.
5. Assess for and maintain optimal hydration status.
   a. Limit intake of fluids (65 to 100 ml/kg/day).
   b. Monitor urinary output.
   c. Observe for signs of fluid overload.
6. Promote and maintain optimal body temperature.
   a. Use radiant warmer.
   b. Keep child covered.
7. Monitor action and side effects of medications.
   a. Diuretics (e.g., furosemide)—decrease fluid overload, increase urinary output

b. Indomethacin—inhibits prostaglandins, promotes closure of PDA
c. Digitalis—increases contractility of heart (monitor serum levels)
8. Monitor response to and side effects of blood transfusions.
9. Promote process of attachment between parents and infant.
10. Provide developmentally appropriate stimulation activities (see section on growth and development, Appendix B).

Preoperative Care

1. Allow parents to vent feelings; despite its being a relatively minor heart surgery, PDA repair is still overwhelming to parents.
2. Prepare child for surgery by obtaining assessment data.
   a. Complete blood count (CBC), urinalysis, serum glucose, BUN
   b. Baseline electrolytes
   c. Blood coagulation
   d. Type and cross match of blood
   e. Chest x-ray study, ECG
3. Because the older child is usually preschool age, prepare him or her accordingly; do not tell the child that surgery will make him or her "feel better," because he or she is usually asymptomatic.

Postoperative Care

1. Monitor child's or infant's cardiac status (see section on cardiovascular assessment, Appendix A).
   a. Vital signs (temperature, apical pulse, respiratory rate, blood pressure)
   b. Arterial blood pressure and central venous pressure (CVP)
   c. Peripheral pulses—quality and intensity
   d. Capillary refill time
   e. Presence of ascites (rare)
   f. Arrhythmias
2. Monitor for and report signs and symptoms of complications.
   a. Atelectasis

   b. Bleeding
   c. Chylothorax
   d. Hemothorax
   e. Pneumothorax
   f. Phrenic nerve damage
   g. Recurrent laryngeal nerve damage
3. Treat chylothorax if present.
   a. Provide and monitor child's intake of medium-chain triglyceride diet.
   b. Monitor for signs of respiratory distress.
4. Provide intensive pulmonary toilet.
   a. Perform postural drainage and percussion.
   b. Change child's position every 2 hours.
   c. Encourage deep breathing and use of spirometer hourly.
   d. Encourage coughing; if child cannot cough, use suction.
5. Provide intensive pain control, because pain with a thoracotomy incision is usually greater than with a median sternotomy.
6. Monitor child's response to medications.
   a. Diuretics
   b. Digitalis
7. Provide emotional support to infant or child during hospitalization.
   a. Use age-appropriate explanations before treatments.
   b. Encourage, through age-appropriate means, child's expression of fears and anxieties (e.g., verbal expression, play, drawings).
   c. Encourage parental expression of feelings.

♠ Discharge Planning and Home Care

1. Instruct parents to observe for and report signs of cardiac or respiratory distress.
2. Instruct parents about the administration of medications.
3. Provide parents with name of physician or nurse to contact for medical or health care follow-up.
4. Instruct parents about principles of infection control and well child care (e.g., use of prophylactic medications before dental care).

5. Encourage and instruct parents about providing developmentally appropriate stimulation activities (see section on growth and development, Appendix B).

CLIENT OUTCOMES

1. Adequate cardiac output will be achieved.
2. Respiratory compromise will be reduced.

REFERENCES

Clyman RI: Patent ductus arteriosus in the premature infant. In Taeusch HW et al, editors: *Schaeffer's diseases of the newborn,* ed 6, Philadelphia, 1991, WB Saunders.

Fryer DC: Patent ductus arteriosus. In Fryer DC, editor: *Nadas' pediatric cardiology,* St Louis, 1992, Mosby.

Huddleston K: Patent ductus arteriosus ligation: performing surgery outside the operating room, *AORN J* 53(1):69, 1990.

Lott, JW: Assessment and management of cardiovascular dysfunction. In Kenner C et al, editors: *Comprehensive neonatal nursing,* Philadelphia, 1993, WB Saunders.

58

Pneumonia

PATHOPHYSIOLOGY

Pneumonia is an inflammation or infection of the pulmonary parenchyma. Pneumonia is attributable to one or more agents: viruses, bacteria, mycoplasmas, and aspiration of foreign substances. The pattern of the illness is dependent on the following: (1) causative agent, (2) age of the child, (3) child's reaction, (4) extent of lesions, and (5) degree of bronchial obstruction. The clinical features of bacterial, viral, and mycoplasmal pneumonia are listed in the box on pp. 384-385.

INCIDENCE

1. Viral pneumonia occurs more frequently than bacterial pneumonia.
2. Staphylococcal pneumonia occurs most frequently during the first 2 years of life—in 30% of children with pneumonia who are less than 3 months old and in 70% of children with pneumonia who are less than 1 year old.
3. Pneumococcal pneumonia accounts for 90% of all lobar pneumonia.
4. Mycoplasmas rarely cause pneumonia in children less than 5 years old; they are associated with 20% of cases of pneumonia diagnosed in patients between 16 and 19 years of age.
5. Pneumonia is more severe and more common in infancy and early childhood.

Clinical Features of Bacterial, Viral, and Mycoplasmal Pneumonia

Bacterial Pneumonia

Staphylococcal, streptococcal, and pneumococcal pneumonia occur most frequently.

Initial symptoms
Mild rhinitis
Anorexia
Listlessness

Progresses to abrupt onset
Fever
Malaise
Rapid and shallow respiratory rate (50 to 80)
Expiratory grunt
Greater than 5 years old—headache and chills
Less than 2 years old—vomiting and mild diarrhea
Increased white blood count
Chest x-ray result—lobar pneumonia

Viral Pneumonia

Causative viruses include influenza virus, adenovirus, rubeola, varicella, human cytomegalovirus, and respiratory syncytial virus.

Initial symptoms
Cough
Rhinitis

Progresses to insidious or abrupt onset
Range of symptoms—mild fever, slight cough, and malaise to high fever, severe cough, and prostration

Viral Pneumonia—cont'd
  Obstructive emphysema
  Scattered rales, rhonchi
  Chest x-ray result—bronchopneumonia
  Decreased white blood count

Mycoplasmal Pneumonia

Initial symptoms
  Fever
  Chills
  Headache
  Anorexia
  Myalgia

Progresses to insidious or abrupt onset
  Rhinitis
  Sore throat
  Dry hacking cough—blood streaked
  Chest x-ray result—areas of
    consolidation

6. Respiratory syncytial virus (RSV) accounts for the largest percentage of viral pneumonia cases.
7. Viral respiratory tract infection is the second leading cause of death in infants and young children.
8. Mycoplasmal pneumonia accounts for 10% to 20% of hospital admissions.

CLINICAL MANIFESTATIONS

Major clinical signs include the following (see box for specific clinical manifestations):
  1. Cough
  2. Dyspnea
  3. Tachypnea
  4. Cyanosis

5. Decreased breath sounds
6. Retractions of chest wall
7. Nasal flaring
8. Abdominal pain (caused by irritation of the diaphragm by the adjacent infected lung)
9. Paroxysmal cough simulating pertussis (common in smaller children)
10. Older child does not appear as ill

COMPLICATIONS

1. Chronic interstitial pneumonia
2. Chronic segmental or lobar atelectasis
3. Airway damage
4. Pleural effusion
5. Pulmonary calcification
6. Pulmonary fibrosis
7. Obliterative bronchitis and bronchiolitis
8. Persistent atelectasis

LABORATORY AND DIAGNOSTIC TESTS

1. Chest x-ray studies—diagnostic; used to visualize the lungs for presence of infection and pulmonary status (to assess lung changes)
2. Blood gas values—to evaluate cardiopulmonary status in terms of oxygenation
3. Complete blood count (CBC) with differential—used to determine presence of anemia, infection, inflammatory process
4. Gram stain of blood—for initial antimicrobial selection
5. Tuberculin skin test—rules out tuberculosis if child does not respond to treatment
6. White blood count (WBC)—leukocytosis with bacterial pneumonia
7. Pulmonary function test—used to evaluate pulmonary function, determine extent and severity of disease, and assist in diagnosis of condition
8. Static spirometry—used to assess amount of inspired air
9. Blood culture—blood specimen obtained to identify causative agents such as viruses and bacteria

10. Culture of pleural fluid—specimen of fluid from pleural space obtained to identify causative agents such as bacteria and viruses
11. Bronchoscopy—used to visualize and manipulate the main branches of the tracheobronchial tree; tissue obtained for diagnostic testing therapeutically used to identify and remove foreign bodies
12. Lung biopsy—during thoracotomy, lung tissue is excised for diagnostic studies

MEDICAL MANAGEMENT

Medical treatment includes improving oxygenation with oxygen and respiratory treatments. Intravenous (IV) antibiotics are used to treat bacterial pneumonia based on culture and sensitivity testing. If pleural effusion occurs, thoracentesis or chest tube drainage may be warranted.

NURSING ASSESSMENT

1. See the section on respiratory assessment in Appendix A.
2. Assess patency of airway.
3. Assess for signs of respiratory distress and response to oxygen therapy.
4. Assess for signs of dehydration.
5. Assess child's response to medications.
6. Assess family's ability to manage home treatment regimen.

NURSING DIAGNOSES

- Ineffective airway clearance
- Impaired gas exchange
- High risk for fluid volume deficit
- High risk for altered body temperature: hyperthermia
- High risk for ineffective management of therapeutic regimen

NURSING INTERVENTIONS

1. Monitor airway and maintain patency.
   a. Place child in semi-Fowler's position.
   b. Provide mist therapy as ordered by physician.
   c. Perform postural drainage, percussion, and vibration as needed and tolerated by the child.
   d. Perform bulb or deep suction as needed.
   e. Provide for adequate rest.

2. Monitor for signs of respiratory distress and response to oxygen therapy.
   a. Monitor respiratory status.
   b. Perform care of mist tent.
   c. Change child's clothing and linens frequently to prevent chilling.
   d. Observe for signs of complications (see section on complications, this chapter).
3. Monitor for and maintain optimal hydration status.
   a. Monitor administration of IV fluids.
   b. Record strict intake and output.
   c. Monitor for dehydration.
4. Monitor child's therapeutic response to and side effects from medications (for bacterial pneumonia—nafcillin, gentamicin, methicillin, oxacillin, penicillin G, erythromycin).
5. Control fever with antipyretics and sponge bath with tepid water.
6. Teach parents how to care for infant on IV and oxygen therapy.

♠ Discharge Planning and Home Care

1. Instruct parents about the administration of medications.
   a. Appropriate dose, route, and time, and completing entire dose
   b. Side effects
   c. Child's response
2. Provide information to parents about measures for infection control and prevention.
   a. Avoid exposure to infectious contacts.
   b. Adhere to immunization schedule.

CLIENT OUTCOMES

1. Child will not have signs or symptoms of respiratory distress.
2. Child will have adequate hydration.
3. Parent will provide comfort to child in spite of IV and/or oxygen therapy.

REFERENCES

Everett D: For a child with pneumonia, there's no place like home, *RN* 53(3):85, 1990.

LeBlanc K, Forestell F: Assessment of the neonatal respiratory system, *AACN: Clin Issues Crit Care Nurs* 1(2):401, 1990.

Sheahan S, Seabolt J: *Chlamydia trachomatis* infections: a health problem of infants, *J Pediatr Health Care* 3(3):144, 1989.

Steele R: Drugs for viral respiratory tract infections, *Choices Resp Manag* 20(5):109, 1990.

Winthrop AL, Waddell T, Superina RA: The diagnosis of pneumonia in the immunocompromised child: use of bronchoalveolar lavage, *J Pediatr Surg* 25(8):878, 1990.

59

Poisoning

INCIDENCE

1. Poisoning is the most prevalent injury in children.
2. It is the fourth leading cause of death in children 1 to 4 years old.
3. The most common poisonings are from nonprescription drugs (e.g., cough and cold preparations, analgesics, and topical agents).
4. Nonpharmaceutical agents ingested are household cleaners, plants, cosmetics, and beauty aids.
5. Most poisonings take place in the home; the most common location is the child's own home, and the second is the grandparents' home.
6. Times of peak incidence are mealtimes, weekends, and holidays.
7. The peak age of incidence is between 1 and 2 years, when a child is autonomous and exploring.

CLINICAL MANIFESTATIONS

The manifestations depend on the agent that is ingested. The following are some examples:

1. Hyperthermia or hypothermia
2. Tachycardia or bradycardia
3. Salivation
4. Diarrhea
5. Seizures
6. Lethargy

7. Dry mouth
8. Dilated pupils
9. Ileus
10. Urinary retention

COMPLICATIONS

1. Cardiac arrest
2. Respiratory arrest
3. Esophageal or tracheal corrosion if caustic substance is ingested

LABORATORY AND DIAGNOSTIC TESTS

1. Blood screen
2. Urine screen

MEDICAL MANAGEMENT

Children who have ingested a poison may require initial stabilization ("A,B,Cs"). If an antidote is appropriate, it should be given. Otherwise, decontamination by decreasing absorption or hastening elimination through the gastrointestinal (GI) system should be instituted, depending on the substance ingested. Treatments include emetic agents like syrup of ipecac, orogastric lavage, activated charcoal, or cathartic lavage.

NURSING ASSESSMENT

1. A detailed history is essential (agent ingested, dose, time of ingestion, underlying problems of the child, age and weight of the child, signs and symptoms produced, treatment rendered).
2. A complete system-by-system assessment must be made (see Appendix A).
3. After the child is stabilized or during a well-child visit around 6 months of age, the status of childproofing the house must be assessed.

NURSING DIAGNOSES

- High risk for injury
- Anxiety
- Knowledge deficit

NURSING INTERVENTIONS

1. Monitor patient during decontamination procedures and until stable.
2. Provide emotional support to child and family (refer to Appendix J, section on supportive care).

♠ Discharge Planning and Home Care

Teach parents about poison-proofing at home and poison management.

1. Make sure that all poisonous substances and medicines remain in their original containers, have child-resistant caps, and are out of reach of children.
2. Have a bottle of syrup of ipecac available.
3. Post poison control center number on telephone.

CLIENT OUTCOMES

1. Child will have minimal injuries related to the poisoning.
2. Parents will ventilate their fears and concerns.
3. Parents will understand the child's developmental level as it relates to childproofing the house and supervising the child appropriately.

REFERENCES

Castiglia PT: Pica, *J Pediatr Health Care* 7:174, 1993.
Swartz MK: Poison prevention, *J Pediatr Health Care* 7:143, 1993.
Woolf AD, Anderson A: The diagnosis and initial management of pediatric poisonings, *Emerg Care Quart* 6(3):7, 1990.

60

Renal Failure: Acute

PATHOPHYSIOLOGY

Acute renal failure (ARF) is the abrupt reduction or cessation of renal function resulting in a variety of physiologic disturbances in homeostasis. The predominant signs of renal failure are (1) oliguria or anuria, (2) electrolyte imbalances, (3) acid and base imbalances, and (4) impaired secretion of waste products (urea and creatinine).

The three types of renal failure are prerenal, intrarenal, and postrenal. Acute prerenal failure results from decreased blood flow to the kidneys. Acute intrarenal failure results from injury to the kidney cells. Acute postrenal failure results from urinary outflow obstruction. The disease processes that result in renal failure are categorized according to type (see the box on p. 394).

The four phases of acute renal failure represent the stages of the clinical course. The onset phase begins with the precipitating event and continues until the patient develops oliguria. The oliguria and anuria (low output) phase continues until the kidney begins to produce urine. The diuretic (high output) phase begins with a sudden onset of diuresis and continues until urine output normalizes. The recovery phase begins with the stabilization of lab values and continues until normal renal function returns.

Causes of Acute Renal Failure

Prerenal (Hypoperfusion)

- Dehydration
- Sepsis
- Shock
- Cardiac failure
- Burns
- Vascular fluid shifts (third-space losses)
- Hemorrhage
- Renal artery thrombosis
- Hypoxic ischemic events
- Medications that cause renal vasoconstriction or hypotension

Intrarenal (Intrinsic)

- Unresolved prerenal failure resulting in kidney cell damage
- Hemolytic-uremic syndrome
- Glomerulonephritis
- Interstitial nephritis
- Septicemia
- Nephrotoxic agents
- Structural kidney abnormalities
- Acute tubular necrosis
- Tubular damage and/or obstruction from a variety of sources
- Renal vasculitis

Postrenal (Obstruction)

- Renal calculi
- Thrombosis
- Developmental structural abnormalities (urethral valves, ureteropelvic junction)
- Tumors (Wilms')
- Inflammation

INCIDENCE

1. Incidence and prognosis vary according to the following factors: age, etiology, associated problems, underlying condition, geographic location, and type of treatment.
2. Prerenal failure accounts for approximately 40% of all cases of ARF in children.
3. Hemolytic-uremic syndrome is the most common cause of ARF in the United States.
4. Approximately 70% of the cases of ARF in infants under 1 year of age occur within the first week of life.

CLINICAL MANIFESTATIONS

In critically ill children, clinical manifestations of ARF are overshadowed by the precipitating disease process. Although patients' symptoms will vary with different disease processes, the most common symptoms associated with ARF are the following:

1. Oliguria and/or anuria
2. Fluid retention and edema—weight gain, periorbital edema, dependent edema, external genitalia swelling, facial edema, ascites, and circulatory congestion
3. Hypertension
4. Electrolyte imbalance
5. Lethargy
6. Weakness
7. Anemia (related to deficient red blood cell [RBC] production and/or RBC destruction)
8. Cardiac arrhythmias (related to hyperkalemia)
9. Tachypnea (related to metabolic acidosis and fluid retention)
10. Seizures (related to hyponatremia and hypocalcemia)
11. Growth failure and muscle wasting (long term)

COMPLICATIONS

1. Fluid balance complications—fluid overload or intravascular volume depletion (from third-space losses)
2. Complications from electrolyte imbalances—cardiac arrest, seizures
3. Cardiovascular complications—congestive heart failure, hypertension, hypotension, arrhythmias, cardiac arrest

4. Neurologic complications—altered level of consciousness, seizures, intracranial bleeding (in newborn infants)
5. Respiratory complications—pulmonary edema, respiratory failure
6. Bleeding (from coagulopathies)
7. Pruritis and skin breakdown
8. Infection
9. Malnutrition (from decreased caloric intake)
10. Untoward side effects from steroids

LABORATORY AND DIAGNOSTIC TESTS

1. Blood tests
   a. Blood urea nitrogen (BUN) and serum creatinine—increased
   b. Serum sodium and calcium—decreased
   c. Serum potassium and phosphorus—increased
   d. Serum pH and bicarbonate (HCO_3)—decreased (metabolic acidosis)
   e. Hemoglobin, hematocrit, platelet count—decreased (with decreased white blood cell and platelet function)
   f. Serum albumin—decreased
   g. Serum glucose—decreased (most common in infants)
   h. Serum uric acid—increased
   i. Blood cultures—positive (with systemic infection)
2. Urine tests
   a. Urinalysis—RBCs and/or casts
   b. Urine electrolytes, osmolality, and specific gravity—vary with disease process and stage of ARF
3. Electrocardiogram (ECG)—changes associated with electrolyte imbalance and heart failure
4. Chest and abdominal x-ray studies—changes associated with fluid retention

MEDICAL MANAGEMENT

1. Determine the type of ARF through evaluation of the child's history, symptoms, and laboratory results.
2. Stabilize the fluid and electrolyte balance.
   a. Administer fluids as needed to maintain adequate circulation.
   b. Administer diuretics to assist in the elimination of excess fluid.

    c. Initiate dialysis (peritoneal or hemodialysis) as indicated for patients with severe fluid retention, electrolyte imbalances, and/or acidosis.

    d. Correct electrolyte imbalances.

       (1) Correct hyperkalemia (Kayexalate, glucose, insulin, calcium gluconate, sodium bicarbonate, dialysis).

       (2) Increase serum sodium, calcium, and glucose with intravenous (IV) infusions.

3. Support cardiovascular function.

    a. Decrease excess fluids.

    b. Control hypertension.

    c. Maintain circulating volume.

4. Prevent infection (antibiotics).

5. Support nutrition (IV nutrition with adequate protein).

6. Control bleeding and anemia (blood product administration).

NURSING ASSESSMENT

1. See the section on genitourinary assessment in Appendix A.

2. Assess for signs and symptoms of fluid volume excess (edema; taut, shiny skin; intake greater than output; and weight gain).

3. Assess for signs and symptoms of decreased cardiac output, fluid volume deficit, and ineffective breathing pattern.

4. Assess for signs and symptoms of these potential collaborative problems: shock, infection, fluid overload, hypertension, heart failure, pulmonary edema, electrolyte imbalances, disseminated intravascular coagulation (DIC), coma, and seizures.

5. Assess for signs and symptoms of infection.

6. Assess child's level of activity and coping response.

7. Assess family's ability to manage their child's long-term care.

NURSING DIAGNOSES

- Fluid volume excess
- High risk for fluid volume deficit
- Decreased cardiac output
- Ineffective breathing pattern

- High risk for injury
- High risk for impaired skin integrity
- High risk for infection
- Activity intolerance
- Pain
- High risk for altered growth and development
- High risk for ineffective management of therapeutic regimen

NURSING INTERVENTIONS

1. Monitor and maintain fluid balance.
   a. Assess hydration status every 4 to 6 hours during acute phase.
   b. Replace fluids lost as a result of interstitial fluid shifts.
   c. Monitor type of fluids and administration rate to avoid fluid overload and cerebral edema while maintaining adequate circulating volume.
   d. Record accurate input and output.
   e. Record daily weights.
   f. Monitor blood pressure and distal perfusion (pulses, capillary refill, temperature, color).
   g. Monitor arterial pressure and central venous pressure (CVP).
   h. Administer diuretics and assess effectiveness.
   i. Monitor and maintain patency of dialysis catheters.
2. Monitor electrolytes and observe for signs of imbalances.
   a. Hyperkalemia—muscular irritability, ECG changes (peaked T wave, wide QRS complex, prolonged PR interval), cardiac arrhythmias
   b. Hypocalcemia—coma, convulsions
   c. Hyponatremia—seizures
   d. Hypoglycemia—seizures
3. Observe for and report signs and symptoms of impending complications.
   a. Shock
   b. Infection
   c. Fluid overload
   d. Hypertension
   e. Heart failure
   f. Respiratory complications—pulmonary edema
   g. Potassium intoxication

    h. Bleeding—DIC
    i. Malnutrition
    j. Anemia
    k. Neurologic disturbance—lethargy, coma, seizures
4. Monitor for therapeutic and untoward responses to administered medications.
5. Prevent infection.
    a. Be aware that patient must cough and deep breathe.
    b. Perform mouth and skin care.
    c. Perform care for all invasive catheters and lines.
    d. Protect child from infectious contacts.
6. Prepare child and family for dialysis if indicated.
    a. Fluid volume overload causing congestive heart failure or pulmonary edema
    b. Intractable hyperkalemia
    c. Intractable acidosis
    d. Severe uremic symptoms
    e. Change in neurologic status
    f. Bleeding
    g. Intractable hypernatremia
    h. Severe calcium imbalances
    i. Inability to support nutritional status because of fluid overload
    j. BUN greater than 100 mg/dl
7. Encourage child and parents to ventilate feelings of concern about child's condition.
8. Provide developmentally appropriate information, and reinforce data provided to child and parents (see Appendix J, section on preparation for procedure/surgery).
9. Monitor for and alleviate child's pain (see Appendix I).

♠ Discharge Planning and Home Care

If ARF has not resolved before discharge, provide child and parents with developmentally appropriate verbal and written instruction regarding home management of the following (see section on home care, Appendix K):
1. Disease process (include expected clinical process and signs of complications)
2. Medications (dose, route, schedule, side effects, and complications)

3. Skin care
4. Nutrition
5. Prevention of infection
6. Follow-up care

CLIENT OUTCOMES

1. Child's fluid and electrolyte balance will be within normal limits.
2. Child will not demonstrate signs and symptoms of impending complications.
3. Child and family will demonstrate sense of mastery in dealing with disease process.

REFERENCES

Baer C, Lancaster L: Acute renal failure, *Crit Care Nurs Q* 14(4):1, 1992.

Behrman R et al: *Nelson textbook of pediatrics*, ed 14, Philadelphia, 1992, WB Saunders.

Feld L, Cachero S, Springate J: Fluid needs in acute renal failure, *Pediatr Clin North Am* 37:337, 1990.

Kennedy J: Renal Disorders. In Hazinski M, editor: *Nursing care of the critically ill child*, ed 2, St Louis, 1992, Mosby.

Rahman M, Hossain M: The bimodal mortality pattern of acute renal failure in children, *Ren Fail* 15(1):55, 1993.

Stork J: Acute renal failure. In Blumer J, editor: *A practical guide to pediatric intensive care*, ed 3, St Louis, 1990, Mosby.

61

Renal Failure: Chronic

PATHOPHYSIOLOGY

Chronic renal failure (CRF) is the long-term deterioration of renal function resulting in the inability to maintain body substances under normal living conditions. Causes of CRF are associated with a variety of congenital and acquired factors including (1) glomerular disease (e.g., pyelonephritis, glomerulonephritis, glomerulouropathy), (2) obstructive uropathies (e.g., reflux), (3) renal hypoplasia (e.g., segmental hypoplasia or dysplasia), (4) inherited renal disorders (e.g., polycystic kidney disease, congenital nephrotic syndrome, Alport syndrome), (5) vascular neuropathies (e.g., hemolytic-uremic syndrome, renal thrombosis), and (6) severe renal trauma.

CRF has been associated with a variety of types of biochemical dysfunction. Sodium and fluid imbalances result from the kidney's inability to concentrate urine. Hyperkalemia results from decreased potassium secretion. Metabolic acidosis results from impaired reabsorption of bicarbonate and decreased ammonia production. Bone demineralization and impaired growth result from secretion of parathyroid hormone, elevation of plasma phosphate (decreasing serum calcium), acidosis (causing calcium and phosphorus release into the bloodstream), and impaired intestinal calcium absorption. Anemia results from impaired red blood cell (RBC) production, decreased RBC life span, and an increased tendency to bleed (due to impaired platelet function). Encephalopathy and neuropathy have been associated with the accumulation of uremic toxins. Altered growth and sexual maturation have been associated with altered nutrition and a variety of biochemical processes.

INCIDENCE

1. The incidence of CRF in children has been estimated at 18.5 per 1 million children.
2. The incidence of end-stage renal failure in children has been estimated at 3 to 6 per 1 million children.
3. Congenital renal and urinary tract malformations (renal hypoplasia, renal dysplasia, obstructive uropathies, and vesicourethral reflux) are the most frequent causes of CRF in children under 5 years of age.
4. Glomerulonephritis is the chief cause of acquired CRF in children.

CLINICAL MANIFESTATIONS

Although the child's symptoms will vary with different disease processes, the most common symptoms associated with CRF are the following:

1. Fluid imbalance
   a. Fluid overload—edema, oliguria, hypertension, congestive heart failure
   b. Vascular volume depletion—polyuria, decreased fluid intake, dehydration
2. Electrolyte imbalance
   a. Hyperkalemia—cardiac rhythm disturbances, myocardial dysfunction
   b. Hypernatremia—thirst, stupor, tachycardia, dry membranes, increased deep tendon reflexes, decreased level of consciousness
   c. Hypocalcemia and hyperphosphatemia—irritability, depression, muscle cramps, paresthesias, psychosis, tetany, Trousseau's sign, Chvostek's sign
   d. Hypokalemia—decreased deep tendon reflexes, hypotonia, electrocardiogram (ECG) changes
3. Uremic neuropathy and encephalopathy
   a. Itching (uremic frost skin deposits)
   b. Muscle cramps and weakness

    c. Slurred speech
    d. Paresthesia of the palms and/or soles
    e. Poor concentration, memory loss
    f. Drowsiness
    g. Signs of elevated intracranial pressure (ICP)
    h. Coma
    i. Seizures
4. Acidosis—tachypnea
5. Anemia and blood cell dysfunction
    a. Pallor
    b. Weakness
    c. Bleeding (stomatitis, bloody stools)
6. Growth dysfunction
    a. Abnormal bone growth
    b. Delayed sexual development
    c. Malnutrition and muscle wasting
    d. Poor appetite
    e. Bone pain
    f. Menstrual irregularities

COMPLICATIONS

1. Fluid balance complications—fluid overload or intravascular volume depletion
2. Complications from electrolyte imbalances—cardiac dysrhythmias, arrest, seizures
3. Cardiovascular complications—congestive heart failure, hypertension, left-ventricular hypertrophy, arrhythmias, cardiac arrest, hypotension (with dehydration)
4. Neurologic complications—altered level of consciousness, increased ICP, seizures
5. Respiratory complications—pulmonary edema, respiratory failure
6. Bleeding
7. Infection
8. Hypoglycemia
9. Hypertensive retinopathy
10. Malnutrition and growth retardation
11. Delayed sexual development
12. Osseous and dental malformations (renal rickets)
13. Mental retardation

LABORATORY AND DIAGNOSTIC TESTS

1. Blood tests
   a. Blood urea nitrogen (BUN) and serum creatinine—increased
   b. Serum potassium—increased (decreased with diuretics and/or restricted intake)
   c. Serum sodium—increased (decreased with hemodilution and/or restricted intake)
   d. Serum calcium—decreased
   e. Serum phosphorus—increased
   f. Serum pH and bicarbonate (HCO_3)—decreased (metabolic acidosis)
   g. Hemoglobin, hematocrit, platelet count—decreased (with decreased white blood cell and platelet function)
   h. Serum glucose—decreased (most common in infants)
   i. Serum uric acid—elevated
   j. Blood cultures—positive (with systemic infection)
2. Urine tests
   a. Urinalysis—RBCs and/or casts
   b. Urine electrolytes, osmolality, and specific gravity—vary with disease process
   c. Twenty-four–hour urine sodium collection—quantifies sodium secretion
3. Electrocardiogram—changes associated with electrolyte imbalance and heart failure
4. Chest and abdominal x-ray studies—changes associated with fluid retention
5. Diagnostic procedures
   a. Renal biopsy
   b. Renal scan
   c. Renal ultrasound
   d. Magnetic resonance imaging (MRI), computed axial tomography (CAT) scan
   e. Voiding cystourethrogram

MEDICAL MANAGEMENT

1. Stabilize the fluid and electrolyte balance.
   a. Administer fluids as needed to maintain adequate circulation.

    b. Administer diuretics to assist in the elimination of excess fluid.

    c. Correct electrolyte imbalances.

       (1) Correct hyperkalemia (Kayexalate, glucose, insulin, calcium gluconate, sodium bicarbonate, dialysis) and restrict dietary potassium.

       (2) Administer calcium (by mouth [po] or intravenous [IV] route) and encourage dietary calcium intake.

       (3) Restrict dietary sodium.

       (4) Correct hypoglycemia.

2. Support cardiovascular function.

    a. Limit excess fluids.

    b. Control hypertension (antihypertensive medication).

    c. Maintain circulating volume.

3. Prevent infection (antibiotics, avoidance of invasive lines).

4. Support nutrition (adequate protein, enteral tube feedings as needed, multivitamins).

5. Control bleeding and anemia (blood products, recombinant human erythropoietin).

6. Initiate dialysis (peritoneal or hemodialysis) as indicated for children with untreatable, severe complications of CRF: fluid retention (cardiac or pulmonary compromise), electrolyte imbalances, acidosis, central nervous system (CNS) dysfunction, bone deformation, and/or bone marrow depression.

7. Initiate renal transplantation as appropriate.

NURSING ASSESSMENT

1. See the section on genitourinary assessment in Appendix A.

2. Assess for signs and symptoms of fluid volume excess (edema; taut, shiny skin; intake greater than output; and weight gain).

3. Assess for signs and symptoms of decreased cardiac output, fluid volume deficit, and ineffective breathing pattern.

4. Assess for signs and symptoms of these potential collaborative problems: shock, infection, fluid overload, hypertension, heart failure, pulmonary edema, electrolyte

imbalances, disseminated intravascular coagulation (DIC), coma, and seizures.
5. Assess for signs and symptoms of infection.
6. Assess child's growth and biopsychosocial and spiritual development.
7. Assess child's level of activity and coping response.
8. Assess family's ability to manage and cope with their child's long-term care and needs.

NURSING DIAGNOSES

- Fluid volume excess
- High risk for fluid volume deficit
- Altered patterns of urinary elimination
- Decreased cardiac output
- Ineffective breathing pattern
- High risk for impaired skin integrity
- High risk for injury
- High risk for infection
- Altered nutrition: less than body requirements
- High risk for ineffective management of therapeutic regimen
- High risk for altered family processes
- High risk for altered growth and development

NURSING INTERVENTIONS

1. Monitor fluid and electrolyte status.
   a. Record accurate intake and output.
   b. Maintain fluid limit.
   c. Monitor hydration status.
   d. Administer diuretics and monitor response.
   e. Administer medications to maintain electrolyte balance.
   f. Monitor for signs of electrolyte imbalances.
   g. Administer dialysis therapy as ordered.
2. Support cardiovascular and pulmonary functioning.
   a. Monitor for fluid volume overload.
   b. Monitor for signs of dehydration.
   c. Monitor for ECG changes related to electrolyte imbalance.
   d. Monitor vital signs, including blood pressure; administer antihypertensives as indicated.
   e. Administer blood products as ordered; assess for signs of transfusion reaction.

3. Maintain skin integrity and prevent infection.
   a. Provide daily bath and frequent mouth care.
   b. Assist the patient with turning as needed; prevent pressure ulceration.
   c. Use bleeding precautions (soft toothbrush, avoidance of needle sticks).
   d. Avoid patient's contact with infectious visitors.
   e. Maintain sterility of all invasive lines, and perform dressing changes and site care as needed and on schedule.
   f. Monitor for signs of infection (fever, lethargy, nausea, vomiting, diarrhea), and begin antibiotic therapy promptly.
4. Promote growth and nutrition (work with dietitian).
   a. Assist patient in finding appetizing choices in a low-potassium, low-sodium, low-phosphorus, high-calcium, high-protein diet.
   b. Monitor patient's growth status by assessing growth trends.
   c. Administer enteral or IV nutrition as needed.
   d. Administer vitamins, calcium supplements, and phosphate binders.
5. Provide psychosocial support to patient and family (see Appendix J, section on supportive care).

♠ Discharge Planning and Home Care

Provide child and parents with developmentally appropriate verbal and written instruction regarding home management of the following (see Appendix K):

1. Disease process (include expected clinical progress and signs of complications)
2. Medications (dose, route, schedule, side effects, and complications)
3. Skin care and bleeding precautions
4. Nutrition (dietary restrictions and supplements)
5. Prevention of infection (wound and/or line care if indicated)
6. Home dialysis therapy (if indicated)
7. Follow-up care and long-term treatment plan
8. Child's developmental needs

CLIENT OUTCOMES

1. Child will maintain electrolyte and fluid balance within appropriate limits.
2. Child will be free of infection.
3. Child and family will adhere to treatment regimen without the occurrence of complications.

REFERENCES

Behrman R et al: *Nelson textbook of pediatrics,* ed 14, Philadelphia, 1992, WB Saunders.

Fine R: Recent advances in the management of the infant, child and adolescent with chronic renal failure, *Pediatr Rev* 11:277, 1990.

Fine R, Saulsky I, Ettenger R: The therapeutic approach to the infant, child and adolescent with end-stage renal disease, *Pediatr Clin North Am* 34:789, 1990.

Innerarity S: Electrolyte emergencies in the critically ill renal patient, *Crit Care Nurs Clin North Am* 2(1):89, 1990.

Kennedy J: Renal disorders. In Hazinski M, editor: *Nursing care of the critically ill child,* ed 2, St Louis, 1992, Mosby.

Knight F et al: Hemodialysis of the infant or small child with chronic renal failure, *ANNA Journal* 20:35, 1993.

62

Renal Transplant

PATHOPHYSIOLOGY

Renal transplant is the treatment of choice for children with irreversible renal failure. Primary diseases that can lead to the need for a renal transplant include acquired diseases such as chronic glomerulonephritis, lupus, pyelonephritis, hemolytic-uremic syndrome, and bilateral Wilms' tumor. It is also the treatment for congenital conditions such as polycystic disease, obstructive uropathy, cystinosis, and Alport syndrome. The mortality rate is higher in children than in adults who have transplants, especially when the kidney is obtained from cadaveric sources. Nevertheless, extended hemodialysis and renal transplant have increased the survival rate of children with irreversible renal failure. The major problem associated with a transplant is rejection of the kidney. Rejection can result from one of a variety of causes: cellular and/or humoral immune response, infection, and noncompliance. Other causes of graft failure include technical failure, renal artery stenosis, and medication toxicity. Long-term consequences of a transplant include retarded bone growth (short stature) and osteodystrophy. Pubertal development proceeds normally after successful transplantation.

INCIDENCE

1. Occurrence is 1 to 3 in a million in children less than 10 years old, and 3 to 5 in a million in children older than 10 years.

2. One-year graft survival rate for living-related transplants is 90%.
3. One-year graft survival rate for cadaver transplants is 80% to 85%.
4. Patient survival rate at 1 year after transplant is 95%.
5. Survival rates are decreased with subsequent grafts.

CLINICAL MANIFESTATIONS

Refer to specific renal condition (e.g., nephrotic syndrome).

COMPLICATIONS (AFTER TRANSPLANT)

1. Hyperacute, acute, or chronic rejection
   a. Fever
   b. Hypertension
   c. Graft tenderness
   d. Oliguria
   e. Proteinuria
   f. Anuria
2. Ureteral obstruction
3. Acute tubular necrosis
4. Bleeding at transplant site
5. Infection (peritonitis, *Candida* infections, cytomegalovirus infections, viral infections)
6. Corticosteroid toxicity
7. Surgical complications (lymphocele)
8. Need for transplant nephrectomy because of irreversible technical complications or hyperacute rejection

LABORATORY AND DIAGNOSTIC TESTS
Preoperative Evaluation

1. Extensive serologic studies, including general survey panel, complete blood count (CBC) with differential, platelets, viral screening, blood culture
2. Meticulous search for infection, including dental exams, sinus films
3. Electrocardiogram (ECG), chest x-ray study, voiding cystourethrogram (VCUG)

4. Urinalysis, urine culture and sensitivity, urine collection for creatinine clearance, and total protein
5. Histocompatibility testing
   a. ABO blood type
   b. Antibody screening
   c. Human leukocyte antigens (HLA) typing (A, B, C, D, DR)

Postoperative Tests

1. Blood urea nitrogen (BUN), creatinine, electrolytes, CBC, glucose
2. Renal scan
3. Cyclosporine levels
4. Urine for protein, creatinine, electrolytes
5. Renal biopsy (diagnostic for rejection)

SURGICAL MANAGEMENT

The operative procedure for kidney transplantation has become fairly standardized. Most often the transplanted kidney is placed extraperitoneally in the iliac fossa; the renal artery and vein are anastomosed to the external or common iliac artery and hypogastric vein. Intraperitoneal placement may be indicated in children for whom the transplanted kidney is too large to fit in the extaperitoneal space. Immunosuppression regimens vary by center, but most include cyclosporine, azathioprine, and corticosteroids to prevent rejection. Rejection is treated with high-dose steroids or polyclonal or monoclonal antibodies. Other medications include nystatin as a prophylactic for *Candida* infection in the mouth, diuretics for hypertension and edema, and antihypertensives, antibiotics, and antacids. The average length of stay following renal transplantation is 2 weeks. Medications must be taken for life, and close medical follow-up is required.

NURSING ASSESSMENT

1. See the section on renal assessment in Appendix A.
2. Assess hydration status.
3. Assess for signs and symptoms of infection.

NURSING DIAGNOSES

- High risk for infection
- Fluid volume excess
- Body image disturbance
- Fear
- Ineffective individual coping

NURSING INTERVENTIONS
Preoperative Care

Prepare donor, recipient, and family for transplantation.
1. Provide information about presurgical routine.
2. Reinforce information given about surgery.
3. Provide age-appropriate preprocedural or preoperative preparation.

Postoperative Care

1. Monitor for and report signs of kidney rejection.
2. Monitor vital signs and report significant changes because they may be indicators of rejection, bleeding, infection, or hypovolemic shock.
   a. Check vital signs every hour for 24 hours; if stable, then check vital signs every 4 hours.
   b. Check graft or fistula for patency.
3. Monitor urinary output; report any significant changes.
   a. Monitor urinary output hourly for 24 hours, then every 2 hours for 48 hours.
   b. Check for increased bleeding or clot formation.
   c. Check for decreased urinary output; then assess possible causes.
      (1) Check for catheter kinking.
      (2) Check for dehydration or hypovolemia.
      (3) Irrigate to remove clots.
4. Observe for drainage on dressing.
   a. Circle extent of drainage.
   b. Notify physician if drainage increases significantly.
5. Observe for child's therapeutic response to or untoward effects of medications.
6. Observe for and report signs and symptoms of possible complications.

♠ Discharge Planning and Home Care

1. Instruct child and family about the therapeutic responses and untoward reactions to medications.
2. Reinforce the necessity of being compliant with medical regimen.
3. Reinforce information provided about nutritional needs.
   a. High-calorie and high-protein diet
   b. Limited sugar
   c. Limited salt
4. Instruct about proper dental care (brushing and flossing).
5. Refer to appropriate community resources, clinics, agencies, or personnel for psychosocial needs.

CLIENT OUTCOMES

1. Child will have normal renal function.
2. Child will remain free of infection.
3. Child and family will understand and remain compliant with medications and follow-up.

REFERENCES

Baluarte HJ et al: Analysis of hypertension in children post renal transplantation—a report of the North American Pediatric Renal Transplant Cooperative Study (NAPRTCS), *Pediatr Nephrol* 8(5):570, 1994.

Fedic T: Immunosuppressive therapy in renal transplantation, *Crit Care Nurs Clin North Am* 2(1):123, 1990.

Fine RN, Tejani A, Sullivan EK: Pre-emptive renal transplantation in children: report of the North American Pediatric Renal Transplant Cooperative Study (NAPRTCS), *Clin Transplant* 8(5):474, 1994.

Sigardson-Poor K, Haggerty L: *Nursing care of the transplant recipient*, Philadelphia, 1990, WB Saunders.

63

Respiratory Distress Syndrome

PATHOPHYSIOLOGY

Respiratory distress syndrome (RDS), or hyaline membrane disease, remains one of the leading causes of neonatal mortality and morbidity. This disease is the result of the absence, deficiency, or alteration of the components of pulmonary surfactant. Surfactant, a lipoprotein complex, is an ingredient of the filmlike surface of each alveolus that prevents alveolar collapse. It is secreted from type II respiratory cells in the alveoli. When surfactant is inadequate, there is alveolar collapse and resulting hypoxia. Pulmonary vascular constriction and decreased pulmonary perfusion then occur, leading to progressive respiratory failure.

INCIDENCE

1. There is an inverse relationship to gestational age: the younger the infants, the greater the incidence of RDS. However, the occurrence of RDS appears to be more dependent on lung maturity than actual gestational age.
   a. Diagnosed in 90% of infants at 26 weeks gestation
   b. Diagnosed in 70% of infants at 30 weeks gestation
   c. Diagnosed in 25% of infants at 34 weeks gestation
   d. Diagnosed in less than 1% to 2% of infants at full term
2. RDS occurs twice as often in male individuals as in female individuals.

3. Incidence increases in full-term infants in the presence of certain factors.
   a. Diabetic mother who delivers at less than 38 weeks gestation
   b. Perinatal hypoxia
   c. Cesarean delivery without labor

CLINICAL MANIFESTATIONS

The following symptoms are observed in the first 6 to 8 hours of life:
1. Tachypnea (greater than 60 breaths per minute)
2. Intercostal and sternal retractions
3. Audible expiratory grunting
4. Nasal flaring
5. Cyanosis as hypoxemia increases
6. Decreasing lung compliance (paradoxical seesaw respirations)
7. Systemic hypotension (peripheral pallor, edema, capillary filling delayed by more than 3 to 4 seconds)
8. Decreased urinary output
9. Decreased breath sounds with rales
10. Tachycardia as acidosis and hypoxemia progress
    RDS is a self-limiting disease. Improvement is typically seen 48 to 72 hours after birth when type II alveolar cell regeneration occurs and surfactant is produced. Presentation and duration of symptoms may be altered with administration of artificial surfactant.

COMPLICATIONS

1. Acid base imbalance
2. Air leaks (pneumothorax, pneumomediastinum, pneumopericardium, pneumoperitoneum, subcutaneous emphysema, pulmonary interstitial emphysema)
3. Pulmonary hemorrhage
4. Bronchopulmonary dysplasia (BPD)—see Chapter 8, Bronchopulmonary Dysplasia
5. Apnea
6. Systemic hypotension
7. Anemia

8. Infection (pneumonia, septicemia)
9. Altered infant development and parenting behaviors

Complications Associated with Intubation

1. Endotracheal tube complications (displacement, dislodgement, occlusion, atelectasis after extubation, palatal grooves)
2. Tracheal lesions (erosion, granuloma, subglottic stenosis, necrotizing tracheobronchitis)

Complications Associated with Prematurity

1. Patent ductus arteriosus (PDA)
2. Intraventricular hemorrhage (IVH)
3. Retinopathy of prematurity (ROP)

LABORATORY AND DIAGNOSTIC TESTS

1. Chest x-ray studies
   a. Diffuse reticulogranular pattern with superimposed air bronchograms
   b. Central lung markings and heart border difficult to see; poor lung inflation
   c. Possible presence of cardiomegaly when other systems also involved (infants of diabetic mothers [IDM], hypoxia, congestive heart failure [CHF])
   d. Large thymic silhouette
   e. Whiteout (uniform granularity) with air bronchogram, indicating severe disease if present in first few hours
2. Arterial blood gases—respiratory and/or metabolic acidosis
3. Complete blood count
4. Serum electrolytes, calcium, sodium (Na^+), potassium (K^+), glucose
   Lecithin-sphingomyelin ratio and phosphatidylglycerol levels are beneficial in determining timing for labor induction or elective cesarean deliveries as a means of preventing RDS.

MEDICAL MANAGEMENT

1. Improve oxygenation and maintain optimal lung volume.
   a. Maintenance of PaO_2 of 50 to 80 mm Hg, $PaCo_2$ of 40 to 50, pH of at least 7.25

b. Surfactant replacement via endotracheal tube (ET)
c. Continuous positive airway pressure (CPAP) via nasal prongs to prevent volume loss during expiration
d. Mechanical ventilation via ET for severe hypoxemia (PaO_2 less than 50 to 60 mm Hg) and/or hypercapnia ($PaCO_2$ greater than 60 mm Hg)
e. Transcutaneous monitoring and pulse oximetry
f. Aerosol administration of bronchodilators
g. Chest physiotherapy
h. Additional cardiorespiratory options (high-frequency ventilation, extracorporeal membrane oxygenation [ECMO], nitric oxide, liquid ventilation)
2. Maintain temperature stabilization.
3. Provide appropriate fluid, electrolyte, and nutritional intake.
4. Monitor arterial blood gas levels, hemoglobin and hematocrit (H&H), and bilirubin.
5. Transfuse blood as needed to maintain hematocrit.
6. Maintain arterial line for monitoring of PaO_2 and blood sampling.
7. Administer medications as indicated.
    a. Diuretics to minimize interstitial edema
    b. $NaHCO_3$ for metabolic acidosis
    c. Antibiotics for associated infection
    d. Analgesics for pain and irritability
    e. Theophylline as a respiratory stimulant
    f. Vasopressors (dopamine, dobutamine)
    g. Corticosteroids to enhance lung maturity
    h. Bronchodilators
8. See Chapter 8 for management of ongoing problems.

NURSING ASSESSMENT

1. See the section on respiratory assessment in Appendix A.
2. Assess child's cardiorespiratory status.
3. Assess child's oxygenation.
4. Assess child's hydration status.
5. Assess child's nutritional status.
6. Assess child's developmental level.
7. Assess infant-family interaction.
8. Assess family's ability to cope with home care needs.

NURSING DIAGNOSES

- Impaired gas exchange
- Ineffective airway clearance
- Ineffective breathing pattern
- Altered nutrition: less than body requirements
- Hypothermia
- Altered tissue perfusion
- Altered growth and development
- Altered parenting
- Fluid volume excess
- High risk for ineffective management of therapeutic regimen

NURSING INTERVENTIONS

1. Maintain cardiorespiratory stability.
   a. Monitor depth, symmetry, and rhythm of respirations.
   b. Monitor rate, quality, and murmurs of heart sounds.
   c. Assess responsiveness to medical interventions: mechanical ventilation, aerosol administration, and surfactant replacement therapy.
   d. Monitor arterial blood gases (ABGs) and lab data.
   e. Monitor PaO_2 through pulse oximetry and/or transcutaneous monitoring.
   f. Monitor blood pressure and fluctuations with activity and treatments.
   g. Administer medications as indicated.
2. Optimize oxygenation.
   a. Monitor correlation between positioning and transcutaneous monitoring (TCM) readings.
   b. Coordinate delivery of routine care and procedures.
   c. Maintain ET or nasal prongs position and patency.
   d. Suction as needed.
   e. Administer sedatives and analgesics as needed.
   f. Maintain temperature stability.
3. Maintain appropriate fluid, nutrient, and caloric intake.
   a. Maintain intravenous (IV) access as needed.
   b. Administer feedings via most appropriate route for medical and developmental status.
   c. Record daily weights and weekly length and head circumference.

   d. Monitor and record intake and output (including blood products, urine, and stool); check pH and specific gravity.
4. Promote normal growth and development.
   a. Maintain therapeutic environment with controlled handling and appropriate stimulation.
   b. Identify individual stress and interaction cues.
   c. Coordinate nursing care and procedures with tolerance level of infant.
   d. Facilitate parent-infant interaction by teaching parents infant cues and encouraging parents to hold and provide some routine care for infant (e.g., feeding and bathing).
   e. Incorporate other immediate family members (siblings) into infant's care as soon as appropriate.

♠ Discharge Planning and Home Care

1. Monitor readiness for discharge (see Chapter 8).
2. Provide appropriate discharge instructions for parents (see Chapter 8).

CLIENT OUTCOMES

1. Infant will have optimal lung functioning with gas exchange and oxygenation sufficient for tissue perfusion and growth.
2. Infant will meet growth and development parameters appropriate for corrected age.
3. Parents are competent in care of their infant.

REFERENCES

Beachy P, Deacon J, editors: *Respiratory disorders in core curriculum for neonatal intensive care nursing,* Philadelphia, 1993, WB Saunders.

Fanaroff AA, Martin RJ: *Neonatal-perinatal medicine: diseases of fetus and infant,* ed 5, St Louis, 1992, Mosby.

Kenner C et al, editors: *Comprehensive neonatal nursing,* Philadelphia, 1993, WB Saunders.

Peters KL: Does routine nursing care complicate the physiologic status of the premature neonate with respiratory distress syndrome? *J Perinat Neonatal Nurs* 6(2):67, 1992.

Urrutia NL: Sorting the complexities of respiratory distress syndrome, *MCN* 16:308, 1991.

64

Respiratory Syncytial Virus

PATHOPHYSIOLOGY

Respiratory syncytial virus (RSV) is a highly contagious pathogen. Its primary effect is on the lower respiratory tract. RSV has an incubation period of 5 to 8 days, after which it usually causes "upper respiratory tract infection symptoms." The primary mode of transmission (similar to that of other respiratory pathogens) is contact with respiratory secretions by direct handling of patients or objects contaminated with the virus.

INCIDENCE

1. Annual epidemics occur during winter and early spring.
2. RSV affects any age group, but most often small children and infants under 2 years of age.
3. It tends to cause more severe illness in very young and debilitated children; infants age 6 weeks to 3 months and those with cardiac problems, pulmonary problems, or immune diseases are generally made most ill by RSV.

CLINICAL MANIFESTATIONS

1. Rhinorrhea and pharyngitis—usually the first symptoms
2. Progression to coughing and wheezing
3. Associated otitis media
4. Lower respiratory tract symptoms: bronchitis, pneumonia, and apnea

5. Air hunger, retractions, increased respiratory rate, and cyanosis
6. Hypoxemia

COMPLICATIONS

1. Respiratory distress leading to respiratory failure
2. Apnea

LABORATORY AND DIAGNOSTIC TESTS

1. Complete blood count (CBC) with differential
2. Chest x-ray studies
3. Nasal washing examination (enzyme immune assay [EIA])
4. Nasopharyngeal viral culture

MEDICAL MANAGEMENT

Treatment of this viral infection is supportive and is based on the severity of symptoms. In mild cases, humidified oxygen and intravenous fluids are administered. Children with significant respiratory distress require endotracheal intubation and mechanical ventilation. Ribavirin, an antiviral drug, may be administered. Ribavirin should be given to those children with congenital heart disease, bronchopulmonary dysplasia, immune deficiency, or respiratory failure.

NURSING ASSESSMENT

1. See the section on respiratory assessment in Appendix A.
2. Assess ability to clear the airway.
3. Assess hydration status.

NURSING DIAGNOSES

- Ineffective breathing pattern
- Impaired gas exchange
- Altered tissue perfusion
- Knowledge deficit

NURSING INTERVENTIONS

1. Suction as needed to clear airway.
2. Implement pulmonary toilet.
3. Position patient with the head of the bed elevated; allow position of comfort.

4. Administer oxygen.
5. Provide adequate fluid intake (intravenous [IV] and oral).
6. Strictly monitor intake and output.
7. Weigh patient daily.
8. Provide small, frequent meals.
9. Take isolation precautions.
10. Encourage parental education.

♠ Discharge Planning and Home Care

1. Instruct parents in pulmonary toilet as indicated.
2. Provide family education regarding the transmission of the virus and prevention of reinfection.

CLIENT OUTCOMES

1. The child will have a return to normal respiratory function.
2. The child will have effective airway clearance.

REFERENCES

Balfour-Lynn IM, Girdhar DR, Aitken C: Diagnosing respiratory syncytial virus by nasal lavage, *Arch Dis Child* 72(1):58, 1995.

Chiocca EM: RSV and the high-risk infant, *Pediatr Nurs* 20:565, 1994.

Singleton RJ et al: Hospitalizations for respiratory syncytial virus infection in Alaska Native children, *Pediatr Infect Dis J* 14(1):26, 1995.

Toms GL: Respiratory syncytial virus—how soon will we have a vaccine? *Arch Dis Child* 72(1):1, 1995.

65

Reye's Syndrome

PATHOPHYSIOLOGY

Reye's syndrome is a noninflammatory encephalopathy that is associated with fatty infiltration of the viscera and for which no other chemical or clinical explanation can be found.

Typically, symptoms are seen following a viral illness, but a definitive cause has not been identified. Viral infections most strongly associated with the onset of Reye's syndrome are influenza type A and type B, and varicella. In addition, the use of aspirin has been strongly linked to the onset of the syndrome, but it is not involved in every case. Even though the American Academy of Pediatrics and the Centers for Disease Control have issued warnings against the use of salicylates in children with possible varicella or influenza infection, the link between salicylates and Reye's syndrome remains a topic of intense discussion.

The widespread organ dysfunctions that accompany Reye's syndrome have led to speculation that the syndrome is the result of a universal mitochondrial insult from an unknown source. Abnormalities related to hepatic failure may occur, including enzyme elevations, coagulation disorders, and alterations in carbohydrate, amino acid, and lipid metabolism. Cerebral edema and neuronal necrosis are possible, and the usual cause of death is severe cerebral edema and brain tissue herniation. Other multisystem failures may occur, including myocardial failure, dehydration and shock, acute renal failure, peptic ulcers, pancreatitis, sepsis, and hypoglycemia.

Morbidity and mortality rates vary greatly from study to study, but overall, mortality rates have decreased dramatically in recent years. Early recognition and improved treatment are the most significant factors contributing to increased survival. The severity of the illness at the time of diagnosis correlates with the likelihood of recovery. Some children survive with profound intellectual and neurologic damage, whereas others have minimal to no sequelae. Psychiatric problems, including attention-focusing problems, anxiety disorders, and depression, are common in survivors. Vocal and speech disorders are also frequently reported disabilities.

INCIDENCE

1. Reye's syndrome is the major cause of noninfectious neurologic death following a viral illness in the pediatric age group.
2. Reye's syndrome occurs in infants and children of all age groups, with the highest incidence in children 5 to 14 years of age.
3. There is no gender preference.
4. Reye's syndrome occurs most frequently in winter months.
5. Reye's syndrome usually appears 5 to 7 days after a viral illness has resolved.

CLINICAL MANIFESTATIONS
Phase I

1. Recovery from a viral illness
2. Improvement of condition

Phase II

1. Acute deterioration about 5 to 7 days following phase I
2. Vomiting
3. Fever
4. Altered mental status that may deteriorate rapidly
5. Tachypnea
6. Hyperpnea
7. Increased intracranial pressure
8. Sluggish pupillary response

9. Seizures
10. Coma

See Table 9 for one of a variety of staging systems that establish criteria to assess the severity of Reye's syndrome.

COMPLICATIONS

1. Encephalopathy
2. Cerebral herniation
3. Hepatic failure
4. Multiple organ failure
5. Gastrointestinal hemorrhage
6. Pancreatitis (severe complication with poor prognosis)

LABORATORY AND DIAGNOSTIC TESTS

1. Serum transaminase values—elevated serum glutamic-oxaloacetic transaminase (SGOT) and serum glutamic-pyruvic transaminase (SGPT), to at least one and a half to two times normal values
2. Prothrombin and partial thromboplastin times—prolonged
3. Serum glucose—decreased
4. Serum amylase—elevated
5. Serum lactic dehydrogenase—elevated
6. Serum ammonia (hyperammonemia)—elevated to at least two times normal levels
7. Serum creatinine phosphokinase—elevated
8. Serum lipase—elevated
9. Serum bilirubin—usually normal
10. Liver biopsy—to define histopathologic features (usually with infants and atypical cases only)
11. Lumbar puncture—to rule out bacterial meningitis or viral encephalitis (controversial), elevated opening pressure
12. Computed tomography (CT) scan—to rule out other causes of encephalopathy
13. Electroencephalogram (EEG)—to predict survival

MEDICAL MANAGEMENT

Medical management is supportive and based on the child's stage of illness. Children with stage I Reye's syndrome must

Table 9. Staging of Reye's Syndrome

Criterion	Stage				
	I	II	III	IV	V
Level of consciousness	Lethargy; follows verbal commands; vomiting; sleepiness	Combative or stuporous; verbalizes inappropriately; disoriented	Coma	Coma; seizures	Coma; no respirations; flaccid paralysis
Posture	Normal	Normal	Decorticate	Decerebrate	Flaccid
Response to pain	Purposeful	Purposeful or nonpurposeful	Decorticate	Decerebrate	None
Pupillary reaction	Brisk	Sluggish	Sluggish	Sluggish	None
Oculocephalic reflex ("doll's eyes")	Normal	Conjugate deviation	Conjugate deviation	Inconsistent or absent	None

Modified from National Institutes of Health Consensus Development Conference, March 1981; Lovejoy FH et al: *Am J Dis Child* 128:136, 1974.

be hospitalized for close observation because progression of symptoms may occur rapidly. Intravenous (IV) hydration with a high-dextrose solution is needed to keep serum glucose levels normal. Children with stage II to V Reye's syndrome require aggressive therapy in a pediatric intensive care unit. Measures to normalize intracranial pressure and provide support to failing systems must be implemented. Restoration of a normal temperature and prevention of infection are priorities. The following medications may be used:

1. Anticoagulants
2. Sedatives
3. Vitamin K—for prothrombin deficiencies
4. Mannitol—osmotic diuretic to control intracranial hypertension
5. Vecuronium—for paralysis of skeletal muscles, to enhance ventilation

NURSING ASSESSMENT

1. See the section on neurologic assessment in Appendix A.
2. Assess respiratory pattern.
3. Assess hydration status.

NURSING DIAGNOSES

- Altered tissue perfusion: cerebral
- Fluid volume deficit
- Hyperthermia
- Altered nutrition: less than body requirements
- Anxiety

NURSING INTERVENTIONS

1. Maintain patency of airway.
   a. Monitor respiratory status.
   b. Check patency of endotracheal tube and airway.
   c. Check ventilator settings.
   d. Irrigate and suction as needed.
2. Monitor neurologic status with serial measures.
   a. Report any deterioration or questionable findings; intervention may be required on an emergency basis.
   b. Monitor level of consciousness.
      (1) General appearance
      (2) Arousability

      (3) Orientation

      (4) Restlessness

  c. Monitor vital signs.

      (1) Respiratory pattern

      (2) Blood pressure

      (3) Heart rate

      (4) Temperature

  d. Check pupils (pupils equal, react to light, accommodate [PERLA]).

  e. Monitor reaction to pain.

  f. Check head circumference (check fontanels).

  g. Use Glasgow Coma Scale (see section on neurologic assessment in Appendix A).

3. Avoid increase in intracranial pressure.

  a. Keep head in midline.

  b. Elevate head of bed 30 to 45 degrees.

  c. Avoid flexed knees.

  d. Avoid using restraints.

  e. Avoid child's crying.

  f. Provide calm, quiet environment.

4. Maintain adequate nutrition and fluid balance.

  a. Monitor nasogastric (NG) tube drainage.

  b. Monitor for residuals before feedings.

  c. Monitor infusion of hypertonic glucose and electrolytes.

  d. Monitor central venous pressure (CVP) and arterial pressure.

  e. Monitor intake and output.

5. Administer medications and monitor child's response.

  a. Therapeutic response

  b. Side effects

6. Monitor for complications.

  a. Atelectasis

  b. Hypoxia

  c. Respiratory disorders

  d. Coma

  e. Seizures

  f. Increased secretion of antidiuretic hormone (ADH)

7. Prevent skin breakdown through frequent skin care, change of position, and use of pressure mattress or sheepskin.

8. Provide lubrication to eyes to prevent drying and ulceration.
9. Use cooling measures.
10. Provide environmental stimulation (e.g., auditory and tactile) because child may be able to hear and feel even though unresponsive.

🏠 Discharge Planning and Home Care

1. Instruct parents about long-term management.
   a. Administration of medications
   b. Level of exercise
   c. Infection control
2. Give anticipatory guidance related to recovery.
   a. Abnormalities present in the early phase of recovery often improve or disappear completely in 6 to 12 months; the most common sequelae are motor and intellectual deficits.
   b. Hearing impairments have been reported and may require individual evaluation.
   c. Voice and speech disorders such as aphonia, slurred speech, and dysfluency may occur; severely impaired voice function does not necessarily imply that the child is intellectually impaired.

CLIENT OUTCOMES

1. The child's neurological function will be maximized.
2. The family will understand the rehabilitation plan.
3. The child's nutritional status will be normalized.

REFERENCES

LaJoie J, Sagy M, Gonzalez R: Reye's syndrome associated with acute myocarditis and fatal circulatory failure, *Pediatr Emerg Care* 7(4):226, 1991.

Levin D, Morriss F: *Essentials of pediatric intensive care,* St Louis, 1990, Quality Medical Publishing.

Mascarella J, Hudson D: Dysimmune neurologic disorders, *AACN Clinical Issues in Critical Care Nursing* 2(4):675, 1991.

Rogers ME: *Textbook of pediatric intensive care,* ed 2, Baltimore, 1992, Williams & Wilkins.

Thomas D: *Quick reference to pediatric emergency nursing,* Gaithersburg, Md, 1991, Aspen.

66

Rheumatic Fever: Acute

PATHOPHYSIOLOGY

Acute rheumatic fever is an inflammatory disease that follows a group A beta-hemolytic streptococcus infection. This disease causes pathologic lesions in the heart, blood vessels, joints, and subcutaneous tissue. The symptoms of rheumatic fever are manifested approximately 1 to 5 weeks after the infection occurs. The initial symptoms, as well as severity of the disease, are widely varied. Arthritis, in the form of migratory polyarthritis, is the most common symptom (75%) that is initially seen. Symptoms can be classified as cardiac and noncardiac and may develop gradually. Diagnosis is based on the revised Jones criteria from the American Heart Association (see the box on p. 431). Two major criteria or one major and two minor criteria indicate an increased possibility of rheumatic fever. Prognosis depends on the severity of cardiac involvement.

INCIDENCE

1. One out of 2000 children between the ages of 5 and 15 years is affected.
2. Crowded living conditions increase the risk of developing acute rheumatic fever.
3. There is increased frequency in male individuals.
4. There is an increased incidence among children who have previously had rheumatic fever.

Revised Jones Criteria

Major Criteria

- Arthritis
- Carditis
- Erythema marginatum
- Subcutaneous nodules
- Sydenham's chorea

Minor Criteria

- Previous history of rheumatic fever
- Arthralgia
- Elevated acute phase reactants
- Prolonged PR interval visible on electrocardiogram
- Fever

Evidence of Streptococcal Infection

- Positive culture
- Scarlatiniform rash
- Elevated streptococcal antibodies

From Stollerman G et al: Jones criteria (revised) for guidance in the diagnosis of rheumatic fever, *Circulation* 32:664, 1965. By permission of the American Heart Association, Inc.

5. A 30% to 67% incidence of heart disease occurs 10 years after an individual has had rheumatic fever.
6. There has been an increase in incidence in the United States and Europe since the late 1980s, possibly as a result of increased virulent strains or changes in medical management of acute pharyngitis.

CLINICAL MANIFESTATIONS

1. Arthritis—painful, warm, red, and swollen; knee, elbow, wrist, ankle most often affected
2. Arthralgia
3. Low-grade fever that usually spikes in late afternoon
4. Chest pain (symptom of carditis)
5. Shortness of breath (symptom of carditis)
6. Tachycardia—especially during rest or sleep
7. Bradycardia
8. Complaints of sore throat
9. Chorea
10. Subcutaneous nodules
11. Abdominal pain (symptom of carditis)
12. Cough (symptom of carditis)

COMPLICATION

Acquired heart disease is the primary complication of acute rheumatic fever.

LABORATORY AND DIAGNOSTIC TESTS

1. Echocardiography—to diagnose pericarditis
2. Pericardiocentesis—to diagnose pericarditis
3. Chest x-ray examination—to detect cardiomegaly
4. Electrocardiogram (ECG)—atrioventricular (AV) block and prolonged PR segment are present in carditis
5. Antistreptolysin O (ASO) titer—increased
6. Antihyaluronidase antibody titers—increased in presence of streptococcal antibodies
7. Nicotinamide adenine dinucleotidase (NADase), anti-NADase, and antideoxyribonuclease (antiDNAse) B—increased in presence of streptococcal antibodies
8. Streptozyme—a streptococcal antibody test can be performed in lieu of ASO titer
9. Erythrocyte sedimentation rate (ESR)—increased with inflammation
10. C-reactive protein—increased with inflammation
11. Throat culture—to diagnose streptococcus
12. White blood count (WBC)—increased with infections

MEDICAL MANAGEMENT

Treatment includes the administration of antibiotics to eliminate any residual streptococci and to prevent recurrent infections. Corticosteroids are used to treat acute cases of carditis. The child is closely observed to detect progressive cardiac abnormalities (valvulitis). The remaining management is symptom related and may include bed rest to conserve energy and decrease pain, aspirin to minimize arthritic pain, and nutritional support.

NURSING ASSESSMENT

1. See the section on cardiovascular and musculoskeletal assessment in Appendix A.
2. Assess for pain.
3. Assess temperature stability.
4. Assess activity level.
5. Assess nutritional status.

NURSING DIAGNOSES

- Activity intolerance
- Pain
- Hyperthermia
- Decreased cardiac output
- Altered family processes
- Anxiety
- Altered nutrition: less than body requirements
- Knowledge deficit

NURSING INTERVENTIONS

1. Conserve child's energy during acute phase of disease.
   a. Maintain bed rest until laboratory results and clinical status improve.
   b. As condition improves, monitor gradual increase in level of activity.
2. Monitor child's response to and possible untoward effects of prescribed medications.
   a. Assess for signs of clinical improvement.
   b. Monitor for side effects of the following medications: aspirin—bleeding tendencies, tinnitus; corticosteroids—cushingoid symptoms, increased weight gain, mood

swings, psychotic behavior; antibiotics (penicillin)—allergic rash, anaphylaxis.
3. Provide pain relief measures (for arthralgia).
   a. Minimize handling.
   b. Use bed cradle for sheets.
   c. Maintain proper body alignment.
   d. Administer aspirin.
   e. Change child's position every 2 hours.
4. Implement age-appropriate safety precautions (for chorea and muscle weakness).
5. Use cooling measures as needed.
6. Support and maintain nutritional status (child may be anorexic during acute phase).
   a. Offer small, frequent meals (include fluids).
   b. Incorporate child's food preferences.
   c. Encourage independence in eating when possible (muscle weakness may impose limits); choose items from menu; arrange foods attractively on tray; arrange meal schedule.
   d. Offer high-quality, nutritious foods.
7. Provide emotional support to child and family.
   a. Encourage parents to ventilate feelings.
   b. Encourage child to share feelings of helplessness, shame, and fear regarding manifestations of disease (e.g., chorea, carditis, and muscle weakness).
   c. Act as child and family advocate and liaison with members of the health care team.
   d. Encourage child's contact with peers.
   e. Encourage involvement in age-appropriate recreational and diversional activities.

🏠 Discharge Planning and Home Care

Instruct parents about methods of secondary prevention.
1. Observe for signs and symptoms of recurrence.
2. Administer prophylactic antibiotics (oral administered on continuous basis; intramuscular (IM) administered once per month) and explain rationale for use.
3. Obtain follow-up throat culture 4 or 5 days after oral penicillin is discontinued, 3 weeks after IM penicillin G benzathine is discontinued.

4. Assist in planning activities if child is to remain in bed after hospitalization.
5. Alert dentist about child's condition before any dental care.

CLIENT OUTCOMES

1. Child will have a return to normal musculoskeletal and cardiac function.
2. Pain will be eliminated.
3. Child and family will understand home care instructions and importance of need for follow-up visits and prophylactic antibiotics.

REFERENCES

Behrman R, Kleigman R: *Nelson essentials of pediatrics,* ed 2, Philadelphia, 1994, WB Saunders.

Grimes D, Woolbert L: Facts and fallacies about streptococcal infection and rheumatic fever, *J Pediatr Health Care* 4(4):186, 1990.

Ingalls J, Salerno C: *Maternal and child health nursing,* ed 7, St Louis, 1991, Mosby.

67

Scoliosis

PATHOPHYSIOLOGY

Scoliosis, a frequently occurring orthopedic problem, is the lateral curvature of the spine, which can occur anywhere along the spine. Curvatures in the thoracic area are the most common, although curves of the cervical and lumbar areas are the most deforming. There are two basic types of scoliosis: functional and structural. Functional scoliosis is secondary to a preexisting problem such as poor posture or unequal leg length. This form of scoliosis can be corrected through exercises or the use of shoe lifts. Structural scoliosis results from the congenital deformity of the spinal column. This condition often occurs in children with myelomeningocele and muscular dystrophy. The structural form of scoliosis can be classified into three basic types: (1) infantile, which occurs during the first year of life (more than 20% of affected children have spontaneous resolution); (2) juvenile, which occurs between 5 and 6 years of age (bracing is used for management); and (3) adolescent, which is not evident until 11 years of age (when skeletal maturation occurs). Management of scoliosis may include nonsurgical and/or surgical methods. Most spinal curvatures do not progress more than 20%. The curvature is flexible initially and becomes rigid with age.

INCIDENCE

1. Familial tendency is noted in one third of diagnosed cases.

2. Male-female ratio of occurrence is 1:6.
3. Adolescent scoliosis is the most common form.

CLINICAL MANIFESTATIONS

Localized lordosis, axial rotation, and lateral curvature of the spine are the major clinical manifestations of scoliosis.

1. Asymmetry of hips
2. Asymmetry of shoulders
3. Shortened trunk
4. Associated skin and soft-tissue changes
5. Patches of hair in sacral area
6. Unequal leg lengths
7. Asymmetrical scapulae
8. Malalignment of trunk and pelvis
9. Asymmetry of flanks
10. Asymmetry of breasts

COMPLICATIONS

1. Urinary problems (most common)
2. Neurologic problems
3. Cardiopulmonary impairment

LABORATORY AND DIAGNOSTIC TESTS

1. Forward bending test—to assess inequality of flank and ribs (screening test)
2. Cobb diagnostic method—to assess angle of curvature
3. Anterioposterior and lateral x-ray studies of spine—to evaluate curvature of spine

MEDICAL MANAGEMENT

1. Curves of less than 20 degrees require evaluation every 3 to 12 months.
2. The Milwaukee brace is used for treatment of lateral curvature of 20 to 40 degrees; the brace consists of neck ring and pelvic girdle, and it must be worn 23 hours a day until curvature is corrected.
3. The orthoplast jacket is a molded plastic jacket that is used for the same purpose as the Milwaukee brace.

SURGICAL MANAGEMENT

A posterior spinal fusion is the treatment of choice for a spinal curve greater than 40% or for progressive worsening of a curve in spite of nonsurgical treatment. Spinal fusion provides a permanent method of halting the progressive worsening of the spine. Several different types of instrumentation are used to stabilize the spine internally, including the Harrington rod, Luque rod (segmental spinal instrumentation), and Dwyer cables. Use of the Luque rod instrumentation is a more recent and preferred technique in the surgical correction of scoliosis. During the surgery, bone chips from the posterior iliac crest are positioned on top of the spine. External immobilization with the use of a body cast is then not needed because greater internal immobilization is achieved with this technique.

NURSING ASSESSMENT

1. See the section on skeletal assessment in Appendix A.
2. Assess for asymmetry of flank, ribs, scapulae, and hips.
3. Assess for malalignment of trunk and pelvis.

NURSING DIAGNOSES

- Knowledge deficit
- High risk for injury
- High risk for impaired physical mobility
- High risk for impaired gas exchange
- High risk for fluid volume deficit
- Pain
- High risk for ineffective management of therapeutic regimen
- High risk for body image disturbance

NURSING INTERVENTIONS
Preoperative Care

1. Prepare child and family before procedures for the sequence of events and sensations that will be experienced.
   a. Complete blood count (CBC)—to assess for anemia
   b. Blood chemistry—to assess for electrolyte imbalances
   c. Coagulation studies (prothrombin)
   d. X-ray skull study

   e. Pulmonary function tests—to assess for pulmonary complications

   f. Arterial blood gas values—to assess for pulmonary complications

   g. Myelography—to rule out genitourinary and neurologic abnormalities

   h. Spinal x-ray studies—to assess curvature of the spine

2. Prepare child for surgery (see Appendix J, section on preparation for procedure/surgery).

3. Orient child to intensive care unit and treatment procedures used postoperatively (e.g., blow gloves and spirometer).

Postoperative Care

1. Monitor for signs and symptoms of potential complications.
   a. Monitor arterial lines.
   b. Monitor temperature, respirations, blood pressure, and pulse every 1 to 2 hours until stable, then every 4 hours.
   c. Auscultate breath sounds; report changes in respiratory status (increased respirations, increased congestion, color change, chest pain, dyspnea).
   d. Monitor for spinal nerve trauma—observe lower extremities for warmth, sensation, movement, pulses, and pain.
   e. Monitor for paralytic ileus.
   f. Monitor dressing for intactness and signs of complications.
     (1) Note bleeding along incision.
     (2) Monitor for signs of infection.

2. Promote proper body alignment.
   a. Turn child every 2 hours (log roll only).
   b. Monitor for reddened areas and pressure.
   c. Keep child flat in bed until doctor orders activity (flat with log rolling only until body jacket arrives [not always ordered with Harrington rod because child is out of bed by 2 to 4 days after surgery]).
   d. Institute passive range of motion (PROM) exercises second postoperative day.

3. Promote pulmonary ventilation.
   a. Monitor vital signs as often as every 2 hours.
   b. Have child cough, turn, and deep breathe as often as every 2 hours.

    c. Use incentive spirometer every 2 hours.

    d. Monitor respiratory status every 2 hours until stable, then every 4 hours.

4. Monitor fluid and electrolyte balance.

    a. Monitor and record intake and output—intravenous (IV) fluids, urine, nasogastric drainage.

    b. Monitor bowel sounds.

    c. Advance diet as tolerated (clear liquid to regular diet).

    d. Monitor for signs and symptoms of dehydration and fluid overload (dehydration—decreased urinary output, increased specific gravity, doughy skin, dry mucous membranes; fluid overload—increased apical pulse [AP], increased respiratory rate, pulmonary congestion, dyspnea, edema [initially of extremities]).

5. Provide pain relief measures as necessary (may have an epidural catheter).

    a. Medicate routinely every 2 to 4 hours for first 72 hours.

    b. Medicate before procedures.

    c. Provide diversional activities and relaxation techniques.

♠ Discharge Planning and Home Care
Postoperative Care

1. Instruct child and family about various aspects of care (vary according to procedure).

    a. Physical restrictions

    b. Use of body cast or jacket (thoracic-lumbar-sacral orthotics [TLSO])

    c. Equipment (e.g., firm mattress), log rolling technique

    d. Signs of infection (increased temperature, odor from cast)

    e. Incision site

2. Encourage child and family to ventilate fears and body image concerns.

3. Refer to community resources (public health nurse, home health nurses). See Appendix K.

4. Encourage adherence to follow-up care regimen (clinic visits for 6 to 12 months postoperatively).

Nonsurgical Interventions

1. Instruct child or adolescent and parents in use of Milwaukee brace or orthoplast jacket.
   a. Application and removal of brace or jacket
   b. Cleaning of brace or jacket
   c. Skin inspection for pressure sores or skin breakdown
   d. Bathing before application
   e. Use of undergarments
2. Instruct child or adolescent and parents in use of exercises, and reinforce instruction.
3. Instruct child or adolescent and parents about participation in sports and recreational activities.
4. Encourage child or adolescent to express feelings of concern and inadequacy concerning brace.
   a. Distortion of body image
   b. Feelings of rejection by peers
5. Initiate community referrals.
   a. School nurse to facilitate school adaptation
   b. Financial assistance to cover costs incurred in treatment of condition
6. Instruct child or adolescent and family about cast care.
   a. Skin care (use alcohol only)
   b. Assessing for sensation and movement
   c. Exercise for unaffected extremities
   d. Assessing for signs of infection (musty odor, drainage on cast)
   e. Petal cast edges

CLIENT OUTCOMES

1. Child will maintain proper body alignment.
2. Child will have minimal pain during the first 72 hours postoperatively.
3. Child and family will understand the various aspects of postoperative home care.

REFERENCES

Bridwell KH: Surgical treatment of adolescent idiopathic scoliosis: the basics and the controversies, *Spine* 19(9):1095, 1994.

Brosnan H: Nursing management of the adolescent with idiopathic scoliosis, *Nurs Clin North Am* 26:17, 1991.

Cotton L: Unit rod segmental spinal instrumentation for the treatment of neuromuscular scoliosis, *Orthop Nurs* 10(5):17, 1991.

Lonstein JE, Winter RB: The Milwaukee brace for the treatment of adolescent idiopathic scoliosis: a review of one thousand and twenty patients, *J Bone Joint Surg Am* 76(8):1207, 1994.

Pinto WC, Avanzi O, Dezen E: Common sense in the management of adolescent idiopathic scoliosis, *Orthop Clin North Am* 25(2):215, 1994.

Puno RM, Mehta S, Byrd JA III: Surgical treatment of idiopathic thoracolumbar and lumbar scoliosis in adolescent patients, *Orthop Clin North Am* 25(2):275, 1994.

U.S. Preventive Services Task Force: Screening for adolescent idiopathic scoliosis: policy statement, *Nurse Pract* 19(9):39, 1994.

Winter S: Preoperative assessment of the child with neuromuscular scoliosis, *Orthop Clin North Am* 25(2):239, 1994.

68

Seizure Disorders

PATHOPHYSIOLOGY

Seizure is a sudden, transient alteration in brain function as a result of abnormal neuronal activity and excessive cerebral electric discharge. This activity can be partial or focal, originating in a specific area of the cerebral cortex, or generalized, involving both hemispheres in the brain. Clinical manifestations vary, depending on the area(s) of brain involvement. The types of seizures affecting children and adolescents are listed in the box on pp. 444-446.

The causes of seizure include perinatal factors, congenital malformations of the brain, genetic factors, infectious disease (encephalitis, meningitis), febrile illness, metabolic disorders, trauma, neoplasms, toxins, circulatory disturbances, and degenerative diseases of the nervous system. Seizures are termed idiopathic when no identifiable cause can be found.

Epilepsy is a disorder characterized by chronic seizures, in which seizures are of primary cerebral origin indicating underlying brain dysfunction. Epilepsy is not a disease in itself.

INCIDENCE

1. At least one seizure will occur in 3% to 5% of all children by the age of 5 years; *most* will occur with fever.
2. Nine percent of the general population will experience seizures at some time in life.
3. One and a half million Americans have active epilepsy.

Types of Seizures: International Classification

Partial (Focal, Local) Seizures
Simple partial seizures
- Consciousness is *not* impaired; may include one or a combination of the following:
    1. Motor signs—twitching of face, hand, or one side of body; usually the same movement with every seizure
    2. Autonomic signs and symptoms—vomiting, sweating, flushing, pupil dilation
    3. Somatosensory or special sensory symptoms—hearing music, feeling of falling in space, parasthesias
    4. Psychic symptoms—déjà vu, fear, panoramic vision

Complex partial seizures
- There is impairment of consciousness, although seizure may begin as simple partial seizure
- May include automatisms or automatic movements—lip smacking, chewing, repetitive picking or other hand movements
- May be without automatisms—staring

Generalized Seizures (Convulsive or Nonconvulsive)
Absence seizures
- Impairment of awareness and responsiveness
- Characterized by staring usually lasting less than 15 seconds

Absence seizures—cont'd
- Abrupt onset and ending, after which child is alert and attentive
- Usually begin between ages 4 and 14 and often resolve by age 18

Myoclonic seizures
- Sudden, involuntary jerks of a muscle or muscle group
- Often observed in healthy people when falling asleep, but when pathologic, involve synchronous jerks of the neck, shoulders, upper arms and legs
- Usually last less than 5 seconds and occur in clusters
- Consciousness lost only momentarily

Tonic-clonic seizures
- Begin with loss of consciousness and a tonic portion, a generalized stiffening of muscles in the limbs, trunk, and face lasting less than a minute
- May involve loss of bladder and bowel control
- Absent respirations and cyanosis
- Tonic portion followed by clonic movements of the upper and lower extremities
- Lethargy, confusion, and sleep in the postictal phase

Atonic seizures
- Sudden loss of tone that may cause eyelids to droop, head to nod, or a fall to the ground
- Brief, and occurring without warning

Continued

> ### Status Epilepticus
> - Usually, generalized tonic-clonic seizures that are repeated
> - Child does not regain consciousness between seizures
> - Potential for respiratory depression, hypotension, and hypoxia
> - Requires immediate emergency medical treatment

CLINICAL MANIFESTATIONS

See box for clinical manifestations.

COMPLICATIONS

1. Aspiration pneumonia
2. Asphyxia
3. Mental retardation

LABORATORY AND DIAGNOSTIC TESTS

1. Electroencephalogram (EEG)—used to help define the type and focus of the seizure
   a. The diagnosis of epilepsy does not depend solely on abnormal EEG findings.
   b. Natural sleep is preferred during EEG, although sedation with monitoring may be indicated.
2. Computed tomography (CT) scan—uses x-ray studies more sensitive than the ordinary to detect differences in tissue density
3. Magnetic resonance imaging (MRI)—produces an image using a magnetic field and radio waves, particularly helpful in demonstrating brain regions (posterior fossa and sellar region) not clearly seen by CT scan

4. Positron emission tomography (PET) scan—for evaluation of intractable seizures to assist in localizing lesions, metabolic alterations, or blood flow in the brain (involves intravenous [IV] injection of radioisotopes)
5. Evoked potentials—used to determine the integrity of sensory pathways in the brain (absent or delayed response may be indicative of pathologic condition)
6. Laboratory tests ordered on basis of child's history and examination
   a. Lumbar puncture for cerebrospinal fluid analysis—used primarily to rule out infection
   b. Complete blood count—used to rule out infection as causative agent; and in those cases in which trauma is suspected, may evaluate hematocrit and platelet count
   c. Electrolyte panel—serum electrolytes, total calcium, and magnesium often ordered for a first-time seizure, and in children less than 3 months of age, in which electrolyte and metabolic causes are more common (a blood glucose test may be especially helpful in the young infant or a child with prolonged seizure to rule out hypoglycemia)
   d. Toxic screen of serum and urine—used to rule out toxic ingestion
   e. Monitoring of levels of antiepileptic drugs—used in the early phase of management and if compliance is in question (see therapeutic levels in section on medical management, this chapter)

MEDICAL MANAGEMENT

Antiepileptic drug therapy is the mainstay of medical management. Single-drug therapy is the most desirable, with the goal of establishing a balance between seizure control and adverse side effects. The drug of choice is based on seizure type, epileptic syndrome, and patient variables. Drug combinations may be needed to achieve seizure control. Complete control is achieved in only 50% to 75% of children with epilepsy.

The mechanisms of action of antiepileptic drugs are complex and have not been well defined. Anticonvulsants may reduce neuronal firing, facilitate the activity of inhibitory amino acids, or reduce slow, rhythmic firing of thalamic neurons. The following are commonly used anticonvulsants:

1. Phenobarbital—indications: myoclonic seizures, tonic-clonic seizures, status epilepticus; therapeutic levels: 15 to 40 mcg/ml
2. Phenytoin (Dilantin)—indications: partial seizures, tonic-clonic seizures, status epilepticus; therapeutic levels: 10 to 20 mcg/ml
3. Carbamazepine (Tegretol)—indications: partial seizures, tonic-clonic seizures; therapeutic levels: 4 to 12 mcg/ml
4. Valproic acid (Depakene)—indications: atypical absence seizures, myoclonic seizures, tonic-clonic seizures, atonic seizures, and especially useful for mixed-seizure disorders; therapeutic levels: 40 to 100 mcg/ml
5. Primidone (Mysoline)—indications: occasionally used to treat tonic-clonic seizures; therapeutic levels: 4 to 12 mcg/ml
6. Ethosuximide (Zarontin)—indications: absence seizures
7. Clonazepam (Klonopin)—indications: absence seizures, tonic-clonic seizures, infantile spasm

NURSING ASSESSMENT

1. See the section on neurologic assessment in Appendix A.
2. Refer to the box on pp. 444-446 for specific types of seizure disorders.

NURSING DIAGNOSES

- High risk for injury
- Body image disturbance
- High risk for ineffective family and individual coping

NURSING INTERVENTIONS
Seizures

1. Protect child from injury.
   a. Do not attempt to restrain child.
   b. If child is standing or sitting so that there is a threat of falling, ease child down to prevent fall.
   c. Do not place anything in child's mouth.
   d. Loosen restrictive clothing.

    e. Prevent child from hitting anything sharp, padding any objects that might be hit and removing any sharp objects from area.

    f. Turn child on side to facilitate airway clearance of secretions.

2. Maintain detailed observation and recording of seizure activity to assist in diagnosis or assessment of medication response.

    a. Time of onset and any precipitating events

    b. Aura (some type of warning that seizure is coming)

    c. Type of seizure or description of motor movements and level of consciousness

    d. Length of seizure

    e. Interventions during seizure (medication or safety measures)

    f. Postictal phase

    g. Vital signs

3. Provide for sleep or rest after seizure.

4. Monitor child's adverse effects to medications.

Status Epilepticus

1. Stabilize patent airway; suction as needed.

2. Provide supplemental 100% oxygen by face mask.

3. Obtain IV access for anticonvulsant or other medication therapy; with the administration of lorazepam, diazepam, phenytoin, or phenobarbital, prepare for respiratory depression and further airway management if needed.

4. Monitor vital signs.

♠ Discharge Planning and Home Care

1. Provide information about seizures and address any misconceptions family may have.

2. Stress importance of regular medication taking and follow-up with physician to monitor growth and development and for any subtle side effects.

3. List steps for family for managing seizures as they occur and when to access emergency medical care.

4. Provide anticipatory guidance regarding safety.

    a. Obtaining medic-alert bracelet

    b. Water safety—swimming only with competent person (knowledgeable in life saving) close

    c. Avoiding unprotected heights

    d. Possible restrictions on operating machinery, hot appliances, or automobiles

5. Assist in understanding process by which a healthy self-concept is developed.
6. Refer to National Epilepsy Foundation for information and support.
7. Refer child and family for support and counseling as needed.

CLIENT OUTCOMES

1. Child will be free of physical injury.
2. Seizure activity will be prevented or controlled.
3. Child will have positive self-esteem and self-image that enhance wellness.

REFERENCES

Devinsky O: Seizure disorders, *Clin Symp* 46(1):2, 1994.

Ferry PC, Banner W, Wolf RA: *Seizure disorders in children,* Philadelphia, 1986, JB Lippincott.

Nypaver MM et al: Emergency department laboratory evaluation of children with seizures: dogma or dilemma? *Pediatr Emerg Care* 8(1):13, 1992.

Penry JK: *Diagnosis, management, quality of life,* New York, 1986, Raven Press Books.

Sagraves R: Antiepileptic drug therapy for pediatric generalized tonic-clonic seizures, *J Pediatr Health Care* 4(6):314, 1990.

69

Short Bowel Syndrome

PATHOPHYSIOLOGY

Short bowel syndrome (SBS) is the syndrome of malabsorption and malnutrition that occurs because of a congenitally malfunctioning bowel or after resection of small bowel necessitated by congenital or acquired conditions (see the box on p. 452). Symptoms of SBS include chronic diarrhea, impaired nutrient absorption, malnutrition, and poor growth and development. Additionally, many affected children are chronically dependent on parenteral nutrition (PN), which can lead to liver dysfunction and disease.

SBS has three characteristic stages:

1. Stage I: immediate postoperative period (7 to 10 days) after enterostomy is created
   a. Irretractable diarrhea with massive water and fluid and electrolyte losses
   b. Dependence on parenteral nutrition
   c. Possible bowel mucosa atrophy
2. Stage II: from 2 weeks to up to 1 year after surgery
   a. Gastric acid hypersecretion leading to quick intestinal transit time and diarrhea, impaired pancreatic enzyme function, and gastric ulcers
   b. At end of stage II, stabilization of diarrhea, and progression of enteral feeds, signaling adaptive hyperplasia of intestinal mucosa

Etiology of Short Bowel Syndrome

Congenital

Multiple intestinal atresias
Gastroschisis
Omphalocele
Cloacal exstrophy
Malrotation and volvulus
Long segment Hirschsprung's disease
Meconium ileus
Intussusception

Acquired

Necrotizing enterocolitis (NEC)
Volvulus
Inflammatory bowel disease
Trauma
Arterial or venous thrombosis
Intussusception

3. Stage III: up to 2 years after surgery (many children do not reach this stage; stomas are usually reanastomosed at this time)
   a. Control of diarrhea
   b. Increased tolerance of enteral nutrition (EN)
   Adaptation of the bowel is dependent on the following:
1. Intestinal length: Most surgeons agree that 40 cm of small bowel without an intact ileocecal valve (ICV) or 15 cm of small bowel with an intact ileocecal valve is necessary for tolerance of enteral feeds.
2. Ileocecal valve: This is very important but not absolutely necessary (depending on bowel length). The ICV slows intestinal transit time, which increases nutrient and fluid absorption. Additionally, the ICV prevents contamina-

tion of the small bowel with colonic flora, therefore decreasing bacterial overgrowth, translocation, and sepsis.

3. Age: Because intestinal length doubles between the second trimester of pregnancy and full term, preterm infants have a greater capacity for adaptation.
4. Individual response: Liver tolerance of chronic parenteral nutrition, number and virulence of infections, and development of bowel obstructions from strictures or adhesions all seem to play an important role in the overall outcome and individual outcome.

Survival rate is reported to be 78% to 94%, with death occurring secondary to liver disease and sepsis. Cost of treatment ranges from $50,000 to $150,000 per patient each year.

CLINICAL MANIFESTATIONS

1. Diarrhea, ranging from acute to chronic
2. Poor tolerance of enteral nutrition
3. Poor and inconsistent growth
4. Malnutrition (poor carbohydrate and fat absorption)
5. Jaundice
6. Anemia

COMPLICATIONS
Early Signs and Symptoms

1. Fluid/electrolyte imbalance
2. Diarrhea
3. Sepsis
4. Gastric acid hypersecretion

Late Signs and Symptoms

1. Nutritional deficiencies, poor growth and development
2. Poor healing
3. Osteopenia
4. Cardiomyopathy
5. Oral aversion
6. Vitamin and mineral deficiency
7. Need for multiple surgeries, particularly for bowel obstructions
8. Gallbladder disease
9. Liver disease

LABORATORY AND DIAGNOSTIC TESTS

1. Complete blood count (CBC) with differential and platelet count—may see increased or decreased white blood count (WBC) with sepsis, decreased platelets, and anemia secondary to liver dysfunction
2. Serum electrolytes, glucose, blood urea nitrogen (BUN), creatinine—to assess fluid and electrolyte imbalances, tolerance of PN
3. Liver function test (LFT)—to assess liver tolerance of PN
4. Dipstick or urinalysis for protein, glucose, blood, and ketones—to assess tolerance of PN
5. Gastric pH—to assess the presence of gastric acid hypersecretion
6. Stool hematest, reducing substances, stool ictotest—to assess tolerance of EN, check for the presence of bile in stool
7. Abdominal x-ray examination—to check for dilated or obstructed loops of bowel
8. Ultrasound of liver and gallbladder—to check for cholestasis and gallstones
9. HIDA scan—to check liver function
10. Liver biopsy—to diagnose liver disease

MEDICAL MANAGEMENT

The medical management of SBS focuses on the minimization of symptoms through medication and diet therapy, with the use of surgical interventions as needed.

Medications

The following medications may be used for the complications indicated.

1. Diarrhea
   a. Loperamide (Imodium)—an antidiarrheal opioid agent that slows transit time, thereby increasing absorption of water and nutrients
   b. Cholestyramine—bile-salt binder to decrease secretory diarrhea
   c. Octreotide acetate (Sandostatin)—decreases secretory diarrhea by inhibiting exocrine and endocrine, gas-

trointestinal (GI) and pancreatic secretions (little is known about effects in infants; decreases insulin and growth hormone levels)

2. Gastric acid hypersecretion: ranitidine (Zantac)—H_2 blocker to increase gastric pH, slow transit time, and prevent ulcers and breakdown at anastomosis site (gastric acid hypersecretion should be temporary [up to 6 months]; these medications may promote bacterial overgrowth of the small intestine)

3. Liver dysfunction
   a. Phenobarbital—increases liver enzyme induction
   b. Ursodiol (Actigall)—increases bile excretion; absorbed in ileum
   c. Cholecystokinin (CCK)—initiates gallbladder contractions

4. Intestinal bacterial overgrowth
   a. Trimethoprim (Bactrim)—antibiotic prophylaxis to "sterilize" the intestine and to prevent bacterial overgrowth, translocation, and sepsis
   b. Metronidazole (Flagyl)—same as trimethoprim

5. Vitamin and mineral deficiency
   a. ADEK drops—fat-soluble vitamin supplementation
   b. Cyanotobalamin (B_{12})—injections usually needed after first few months
   c. Mineral supplements—zinc aids in healing; selenium plays a role in antioxidant system

Nutritional Interventions

1. Stage I
   a. Provide parenteral nutrition in a central venous catheter to provide sufficient calories, proteins, and amino acids for healing and sustained growth.
   b. Replace electrolytes lost in abnormal quantities, particularly sodium.
   c. Provide gut-priming feedings at rates as low as 1 cc/hr to prevent mucosal atrophy.

2. Stages II and III
   a. Provide early enteral feedings with an elemental formula such as Alimentum (Ross Laboratories, Columbus, Ohio), Pregestimil (Mead Johnson, Evansville, Ind.), or human breast milk.

   b. Begin enteral feedings with a continuous infusion into the stomach through either an orogastric or gastrostomy tube.

   c. Begin oral motor stimulation program.

   d. Increase feedings until stool output increases to about 30 to 35 cc/kg/day and/or significant malabsorption occurs.

   e. Provide mineral supplements such as zinc and selenium.

   f. Delete copper and manganese if liver dysfunction occurs.

   g. Introduce strained baby foods as tolerated when developmentally appropriate.

SURGICAL MANAGEMENT

Surgical interventions are designed to slow transit time, increase mucosal surface area, or increase intestinal length.

Indications for surgical intervention include poor tolerance of EN; numerous complications of PN such as multiple catheter-related infections, limiting venous access; and liver dysfunction and disease. The following surgical options may be used.

1. Surgeries to slow intestinal transit time

   a. Intestinal valve—the creation of an intestinal valve to slow transit time (clinical experience is limited)

   b. Reversed intestinal segment—the interposition of a segment of bowel in which peristalsis is opposite (limited to patients who have longer small bowel length)

   c. Colon interposition—the interposition of a piece of colon between two segments of small bowel; this may slow transit time by virtue of the colon's inherent slow peristalsis, increasing absorption of fluids and electrolytes (small number of cases reported)

   d. Intestinal pacing—the application of electrical signals to the distal region of the small bowel to initiate retrograde peristalsis, thereby slowing transit time (no successful clinical reports)

2. Surgeries to increase mucosal surface area

   a. Tapering enteroplasty—reduces the caliber of dilated small bowel while preserving intestinal length; this should theoretically increase peristalsis and decrease bacterial overgrowth (clinical experience is limited)

    b. Neomucosa—the transplant or patch of intestine with new mucosa that has been grown from a cut edge of normal bowel (experimental)

3. Surgeries to increase intestinal length
   a. "Bianchi" intestinal lengthening procedure—the division of a segment of dilated bowel and creation of an end-to-end anastomosis resulting in a doubling of length
   b. Small bowel transplant—has had limited success (reserved for end-stage liver disease)
   c. Multiorgan transplant (liver and small bowel)—has had limited success (reserved for end-stage liver disease)

NURSING ASSESSMENT

1. See the section on gastrointestinal assessment in Appendix A.
2. Assess for fluid and electrolyte imbalances.
3. Assess hydration status.
4. Assess child's tolerance of PN.
5. Assess child's readiness for and tolerance of enteral nutrition.
6. Assess child for presence of pain.
7. Assess for signs and symptoms of infection.
8. Assess child's height and weight, head circumference, and pattern of growth.
9. Assess child's response to medications.
10. Assess family's response to hospitalization and child's condition.
11. Assess family's readiness for discharge and ability to manage home treatment regimen.

NURSING DIAGNOSES

- Fluid volume deficit
- Pain
- High risk for infection
- Altered nutrition: less than body requirements
- Altered growth and development
- Altered family processes
- High risk for ineffective management of therapeutic regimen

NURSING INTERVENTIONS

1. Assess for fluid and electrolyte imbalances, hydration status, and tolerance of PN.
   a. Monitor vital signs, perfusion, and mucous membranes.
   b. Monitor urine output and dipstick.
   c. Monitor serum and urine electrolytes and serum glucose.
   d. Monitor serum nutritional lab tests.
2. Monitor readiness for and tolerance of enteral nutrition.
   a. Record and monitor intake, stool output, and emesis.
   b. Measure abdominal growth.
   c. Hematest stool.
   d. Test stool for reducing substances.
3. Monitor for verbal and nonverbal pain behaviors; administer nonpharmacologic and pharmacologic pain measures.
4. Assess for any signs or symptoms of infection.
   a. Monitor serum CBC, differential, and platelets.
   b. In newborn infants, monitor for increased temperature and glucose instability.
   c. In older children, monitor for poor feeding, increased temperature, and irritability.
5. Monitor for growth deficiencies.
   a. Record daily weights.
   b. Record weekly length and head circumference.
   c. Plot growth parameters on growth chart.
   d. Monitor serum lab results, assessing nutritional status.
6. Monitor for therapeutic and adverse effects of medications.
7. Monitor for appropriate growth and development.
   a. Initiate developmental evaluation and treatment plan.
   b. Initiate oral stimulation program.
   c. Encourage age-appropriate use of toys and activities.
   d. Encourage contact with peers (older children).
8. Support the family.
   a. Involve parents and family in patient's care.
   b. Encourage therapeutic communication.
   c. Consider evaluation and support from social worker.

 d. Assist family in identifying and utilizing resources and support systems.
9. Educate family on patient care and discharge planning.

♠ Discharge Planning and Home Care

1. Instruct family about administration of nutrition.
   a. PN—how to obtain and administer; catheter care
   b. EN—how to obtain, mix, and administer
2. Instruct family about medications—administration, and desired and undesired effects.
3. Instruct family about care of the central venous catheter.
4. Instruct family about ostomy care (if applicable).
5. Arrange follow-up appointments, with specialists and primary care physician.
6. Arrange any developmental and/or oral stimulation program follow-up.
7. Employ family support strategies.
   a. Assist family in identifying support systems.
   b. Encourage open communication.
   c. Encourage family to participate in child's care.

CLIENT OUTCOMES

1. Patient is able to be weaned from PN to EN.
2. Patient is free of infections.
3. Family is able to adhere to treatment regimen.

REFERENCES

Rossi R: Endoscopic examination of the colon in infancy and childhood, *Pediatr Clin North Am* 35:331, 1989.

Thompson J: The current status of surgical therapy for the short bowel syndrome, *Contemp Surg* 33(12):27, 1988.

Warner B, Ziegler M: Management of the short bowel syndrome in the pediatric population, *Pediatr Clin North Am* 40:1335, 1993.

Wessel J: Short bowel syndrome. In *Nutritional care for high risk newborns*, Chicago, 1994, Precept Press.

Wise B: Neonatal short bowel syndrome, *Neonatal Network* 11(7):9, 1992.

70

Sickle Cell Anemia

PATHOPHYSIOLOGY

Sickle cell anemia, or homozygous sickle cell disease (Hb SS), is an inherited autosomal recessive disorder. The basic defect is a mutant autosomal gene that effects a substitution of valine for glutamic acid on the hemoglobin chain. The result is a person with the disease or with sickle cell trait (heterozygous gene Hb AS). There are other variants of sickle cell anemia, with Hb SC, Hb SB thalassemia, Hb SD, and Hb SE being the most common. Sickled red blood cells are crescent shaped, have decreased oxygen-carrying capacity, and have a greater destruction rate than do normal red blood cells. In addition, the life span of sickled cells is diminished to 16 to 20 days. Sickle cells are extremely rigid because of the gelled hemoglobin, cellular dehydration, and an inflexible membrane. The rigid cells become trapped in the circulatory system, leading to a vicious cycle of infarction and progressive sickling.

Splenic hypofunction and, later, splenic atrophy result in reticuloendothelial failure and a 600-times-greater incidence of infection in children with sickle cell disease than in the normal population. Red blood cells with Hb S increase after the child is 6 months of age, resulting in chronic anemia.

Sickle cell crises result from physiologic changes that result in a decrease in oxygen available to the hemoglobin.

> ## Early Detection: Newborn Screening Programs
>
> - Morbidity and mortality can be significantly reduced with newborn screening and early intervention.
> - Screening should include both pre-natal maternal and neonatal screening.
> - Public education is critical for effective neonatal screening. Target groups include day care centers, schools, and the media.

Sickling of cells results in clumping of red blood cells in the vessels, decreased oxygen transport, and increased destruction of red blood cells (erythropoiesis). Ischemia, infarcts, and tissue necrosis result from the obstruction of vessels and decreased blood flow. Three types of crises occur: (1) vasoocclusive (painful); (2) splenic sequestration; and (3) aplastic. Sickle cell crises occur less frequently with age. Mortality in the first years of life is usually caused by infection and sequestration crisis (see the box above).

INCIDENCE

1. Incidence of sickle cell disease among black individuals is estimated at 1 in 400.
2. Sickle cell trait occurs in one of every 10 black Americans.
3. Twenty-five percent of deaths occur before age 5 years.
4. With new treatments, 85% of affected individuals survive to the age of 20 years; 60%, beyond 50 years.

CLINICAL MANIFESTATIONS

1. Vasoocclusive crisis (painful crisis), resulting from ischemia in tissue distal to occlusion
   a. Irritability

    b. Vomiting
    c. Fever
    d. Anorexia
    e. Pain in joints
    f. Dactylitis (hand-and-foot syndrome)—range of motion decreased and extremities inflamed
    g. Leg ulcers
    h. Cerebrovascular accidents (CVA)
    i. Ocular hemorrhages
    j. Proliferative retinopathy
    k. Acute chest syndrome
2. Sequestration crisis (usually seen in children less than 5 years old), due to frequent infarctions from sickling (splenic atrophy follows)
    a. Rapid and massive enlargement of spleen (splenomegaly)
    b. Rapid fall in hemoglobin level
    c. Enlargement of liver
    d. Circulatory collapse and shock
    e. Tachycardia, dyspnea, pallor, and weakness (common)
3. Aplastic crisis, resulting from rapid destruction of red blood cells, especially during an infection when the strong compensatory mechanism is depressed
    a. Weakness
    b. Pallor of mucous membranes
    c. Scleral icterus
    d. Anorexia
    e. Increased susceptibility to infection
    f. Tachycardia
    g. Decreased reticulocyte count

COMPLICATIONS

1. Sleep loss
2. Delayed onset of puberty
3. Impaired fertility
4. Priapism
5. Gallstones
6. Leg ulcers
7. Chronic heart, liver, and kidney disease
8. Osteomyelitis

9. Depression, isolation, and low self-esteem
10. Enuresis
11. High risk for drug addiction
12. Strained parent-child relationships
13. Cerebrovascular accidents

LABORATORY AND DIAGNOSTIC TESTS

1. Hemoglobin electrophoresis, preferably at birth on all infants as part of newborn screening—this test can quantify the percentage of hemoglobin S present
2. Fetal blood or fetal cells—these tests make prenatal diagnosis possible between 9 and 11 weeks gestation

MEDICAL MANAGEMENT

Although there is currently no cure for sickle cell anemia, medical management may help reduce the crisis. Administration of prophylactic penicillin to prevent septicemia should be initiated in the newborn period. Additional immunizations required are (1) pneumococcal vaccine at 2 years of age with a booster at 4 to 5 years and (2) influenza vaccine.

Hypertransfusion programs for children who have had CVAs, progressive pulmonary disease, and possibly debilitating vasoocclusive crisis (controversial) is a current treatment. The iron overload leads to iron deposits on organs, with the following complications occurring: cardiomyopathy, cirrhosis, insulin-dependent diabetes mellitus (IDDM), hypothyroidism, hypoparathyroidism, delayed growth, and delayed sexual development. Deferoxamine (Desferal) administered either subcutaneously or by continuous intravenous transfusion chelates the iron so that it can be excreted through the urine or bile to help reduce these complications.

Analgesics are used to control pain during a crisis period. Antiobotics may be used, because infection can trigger the crisis.

NURSING ASSESSMENT

See the sections on cardiovascular assessment and respiratory assessment in Appendix A and the section on pain assessment in Appendix I.

NURSING DIAGNOSES

- Altered tissue perfusion: renal, cerebral, and peripheral
- Pain
- High risk for fatigue
- High risk for infection
- High risk for fluid volume excess
- High risk for injury
- Altered growth and development
- High risk for ineffective family coping: compromised
- High risk for ineffective individual coping: compromised
- High risk for ineffective management of therapeutic regimen

NURSING INTERVENTIONS

1. Prevent or minimize effects of sickle cell crisis.
   a. Be aware that early assessment and action are *keys* to prevention of and intervention in crisis episode.
   b. Avoid cold and vasoconstriction during pain episode; cold promotes sickling.
   c. Provide for and promote hydration (one and one half to two times maintenance).
      (1) Maintain strict intake and output.
      (2) Assess for signs of dehydration.
   d. Promote oxygenation of tissues; monitor for signs of hypoxia—cyanosis; hyperventilation; increased apical pulse, respiratory rate, and blood pressure; and mental confusion.
2. Provide frequent rest periods to decrease oxygen expenditure.
3. Monitor use of oxygen equipment.
4. Administer and monitor use of blood products and chelation therapy; assess for signs of transfusion reactions—fever, restlessness, cardiac dysrhythmias, chills and shaking, nausea and vomiting, chest pain, red or black urine, headache, flank pain, and signs of shock or renal failure.
5. Monitor for signs of circulatory overload—dyspnea, increased respiratory rate, cyanosis, chest pain, and dry cough.

6. Relieve or minimize pain.
   a. Moist heat for first 24 hours
   b. Whirlpool or walking tank, especially if swelling has occurred
   c. Therapeutic exercises
   d. Administration of analgesics as ordered based on pain assessment
   e. Use of nonpharmacologic methods such as guided imagery (see Appendix I)
7. Prevent infection.
   a. Assess for signs of infection—fever, malaise or irritability, and inflamed and swollen soft tissue and lymph nodes.
   b. Be aware that children are particularly susceptible to pneumococcal sepsis and pneumonia (children less than 3 to 4 years of age) and salmonella osteomyelitis.
8. Monitor for signs of complications.
   a. Vascular collapse and shock
   b. Splenomegaly
   c. Bone and joint infarction
   d. Leg ulcers
   e. Strokes
   f. Blindness
   g. Chest pain or dyspnea
   h. Delay in growth and development
9. Provide age-appropriate explanation to the child about hospitalization and procedures.
10. Provide emotional support to child and family.
    a. Encourage performance of normal activities.
    b. Encourage networking with other children and families who have sickle cell anemia.
11. Encourage parents to screen their family members.
    a. Newborn screening for hemoglobinopathies
       (1) Identification at birth makes possible early prophylaxis against infections.
       (2) Use of prophylactic penicillin is recommended beginning in the newborn period (4 months of age).
    b. Screening of siblings for disease and trait

♠ Discharge Planning and Home Care

1. Provide genetic counseling.
2. Counsel child on appropriate play, leisure activities, and sports participation (to prevent hypoxia resulting from strenuous physical exertion and excessive life stress).
3. Provide parent teaching and anticipatory guidance about the prevention of infection to ensure that the child is seen by a physician at the first signs of illness; teach parents procedure for taking temperature and methods to decrease temperature.
4. Provide parents with information about routine immunization, as well as about *Streptococcus pneumoniae* vaccine at 2 years of age and influenza vaccines.

CLIENT OUTCOMES

1. Child and family will understand the importance of medical follow-up and when to seek medical attention.
2. The child will have minimal vasoocclusive, sequestration, and aplastic crises.
3. The family will seek genetic counseling for other children.

REFERENCES

Abboud MR et al: Bone marrow transplantation for sickle cell anemia, *Am J Pediatr Hematol/Oncol* 16(1):86, 1994.

Barbarin OA, Whitten CF, Bonds SM: Estimating rates of psychosocial problems in urban and poor children with sickle cell anemia, *Health Soc Work* 19(2):112, 1994.

Cohen A: Current status of iron chelation therapy with deferoxamine, *Semin Hematol* 27(2):36, 1990.

Cohen MJ et al: Neuropsychological impairment in children with sickle cell anemia and cerebrovascular accidents, *Clin Pediatr* 33(9):517, 1994.

Sporrer KA et al: Pain in children and adolescents with sickle cell anemia: a prospective study utilizing self-reporting, *Am J Pediatr Hematol/Oncol* 16(3):219, 1994.

Zwerdling T, Kalinyak K, Rucknagel D: Sarcoidosis in a child with sickle cell anemia, *Am J Pediatr Hematol/Oncol* 16(3):278, 1994.

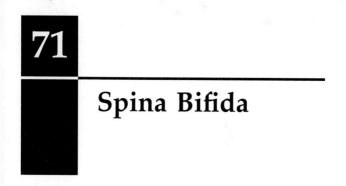

Spina Bifida

PATHOPHYSIOLOGY

There are two distinct types of failure of fusion of the vertebral laminae of the spinal column: spina bifida occulta and spina bifida cystica.

Spina bifida occulta is a defect in closure in which the meninges are not exposed on the surface of the skin. The vertebral defect is small, usually involving the lumbosacral region. External abnormalities (present in 50% of cases) may include a hair tuft, nevus, or hemangioma. A pilonidal sinus may require surgical closure if it becomes infected.

Spina bifida cystica is a defect in closure that results in protrusion of the spinal cord and/or its coverings. *Meningocele* is a protrusion that includes the meninges and a sac containing cerebrospinal fluid (CSF); it is covered by normal skin. No neurologic abnormalities are present, and the spinal cord is not involved. Hydrocephalus occurs in 20% of cases. A meningocele usually is in the lumbosacral or sacral area.

Myelomeningocele is a protrusion of the meninges and a portion of the spinal cord, as well as a sac containing CSF. The lumbar or lumbosacral area is most often affected. The lumbosacral area is affected in 42% of cases; the thoracolumbar, in 27%; the sacral, in 21%; and the thoracic or cervical, in 10%. Infants with a myelomeningocele are prone to injury during the birth process. Hydrocephalus occurs in most affected children (85% to 90%); about 60% to 70% have a normal intelligence quotient. Children with both myelo-meningocele and hydrocephalus have other central nervous system (CNS) malformations, of which Arnold-Chiari deformity is the most common.

The specific cause of spina bifida is unknown. Multiple factors such as heredity and environment are thought to interact to produce these defects. The neural tube is normally complete 4 weeks after conception. The following have been identified as causative factors: low levels of maternal vitamins, including folic acid; the taking of clomiphene and valproic acid; and hyperthermia during pregnancy. It is estimated that nearly 50% of neural tube defects could be prevented if women took preconception vitamins including folic acid.

Advances in the interdisciplinary care provided has improved the long-term outcomes for affected children. Treatment improvement, with the use of medications and neurosurgery, has contributed to extending their lifespan.

Diminished self-esteem is characteristically common to children and adolescents with this condition. Adolescents express concerns about sexual adequacy, social mastery, peer relationships, and physical maturity and attractiveness. The severity of disability is more directly related to *self-perception* of the disability than to the actual disability of the adolescent.

INCIDENCE

1. Annually, approximately 2500 infants are born with neural tube defects.
2. In the United States, the incidence is 1 in 1000 live births.
3. The risk of the disorder occurring increases 4% with the second child.
4. Female individuals are more often affected than male individuals.

CLINICAL MANIFESTATIONS

A varying degree of dysfunction impacting the skeleton, skin, and genitourinary tract results from spina bifida, depending on the portion of the spinal cord involved.

1. Motor, sensory, reflex, and sphincter abnormalities—may occur in varying degrees
2. Flaccid paralysis of legs; loss of sensation and reflexes

3. Hydrocephalus
4. Scoliosis
5. Bladder and bowel functions varying from normal to ineffective

COMPLICATIONS

Birth-related complications of spina bifida include the following:

1. Cerebral palsy
2. Mental retardation
3. Optic atrophy
4. Epilepsy
5. Osteoporosis
6. Fractures (caused by decreased muscle mass)
7. Painless ulcerations, injuries, decubiti

LABORATORY AND DIAGNOSTIC TESTS

1. Diagnostic examinations: chest x-ray studies, ultrasound, computed tomography (CT) scanning, magnetic resonance imaging (MRI), amniocentesis
2. Antenatal period testing: serum alpha fetoprotein between 16 and 18 weeks of gestation, ultrasound exam of fetus, amniocentesis if other tests are inconclusive
3. Routine preoperative testing: complete blood count (CBC), urinalysis, culture and sensitivity (C and S), type and cross match, chest x-ray examination

MEDICAL AND SURGICAL MANAGEMENT

Surgical repair of myelomeningocele is performed in the neonatal period to prevent rupture. Surgical repair of the spinal lesion and shunting of CSF in infants with hydrocephalus is performed at birth. Skin grafting is necessary if the lesion is large. Prophylactic antibiotics are administered to prevent meningitis. Nursing interventions will depend on the presence and extent of dysfunction of various body systems.

The following medications may be used:

1. Antibiotics—used prophylactically to prevent urinary tract infections (selection depends on C and S)

2. Anticholinergics—used to increase bladder tone
3. Stool softeners and laxatives—used for bowel training and evacuation of stool

NURSING ASSESSMENT

1. See the sections on musculoskeletal and neurologic assessments in Appendix A.
2. Assess parents' interactions with their infant and ability to cope with their child's condition.
3. Assess extent of motor and sensory involvement, and presence of reflexes.
4. Assess for signs and symptoms of dehydration or fluid overload.
5. Assess parents' need for preoperative and postoperative information and support.
6. Assess for wound drainage and signs of infection.
7. Assess parents' and child's ability to manage home treatment regimen.

NURSING DIAGNOSES

- Impaired physical mobility
- High risk for infection
- High risk for injury
- Altered patterns of urinary elimination: total incontinence
- Bowel incontinence
- Impaired skin integrity
- Body image disturbance
- Altered sexuality patterns
- Altered family processes
- Altered growth and development
- Altered nutrition: more than body requirements
- High risk for ineffective management of therapeutic regimen

NURSING INTERVENTIONS
Preoperative Care

1. Encourage parental expression of grief over loss of "perfect" child.
   a. Feelings related to guilt, self-blame
   b. Feelings of anger about child's condition
   c. Feelings of inadequacy for procreating the infant

d. Feelings of being overwhelmed with the situation and the unknown
2. Provide emotional support to parents (see Appendix J, section on supportive care).
3. Monitor infant's vital signs and neurologic status.
   a. Temperature, apical pulse, respiratory rate, and blood pressure as often as every 2 hours
   b. Neurologic assessment (see section on neurologic assessment, Appendix A)
4. Promote optimal preoperative hydration and nutritional status.
   a. Monitor for dehydration or fluid overload.
   b. Monitor administration of maintenance fluids (by mouth [po] or intravenous [IV] route).
   c. Monitor and record intake and output.
   d. Record daily weight.
5. Maintain integrity of defect; prevent further injury.
   a. Monitor for signs and symptoms of infection—fever, drainage, odor, swelling, and redness.
   b. Maintain child in prone position.
   c. Maintain sterility of dressing.
6. Prepare parents and infant for surgery (refer to institutional manual for specific guidelines).

Postoperative Care

1. Maintain nutritional and fluid intake.
   a. Assess for signs of dehydration or fluid overload.
   b. Monitor for bowel sounds.
   c. Monitor administration of IV fluids.
   d. Monitor and record intake and output.
   e. Record daily weight.
2. Monitor for signs and symptoms of infections.
   a. Fever (obtain blood C and S when infant is febrile)
   b. Drainage from surgical site
   c. Redness and inflammation
3. Promote healing of surgical site; use sterile technique when changing and reinforcing dressing.
4. Monitor vital signs and neurologic status.
   a. Monitor temperature, pulse, respirations, and blood pressure.

    b. Perform neurologic assessment (see section on neurologic assessment, Appendix A).

    c. Monitor head circumference.

5. Provide emotional support to parents (see Appendix J, section on supportive care).

🏠 Discharge Planning and Home Care

1. Instruct parents about long-term management of bowel and bladder training.

    a. Bladder training

      (1) Prevention of bladder infections

      (2) Modification of diet for bladder control

      (3) Prevention of decubiti, increasing range of motion (ROM) and mobility, and importance of skin care

      (4) Surgical procedures: augmentation, enterocystoplasty, artificial urinary sphincter, urethral sling, abdominal stoma, urinary diversion

      (5) Methods for assessing renal functioning: urine cultures, serum electrolytes, renal scans, intravenous pyelograms, ultrasounds

    b. Bowel training—to implement regular evacuation program

      (1) High-fiber diet with bulking agents

      (2) Use of stool softeners (i.e., glycerin)

      (3) Use of digital stimulation

      (4) Use of laxatives (casanthranol [Peri-Colace])

2. Provide information to parent and child about techniques to facilitate mobility and independence.

    a. Use of casting, corrective appliances (encouraged not only to provide mobility and independence but also to prevent osteoporosis and contractures)

    b. Use of wheelchairs and assistive devices

    c. Physical therapy regimen

    d. Surgical procedures on soft tissue, bone

3. Provide education to parents about normal growth and development and deviations from the norm.

    a. Call attention to the special problems and needs of the disabled child.

    b. Act as liaison with parents, teachers, and school to establish developmentally and intellectually appropriate expectations.

4. Instruct adolescents and provide information about areas of concern.
   a. Sexual counseling (based on evaluation of genital responsiveness)
   b. Vocational counseling and weight control measures as needed

CLIENT OUTCOMES

1. Child will be well hydrated and will maintain weight within normal parameters.
2. Child will be free of infection.
3. Child and parents will demonstrate ability to maintain long-term home care and be free of complications.

REFERENCES

Behrman R, editor: *Nelson textbook of pediatrics,* ed 14, Philadelphia, 1992, WB Saunders.

Centers for Disease Control: Economic burden of spina bifida—United States, 1980-1990, *MMWR* 38(15):264, 1989.

Centers for Disease Control: Recommendations for the use of folic acid to reduce the number of cases of spina bifida and other neural tube defects, *MMWR* 41:1, 1992.

Centers for Disease Control: Prevention program for reducing risk for neural tube defects—South Carolina, 1992-1994, *MMWR* 44(8):141, 1995.

King J, Currie D, Wright E: Bowel training in spina bifida: importance of education, patient compliance, age, and anal reflexes, *Arch Phys Med Rehabil* 75:243, 1994.

Rudolph A, editor: *Rudolph's pediatrics,* ed 19, East Norwalk, Conn, 1991, Appleton & Lange.

72

Sudden Infant Death Syndrome

PATHOPHYSIOLOGY

Sudden infant death syndrome (SIDS) is defined as "the sudden death of an infant under 1 year of age which remains unexplained after a thorough case investigation, including performance of a complete autopsy, examination of the death scene, and review of the clinical history" (National Institute of Child Health and Human Development [NICHD]). The autopsy reports the following findings. External examination reveals a body that appears well developed and nourished. There is a small amount of mucous, watery, or bloody secretions present at the nares. Cyanosis of the lips and nail beds is almost always present. The internal examination findings indicate a subacute inflammation of the upper respiratory tract and petechiae on the pleura, pericardium, and thymus (this is found in 80% of the cases). There is pulmonary edema and congestion. The autopsy reveals symptoms of chronic hypoxemia including brainstem changes; persistence of brown fat, especially around the adrenals; and hepatic erythropoiesis. Some of these autopsy findings are demonstrated in about 80% of SIDS cases, and their absence does not exclude the diagnosis. Risk factors associated with the incidence of SIDS are listed in the box on p. 475.

The pathophysiology of SIDS is unclear, but current research focuses on the following explanations:
1. Abnormalities of the central nervous system(CNS)—particularly delayed myelination or gliosis (or scarring) in the respiratory control areas of the brainstem

Risk Factors

Infant

- Prematurity, particularly with birth weight <2500 g
- Low birth weight for gestational age
- African American and Native American heritage
- Male gender (risk increased by 50%)
- Multiple births
- Low Apgar scores
- Central nervous system disturbances
- Respiratory disorders such as bronchopulmonary dysplasia
- Neonatal intensive care history

Familial

- Low SES
- Low educational level

Maternal

- Young married mother < 20 years old
- History of smoking during pregnancy
- History of drug abuse (including marijuana, methadone, cocaine, heroin, or psychedelics)
- High parity
- Low interpregnancy interval
- Anemia

2. Primary cardiac arrhythmias, particularly bradycardia secondary to a decrease in vagal nerve tone and bradycardia occurring simultaneously with central apnea

3. Airway obstruction—from pharyngeal collapse, which could be exacerbated by the prone sleeping position

4. Impaired temperature regulation and its effects on the respiratory pattern, chemoreceptor sensitivity, and cardiac control
5. Possible infectious agents—viral septicemia

INCIDENCE

1. Sudden infant death syndrome is the most common cause of death before 1 year of age.
2. SIDS occurs in 2 of every 1000 live births in the general public.
3. Age range of peak incidence is 2 to 3 months; it is uncommon before 2 weeks of age or after 6 months of age.
4. It has seasonal occurrence in the winter months, particularly January.
5. Occurrence of death is most frequently between midnight and 9 A.M.
6. Ethnic distribution is as follows: 2.5 to 6.0 of every 1000 live births for Native Americans and African Americans; and 1.0 to 2.5 of every 1000 live births for Asians, whites, and Latinos.
7. SIDS accounts for an estimated 7000 to 10,000 infant deaths per year worldwide.

NURSING ASSESSMENT

1. Assess the infant, familial, and maternal risk factors (see the box on p. 475) associated with SIDS.
2. Assess family's ability to manage in-home apnea monitoring.
3. Assess family's need for support and resources during the acute grieving period.

NURSING DIAGNOSES

- Altered family processes
- High risk for dysfunctional grieving
- High risk for ineffective management of therapeutic regimen

NURSING INTERVENTIONS
Prevention

1. Complete a thorough history and physical examination to determine the presence of risk factors.

SIDS Resources

National Sudden Infant Death Syndrome
Foundation
10500 Little Patuxent Parkway, Suite 420
Columbia, MD 21044
(800) 638-7437

Sudden Infant Death Syndrome Clearing
House
8201 Greensboro Drive, Suite 600
McClean, VA 22102
(703) 821-8955

American Sudden Infant Death
Syndrome Institute
275 Carpenter Drive, Suite 100
Atlanta, GA 30328
(800) 232-SIDS

2. Perform newborn teaching with parents before discharge, stressing the need for follow-up care with a pediatrician and the use of the American Academy of Pediatrics (AAP) 1992 guidelines on sleeping position.
3. Monitor ability of family members to participate in in-home apnea monitoring and use of cardiopulmonary resuscitation (CPR) when applicable.
4. Refer family to appropriate community-based support group (i.e., Compassionate Friends, Candlelighters).

Care after SIDS

Support the family during the acute grieving period.
1. Counsel parents and reassure them that they are not responsible for the infant's death.
2. Encourage parents to express their feelings of guilt and remorse.

3. Employ therapeutic listening skills to assist parents in the grieving process.
4. Allow sufficient privacy for parents to be alone with infant as needed.

🏠 Discharge Planning and Home Care

1. During bereavement period, refer family to appropriate resources to deal with issues such as chronic grief (see the box on p. 477).
2. Follow up with phone call and sympathy card from staff.

CLIENT OUTCOMES

1. Family will be knowledgeable about community resources.
2. Family will demonstrate appropriate grieving behaviors.

REFERENCES

Andrews M et al: Home apnea monitoring in the intermountain west, *J Pediatr Health Care* 1(5):255, 1987.

Davis N, Sweeney L: Infantile apnea monitoring and SIDS, *J Pediatr Health Care* 3(2):67, 1989.

Goldberg J: The counseling of SIDS parents, *Clin Perinatol* 19(4):927, 1992.

Grether J, Schulman J, Croen L: Sudden infant death syndrome among Asians in California, *J Pediatr* 116(4):525, 1990.

Guntheroth W, Lohmann R, Spiers S: Risk of sudden infant death syndrome in subsequent siblings, *J Pediatr* 116(4):520, 1990.

Haglund B, Crattingius S: Cigarette smoking as a risk factor for sudden infant death syndrome: a population based study, *Am J Public Health* 80(1):29, 1990.

Hoffman H, Hillman L: Epidemiology of the infant sudden death syndrome: maternal, neonatal, and postneonatal risk factors, *Clin Perinatol* 19(4):717, 1992.

Katwinkel J, Brooks J, Myerberg D: Report of the American Academy of Pediatrics' ad hoc committee to examine the effect of infant positioning on the incidence of SIDS, *Pediatrics* 89:1120, 1992.

Ponsonby A et al: Factor potentiation the risk of sudden infant death syndrome associated with the prone position, *New Engl J Med* 329(6):377, 1993.

Shannon D: Prospective identification of the risk of SIDS, *Clin Perinatol* 19(4):861, 1992.

Spiers P, Guntheroth W: Recommendations to avoid the prone sleeping position and recent statistics for sudden infant death syndrome in the United States, *Arch Pediatr Adolesc Med* 148:141, 1994.

Swoiskin S: Sudden infant death: nursing care for the survivors, *J Pediatr Nurs* 1(1):33, 1986.

Valdes-Dapena M: The sudden infant death syndrome: pathologic findings, *Clin Perinatol* 19(4):701, 1992.

Willinger M, James L, Catz C: Defining the sudden infant death syndrome (SIDS): deliberations of an expert panel convened by the National Institute of Child Health and Human Development, *Pediatr Pathol* 11:677, 1991.

73

Tetralogy of Fallot

PATHOPHYSIOLOGY

Tetralogy of Fallot is a cyanotic congenital heart defect composed of four structural defects: (1) ventricular septal defect; (2) pulmonic stenosis, which may be infundibular, valvular, supravalvular, or a combination of these, causing obstruction of the blood flow into the pulmonary arteries; (3) right-ventricular hypertrophy; and (4) varying degrees of overriding of the aorta. The ventricular septal defect is invariably large. In patients with tetralogy of Fallot, the diameter of the aorta is larger than normal, whereas the pulmonary artery is smaller than normal. Congestive heart failure (CHF) rarely occurs because the chamber pressures of the right and left ventricles are equal due to the presence of the septal defect. Hypoxia is the primary problem. The degree of cyanosis is related to the severity of the anatomic obstruction to the blood flow from the right ventricle into the pulmonary artery, as well as to the physiologic status of the child.

Most children with tetralogy of Fallot are candidates for surgical repair, which is usually performed when the child is 1 to 4 years old. Shunt procedures may be performed before total correction as palliative measures to correct hypoxia secondary to inadequate pulmonary flow. Blalock-Taussig and Waterston-Cooley are examples of preliminary shunt procedures. Surgical correction is indicated for children with severe hypoxia and polycythemia (hematocrit [Hct] greater than 60%). Surgical risk is associated with the diameter of the pulmonary arteries; risk is less than 10% if the diameter of the pulmonary arteries is at least one third of the aortic diameter.

INCIDENCE

1. Tetralogy of Fallot affects male and female individuals equally.
2. There is a higher incidence with older maternal age.
3. Few patients survive beyond 20 years without surgery.
4. Tetralogy of Fallot accounts for 10% of all congenital defects.
5. It accounts for 50% of individuals with an inoperative congenital heart defect with decreased pulmonary blood flow beyond infancy.
6. There is a 5% mortality rate (slightly higher in infants) for patients who undergo cardiac repair; 10% for patients with shunts.
7. Ten percent of survivors have unsatisfactory results.

CLINICAL MANIFESTATIONS

1. Cyanosis—appears after several months of age; rarely seen at birth; becomes progressively more severe
2. Hypercyanotic spells
   a. Increased rate and depth of respiration
   b. Acute cyanosis
   c. Central nervous system irritability that can progress to limpness and syncope and ultimately result in seizures, cardiovascular accident (CVA), and death (occurs in 35% of cases)
3. Clubbing
4. Initially normal blood pressure—can increase after several years of marked cyanosis and polycythemia
5. Classic squatting position—decreases venous return from lower extremities and increases pulmonary blood flow and systemic arterial oxygenation
6. Failure to thrive
7. Anemia—contributes to worsening of symptoms
   a. Decreased exercise tolerance
   b. Increased dyspnea
   c. Increased frequency of paroxysmal hyperpnea

8. Acidosis
9. Murmur (systolic and continuous)
10. Ejection click after first heart sound
11. Knee or head-to-chest position assumed during spells or after exercise

COMPLICATIONS

The following are complications of the condition:
1. Pulmonary vascular disease
2. Deformity of the right pulmonary artery
   The following complications may occur after Blalock-Taussig anastomosis:
1. Bleeding—especially prominent in children with polycythemia
2. Cerebral embolism or thrombosis—risk greater in polycythemia, anemia, or sepsis
3. Congestive heart failure if the shunt is too large
4. Early occlusion of the shunt
5. Hemothorax
6. Persistent right-to-left shunt at the atrial level, especially in infants
7. Persistent cyanosis
8. Phrenic nerve damage
9. Pleural effusion

LABORATORY AND DIAGNOSTIC TESTS

1. Chest x-ray study—indicates increase or decrease in pulmonary flow; no heart enlargement evident
2. Electrocardiogram (ECG)—indicates right-ventricular hypertrophy, left-ventricular hypertrophy, or both
3. Arterial blood gas (ABG) values—reflect obstructive pulmonary blood flow (increased partial pressure of carbon dioxide [PCO_2], decreased partial pressure of oxygen [PO_2], and decreased pH)
4. Hematocrit (Hct) or hemoglobin (Hb)—monitors viscosity of blood and detects iron deficiency anemia
5. Echocardiogram—detects septal defect, aortic position, and pulmonic stenosis
6. Cardiac catheterization—increased systemic pressures in right ventricle; decreased pulmonary artery pressures with decreased arterial hemoglobin saturation

7. Platelet count—decreased
8. Barium swallow test—demonstrates displacement of trachea to left of midline
9. Radiogram of abdomen—detects existence of other possible congenital anomalies

MEDICAL MANAGEMENT

The following medications may be used:

1. Antibiotics—selection dependent on the results of the culture and sensitivity (C and S); sometimes used for prophylaxis
2. Diuretics (e.g., furosemide [Lasix])—used to promote diuresis; decrease fluid overload; used in the treatment of edema associated with CHF
3. Digitalis—increases the force of contraction of the heart, the stroke volume, and cardiac output and decreases cardiac venous pressures; used to treat CHF and selected cardiac arrhythmias (rarely given before correction unless shunt too large)
4. Iron—to manage anemia
5. Propranolol (Inderal), a beta blocker—reduces heart rate and decreases force of contraction and myocardial irritability; used to prevent or treat hypercyanotic spells
6. Morphine, an analgesic—increases pain threshold; also used to treat hypercyanotic spells by depressing the respiratory center and cough reflex
7. Sodium bicarbonate ($NaHCO_3$), a potent systemic alkalizer—used to treat acidosis by replacing bicarbonate ions and restoring buffering capacity of body

SURGICAL MANAGEMENT
Palliative Measures

Blalock-Taussig anastomosis. A Blalock-Taussig subclavian-pulmonary anastomosis is the palliative intervention generally recommended for children who are unsuitable for corrective surgery. The subclavian artery opposite the side of the aortic arch is ligated, divided, and anastomosed to the contralateral pulmonary artery. The advantages of this shunt are the ability to construct very small shunts, which grow with the child, and the fact that it is easy to remove the shunt during definitive repair. The modified Blalock-Taussig anastomosis is essentially the same, but using a prosthetic material, usually polytetrafluoroethylene. With this shunt, the size can be better controlled, and it is easier to remove since most complete repairs are performed at a young age.

The hemodynamic consequence of the Blalock-Taussig shunt is to allow systemic blood to enter the pulmonary circulation through the subclavian artery, increasing pulmonary blood flow under low pressure, thus avoiding pulmonary congestion. This blood flow allows stabilization of the cardiac and respiratory status until the child grows enough for corrective surgery to be safe. Collateral circulation will develop to ensure adequate arterial flow to the arm, although a blood pressure will not be obtainable in that arm.

Waterston-Cooley anastomosis. Waterston-Cooley anastomosis is a palliative procedure used for infants with defects associated with decreased pulmonary blood flow, such as tetralogy of Fallot. It is a closed-heart procedure in which the posterior ascending aorta is sewn directly to the anterior of the right pulmonary artery, creating a fistula. Although this shunt is difficult to remove during definitive repair, it has generally replaced the Potts-Smith-Gibson, or Potts, anastomosis, which is a side-to-side shunt between the descending aorta and left pulmonary artery, because it is technically the easiest to create.

The desired hemodynamic response is for the blood from the aorta to flow into the pulmonary artery and thus increase the pulmonary blood flow. This procedure should relieve anoxia, cyanosis, and clubbing. A machine-type of murmur is produced.

Definitive Repair

Complete repair of tetralogy of Fallot used to be postponed until the preschool years but now can be safely accomplished in 1- and 2-year-old children. Indications for surgery at a young age include severe polycythemia (hematocrit greater than 60%), hypercyanotic ("tet") spells, hypoxia, and decreased quality of life. A median sternotomy incision is made, and cardiopulmonary bypass is established, with deep hypothermia added for some infants. If a previous shunt is in place, it is removed. Unless the repair cannot be completed through the right atrium, a right ventriculotomy is avoided because of the potential for impaired ventricular function. Right-ventricular outflow obstruction is resected and widened, using Dacron with pericardial backing. Care is taken to avoid pulmonary insufficiency. The pulmonary valve is incised. The ventricular septal defect is closed with a Dacron patch to complete the operation. In cases of severe right-ventricular outflow tract obstruction, a conduit may be inserted.

NURSING ASSESSMENT

1. See the section on cardiovascular assessment in Appendix A.
2. Assess child's level of activity and acquisition of developmental milestones (preoperatively).
3. Assess for changes in cardiopulmonary status.
4. Assess for signs and symptoms of potential collaborative problems (complications): bleeding, congestive heart failure, arrhythmias, persistent pulmonary regurgitation, low cardiac output, pulmonary hypertension, pleural effusion, electrolyte imbalances, fluid overload, hepatomegaly, and neurologic complications.
5. Assess for postoperative pain.

NURSING DIAGNOSES

- Activity intolerance
- Anxiety
- Fear
- Decreased cardiac output
- Altered tissue perfusion
- Fluid volume excess
- High risk for infection
- High risk for injury
- Altered family processes
- Ineffective individual coping
- Altered nutrition: less than body requirements
- High risk for altered growth and development
- High risk for ineffective management of therapeutic regimen

NURSING INTERVENTIONS
Maintenance Care

1. Monitor for changes in cardiopulmonary status.
2. Monitor and maintain hydration status.
   a. Input and output; specific gravity
   b. Signs of dehydration
3. Monitor child's response to medications (see section on medical management, this chapter).
   a. Iron—for iron deficiency anemia and polycythemia
   b. Antibiotics—administered before, during, and after surgery as prophylaxis against subacute bacterial endocarditis
   c. Diuretics (furosemide)—for CHF before or after surgery
   d. Digitalis—for CHF before or after surgery
   e. Morphine—to alleviate hypercyanotic spells
   f. Propranolol—to alleviate hypercyanotic spells (long-term management)
   g. Sodium bicarbonate—if documented acidosis develops
4. Provide foods high in iron (to treat iron deficiency anemia) and protein (to promote healing).
   a. Cereals, egg yolk, and meat
   b. Supplemental iron
5. Provide oxygen supplementation as needed and monitor child's response.
   a. Monitor respiratory status.
   b. Monitor color.
   c. Use and maintain respiratory equipment (oxygen mask, ventilator, or tent).
6. Protect child from potential infectious contacts, and promote preventive practices (to prevent subacute bacterial endocarditis).
   a. Screen visitors for infections.
   b. Instruct child and family about good dental care.
      (1) Brushing and flossing of teeth
      (2) Frequent dental checkups for detection of caries and gingival infections
      (3) Importance of antibiotic prophylaxis for dental extractions

    c. Provide close surveillance for and timely reporting of fever and abrasions for antibiotic prophylaxis.
7. Monitor for signs of complications and child's response to treatment regimen.
    a. Acidosis
    b. Anemia
    c. Brain abscess
8. Observe for phrenic nerve damage and diaphragmatic paralysis.
9. Observe for respiratory complications.

Preoperative Care

1. Prepare child for surgery by obtaining assessment data.
    a. Complete blood count (CBC), urinalysis, serum glucose, and blood urea nitrogen (BUN)
    b. Baseline electrolytes
    c. Blood coagulation
    d. Type and cross match for blood
    e. Chest x-ray study and ECG
2. Use age-appropriate explanations for preparation of child (see Appendix J, section on preparation for procedure/surgery).
3. Do not take blood pressure readings or make arterial punctures in potential shunt arm.

Postoperative Care

Blalock-Taussig or Waterston-Cooley anastomosis

1. Assess child's clinical status.
    a. Immediately after surgery, expect arm with involved subclavian artery to be cool and without blood pressure (Blalock-Taussig anastomosis).
        (1) Flush blood pressure should equal mean arterial blood pressure (no blood pressure readings in shunt arm).
        (2) Note pulse pressure; wide pulse pressure indicates a large shunt.
    b. Note pulses; bounding pulses indicate large shunt.
    c. Note cyanosis; hypoxemia or signs of acidosis indicate early occlusion of shunt.
    d. Assess for Horner's syndrome.

2. Monitor the child for any postoperative complications (Waterston-Cooley anastomosis).
   a. Bleeding
   b. CHF if the shunt is too large
   c. Increased pulmonary blood flow and pulmonary hypertension
3. Monitor child's response to administered medications— digitalis and diuretics are administered if needed.
4. Monitor and maintain fluid and electrolyte balance.
   a. Monitor for signs of dehydration—lack of tearing, doughy skin, specific gravity greater than 1.020, and decrease in urine output or body weight.
   b. Monitor fluids at 50% to 75% of maintenance volume during first 24 hours ($1000 \ ml/m^2$, then $1500 \ ml/m^2$).
5. Promote and maintain optimal respiratory status.
   a. Perform percussion and postural drainage every 2 to 4 hours.
   b. Use suction as needed.
   c. Use spirometer every 1 to 2 hours for 24 hours, then every 4 hours.
6. Monitor and alleviate child's pain (see Appendix I).

Tetralogy of Fallot corrective surgery

1. Monitor child's clinical status, and monitor for postoperative complications.
   a. Arrhythmias
      (1) Right bundle branch block caused by right ventriculotomy or ventricular septal defect repair
      (2) Complete heart blocks
      (3) Supraventricular arrhythmias
      (4) Ventricular tachycardia
   b. Congestive heart failure caused by incision of the right ventricle, which decreases the pumping ability of the heart (more common if pulmonary hypertension is present)
   c. Hemorrhage caused by low platelet count in children with polycythemia
   d. Low cardiac output (most common cause of death)
   e. Neurologic complications caused by thromboemboli

    f. Persistent pulmonary regurgitation

    g. Residual ventricular septal defect (affects 10% of patients)

2. Monitor child's response to medications.

    a. Pressors for low cardiac output

    b. Digitalis and diuretics several weeks to months after surgery to control CHF

3. Monitor child's cardiac function hourly for 24 to 48 hours, then every 4 hours.

    a. Vital signs, including rectal temperature

    b. Color

    c. Peripheral pulses and capillary refill time

    d. Arterial blood pressure and central venous pressure (CVP)

    e. Hepatomegaly

    f. Periorbital edema

    g. Pleural effusion

    h. Pulsus paradoxus

    i. Heart sounds

    j. Ascites (rare)

4. Monitor for cardiac arrhythmias.

5. Monitor for signs and symptoms of hemorrhage.

    a. Assess child's chest tube output every hour.

    b. Assess for bleeding from other sites.

    c. Maintain strict intake and output.

    d. Assess for ecchymotic lesions and petechiae.

6. Monitor and maintain child's fluid and electrolyte balance.

    a. Intravenous (IV) fluids infused at 50% to 75% of maintenance volume for first 24 hours (1000 ml/m^2, then 1500 ml/m^2)

    b. Signs and symptoms of dehydration

7. Monitor and maintain child's respiratory status.

    a. Perform chest physiotherapy.

    b. Place child in semi-Fowler's position.

    c. Humidify air.

    d. Monitor for chylothorax.

    e. Provide adequate pain medications.

8. Provide for child's and family's emotional needs (see Appendix J, section on supportive care).

9. Monitor and alleviate child's pain (see Appendix I).
10. Provide developmentally appropriate stimulation and/or activities (see Appendix B).

♠ Discharge Planning and Home Care

1. Make family aware that antibiotic prophylaxis for dental work and surgery is required.
2. Instruct family about exercise limitations, if such limitations continue.
3. Instruct parents about the administration of medications and child's response to them.
4. Instruct parents about the use of cardiopulmonary resuscitation (CPR).
5. Instruct parents about parenting skills.
   a. Need to maintain usual expectations for behavior and misbehavior
   b. Continuance of disciplinary measures
   c. Methods and strategies to assist child in living normally and dealing with concerns
6. Instruct parents about infection control measures.

CLIENT OUTCOMES

1. Child's vital signs will be within normal limits for age.
2. Child will participate in physical activities appropriate for age.
3. Child will be free of postoperative complications.

REFERENCES

Adams F, Emmanouilides G, Riemenschneider T: *Heart disease in infants, children, and adolescents,* ed 4, Baltimore, 1989, Williams & Wilkins.

Byrd L, Bruton-Maree N: Tetralogy of Fallot, *AANA J* 57(2):169, 1989.

Hazinski M: *Nursing care of the critically ill child,* ed 2, St Louis, 1992, Mosby.

Maloney S: Tetralogy of Fallot: using pulmonary allograft conduits to reconstruct the right ventricular outflow tract, *JORN* 50(3):554, 1989.

McAnear S: Parental reaction to chronically ill child, *Home Healthcare Nurse* 8(3):85, 1990.

Redington A: Determinants of short- and long-term outcome in the surgical correction of tetralogy of Fallot, *Curr Opin Pediatr* 5(5):619, 1993.

Starnes V et al: Current surgical management of tetralogy of Fallot, *Ann Thorac Surg* 58(1):211, 1994.

74

Urinary Tract Infections

PATHOPHYSIOLOGY

Urinary tract infection (UTI) is the bacterial colonization of any segment of the urinary tract. The number of organisms in the urine is greater than can be accounted for by the method of collection. The most common diagnostic criterion for UTI is the presence of at least 100,000 bacterial colonies in 1 ml of a clean midstream urine catch obtained on two consecutive cultures. The presence of urine and stool surrounding the urinary meatus allows the bacteria to proliferate and ascend upward to the urethra. Children at risk are those with underlying defects of the urinary system, chronic disease, and neurologic disorders. UTI is second in frequency of occurrence to upper respiratory tract infections.

INCIDENCE

1. The female-male ratio is 9:1.
2. Age range of peak incidence in girls is 7 to 11 years.
3. Age range of peak incidence in boys is 2 to 6 years.
4. Ninety percent of the infecting organisms are *Eschrichia coli.*
5. Fifty-seven percent of male individuals and 37% of female individuals with UTI have an underlying abnormality.
6. Incidence of symptomatic UTI is lower than that of asymptomatic UTI.

7. Thirty percent to 80% of people with UTI experience reinfection within 1 year.
8. UTI rarely leads to permanent damage, end-stage renal disease, or chronic pyelonephritis.
9. Uncircumcised boys experience 2 to 3 UTIs in childhood.

CLINICAL MANIFESTATIONS
Infants (Initially Seen with Vague Symptoms)

1. Colic
2. Jaundice
3. Poor eating
4. Vomiting
5. Fever
6. Lethargy
7. Irritability
8. Increased number of wet diapers
9. Growth retardation

Preschool Children

1. Fever (most common)
2. Weak urinary stream or dribbling
3. Foul-smelling urine
4. Hematuria
5. Enuresis
6. Abdominal pain

School-Age Children

1. Dysuria
2. Frequency
3. Urgency

All Ages

1. Abdominal distention
2. Dehydration
3. Flank pain
4. Costovertebral angle tenderness
5. Chills and fever
6. Constipation

COMPLICATIONS

1. Reinfection
2. Chronic pyelonephritis

LABORATORY AND DIAGNOSTIC TESTS

1. Urine culture—to determine presence and amount of microorganisms (obtain midstream urine)
2. Suprapubic aspiration—to obtain sterile urine
3. Intravenous pyelogram (IVP)—to visualize kidney and bladder
4. Voiding cystourethrogram (VCUG)—to establish presence of vesicoureteral reflux and abnormalities
5. Cystoscopy—to visualize interior of bladder and urethra (not routinely performed)
6. Retrograde pyelography—to visualize contour and size of ureters and kidneys
7. Cystometry—to assess filling capacity of bladder and effectiveness of detrusor reflux

MEDICAL MANAGEMENT

Before treatment is initiated, a diagnosis needs to be made based on the child's symptoms and results of the culture and sensitivity identifying the organism. Most of the commonly acquired UTIs can be effectively treated with 7 to 14 days of antibiotic therapy. The most commonly used antibiotics are trimethoprim, sulfamethoxazole, nitrofurantoin, amoxicillin, sulfisoxazole, cefaclor, and ampicillin.

NURSING ASSESSMENT

1. See the section on genitourinary assessment in Appendix A.
2. Assess urine output for frequency, urgency, presence of odor, and dysuria.
3. Assess for elevated temperature.
4. Assess for pain.
5. Assess for behavior changes.

NURSING DIAGNOSES

- Altered patterns of urinary elimination
- Hyperthermia

- Pain
- High risk for ineffective management of therapeutic regimen
- High risk for injury

NURSING INTERVENTIONS

Monitor child's therapeutic response to and untoward effects of medication.

1. Obtain urinalysis including culture and sensitivity test before administration of drugs.
2. Repeat urinalysis 48 to 72 hours after antibiotics are initiated and 1 week after therapy has ended.
3. Encourage intake of fluids according to norms.
   a. First 10 kg—100 ml/kg/24 hr
   b. Second 10 kg—150 ml/kg/24 hr
   c. Greater than 20 kg—170 ml/kg/24 hr

♠ Discharge Planning and Home Care

The prime concern is to prevent reinfection.

1. Instruct family and child about importance of completing 7 to 14 days of antibiotic treatment.
2. Instruct child to void frequently (retention of urine serves to maintain infection).
3. Instruct about proper perineal cleaning (e.g., anterior-to-posterior wiping).
4. Instruct about avoidance of bubble baths.

CLIENT OUTCOMES

1. The child will be free of the signs and symptoms of UTI.
2. The child will not experience recurrent UTIs.
3. The child and family will adhere to the treatment regimen.

REFERENCES

Herzog L: Urinary tract infections and circumcision: a case-control study, *Am J Dis Child* 143(3):348, 1989.

Khan, A: Efficacy of single-dose therapy of urinary tract infections in infants and children: a review, *J Natl Med Assoc* 86(9):690, 1994.

Wilson D, Killion D: Urinary tract infections in the pediatric patient, *Nurs Pract* 14(7):38, 1989.

75

Ventricular Septal Defect and Repair

PATHOPHYSIOLOGY

Ventricular septal defect (VSD) is characterized by a septal communication that allows direct blood flow between the ventricles, usually from left to right. The defects may vary from 0.5 to 3.0 cm in diameter. Approximately 20% of the ventricular septal defects seen in children are simple (i.e., small). Many of them close spontaneously. Approximately 50% to 60% of affected children have a moderate-size defect and show symptoms in late childhood. This defect is frequently associated with other cardiac defects. The altered physiology can be described as follows:

1. Pressure is greater in the left ventricle and promotes the flow of oxygenated blood through the defect to the right ventricle.
2. Increased blood volume is pumped into the lungs, which eventually may become congested with blood, and may result in increased pulmonary vascular resistance.
3. If the pulmonary resistance is great, right-ventricular pressure may increase, causing a reversal of the shunt, with the unoxygenated blood flowing from the right ventricle to the left, producing cyanosis (Eisenmenger's syndrome).

In a child with a simple ventricular septal defect, the clinical picture may include the presence of a murmur, mild exercise intolerance, fatigue, dyspnea during exertion, and severe repeated respiratory tract infections. The seriousness of the condition depends on the size of the shunt and the degree of pulmonary hypertension. If the child is asymptomatic, no treatment is required; however, if congestive heart failure (CHF) develops or the child risks pulmonary vascular change or demonstrates extreme shunting, surgical closure of the defect is indicated. The surgical risk is approximately 3%, and the ideal age range for surgery is 3 to 5 years.

With a larger defect, the child will show the same symptoms, but they will be more severe and may appear within the first month of life.

INCIDENCE

1. The male-female ratio with the defect is 1:1.
2. An increase in ventricular septal defects is seen in children with Down syndrome and Holt-Oram syndrome.
3. The surgical risk is from 10% to 25%, depending on the types of complications involved, defect size, the age of the patient, and degree of pulmonary vascular resistance.

CLINICAL MANIFESTATIONS

1. Characteristic sign is a loud, harsh, pansystolic murmur that is generally heard best at the left lower sternal border.
2. Severe overloading of the right ventricle causes hypertrophy and obvious cardiac enlargement.
3. With increased pulmonary vascular resistance, dyspnea and frequent respiratory infections are common.
4. Signs of cyanosis are possible, including assuming a squatting position and decreased venous return.

COMPLICATIONS

1. CHF
2. Infective endocarditis
3. Development of aortic insufficiency or pulmonary stenosis.
4. Progressive pulmonary vascular disease
5. Damage to the ventricular conduction system

LABORATORY AND DIAGNOSTIC TESTS

1. Cardiac catheterization demonstrates an abnormal communication between the ventricles.

2. An electrocardiogram (ECG) and x-ray examination reveal left-ventricular hypertrophy.
3. Complete blood count (CBC) is part of routine preoperative testing.
4. Routine prothrombin time (PT) and partial thromboplastin time (PTT) preoperative testing may reveal bleeding tendencies (usually normal).

MEDICAL MANAGEMENT

Vasopressors or vasodilators are the medications used for children with a ventricular septal defect and severe CHF.

1. Dopamine (Intropin)—has a positive inotropic effect on the myocardium, resulting in increased cardiac output and increased systolic and pulse pressures; has minimal or no effect on diastolic pressure; used to treat hemodynamic imbalance caused by open-heart surgery (dosage regulated to maintain blood pressure and renal perfusion)
2. Isoproterenol (Isuprel)—has a positive inotropic effect on myocardium, resulting in increased cardiac output and work; decreases both diastolic and mean pressures while increasing systolic pressure

SURGICAL MANAGEMENT: VENTRICULAR SEPTAL DEFECT REPAIR

Early repair is preferable if the defect is large. Infants with CHF may require complete or palliative surgery in the form of pulmonary artery banding if they cannot be stabilized medically. Because of the irreversible damage secondary to pulmonary vascular disease, surgery should not be postponed past the preschool years or if progressive pulmonary vascular resistance is present.

A median sternotomy is made and cardiopulmonary bypass is established, with the use of hypothermia for some infants. For a membranous defect high in the septum, a right-atrial incision allows the surgeon to repair the defect by working through the tricuspid valve. Otherwise, a right or left ventriculotomy is necessary. Generally, a Dacron or pericardial patch is placed over the lesion, although direct suturing may be used if the defect is minimal.

Previous banding is removed, and any deformities caused by it are repaired.

Surgical response should include a hemodynamically normal heart, although any damage caused by pulmonary hypertension is irreversible. Complications include the following:

1. Potential aortic insufficiency (particularly if present preoperatively)
2. Arrhythmias
   a. Right bundle branch block (right ventriculotomy)
   b. Heart block
3. CHF, especially in children with pulmonary hypertension and left ventriculotomy
4. Hemorrhage
5. Left-ventricular dysfunction
6. Low cardiac output
7. Myocardial damage
8. Pulmonary edema
9. Residual intraventricular septal defects if repair not complete because of multiple ventricular septal defects

NURSING ASSESSMENT

1. See the section on cardiovascular assessment in Appendix A.
2. Assess for complications.
   a. Diastolic murmur—indicates aortic insufficiency
   b. Widening pulse pressure—indicates aortic insufficiency
   c. Arrhythmias
   d. CHF
   e. Bleeding
   f. Low cardiac output, especially during first 24 hours after surgery

NURSING DIAGNOSES

- Anxiety
- Activity intolerance
- Decreased cardiac output
- Altered tissue perfusion
- Fluid volume excess
- High risk for infection
- High risk for injury

- Altered family processes
- High risk for altered growth and development
- High risk for ineffective management of therapeutic regimen

NURSING INTERVENTIONS
Preoperative Care

1. Prepare child with age-appropriate explanations before surgery (see Appendix J, section on preparation for procedure/surgery).
2. Monitor child's baseline status.
   a. Vital signs
   b. Color of mucous membranes
   c. Quality and intensity of peripheral pulses
   d. Capillary refill time
   e. Temperature of extremities
3. Assist and support child during preoperative laboratory and diagnostic tests.
   a. CBC, urinalysis, serum glucose, and blood urea nitrogen (BUN)
   b. Serum electrolytes—sodium, potassium, and chloride
   c. PT, PTT, and platelet count
   d. Type and cross match of blood
   e. Chest x-ray examination
   f. ECG

Postoperative Care

1. Monitor child's postoperative status as often as every 15 minutes for first 24 to 48 hours.
   a. Vital signs
   b. Color of mucous membranes
   c. Quality and intensity of peripheral pulses
   d. Capillary refill time
   e. Periorbital edema
   f. Pleural effusion
   g. Pulsus paradoxus or decreased pulse pressure
   h. Arterial pressures
   i. Cardiac rhythms
2. Monitor for hemorrhage.
   a. Measure chest tube output hourly.
   b. Assess for clot formation in chest tube.

    c. Assess for ecchymotic lesions and petechiae.

    d. Assess for bleeding from other sites.

    e. Record blood output for diagnostic studies.

    f. Monitor strict intake and output.

    g. Administer fluids at 50% to 75% of maintenance volume during first 24 hours.

    h. Administer blood products as indicated.

3. Monitor child's hydration status.
   a. Skin turgor
   b. Moistness of mucous membranes
   c. Specific gravity
   d. Daily weights
   e. Urine output
4. Monitor for signs and symptoms of CHF.
5. Maintain skin temperature at 36° to 36.5° C and rectal temperature at 37° C.
6. Monitor and maintain child's respiratory status.
   a. Have child turn, cough, and deep breathe.
   b. Perform chest physiotherapy.
   c. Humidify air.
   d. Monitor for chylothorax.
   e. Provide pain medications as needed.
7. Monitor for complications (see section on complications, this chapter).
8. Observe for skin breakdown (e.g., back of head).
9. Monitor and alleviate child's pain (see Appendix I).
10. Provide opportunities for child to express feelings through age-appropriate means (see section on growth and development, Appendix B).
11. Provide emotional support to parents (see Appendix J, section on supportive care).

♠ Discharge Planning and Home Care

Provide instruction to parents about the following (see Appendix K):

1. Medications
2. Time intervals for follow-up care
3. Indications for contacting physician
4. Procedures for treatments
5. Contacting social service
6. Contacting Visiting Nurses Association

CLIENT OUTCOMES

1. Child's vital signs are within normal limits for age.
2. Child will participate in physical activities appropriate for age.
3. Child will be free of postoperative complications.

REFERENCES

Adams F, Emmanouilides G, Riemenschneider T: *Moss' heart disease in infants, children and adolescents,* ed 4, Baltimore, 1989, Williams & Wilkins.

Foldy S et al: Perioperative nursing care for congenital cardiac defects, *Crit Care Nurs Clin North Am* 1(2):289, 1989.

Gersony W: Ventricular septal defect and left sided obstructive lesions in infants, *Curr Opin Pediatr* 6(5):596, 1994.

Meijboom F et al: Long term follow-up after surgical closure of ventricular septal defect in infancy and childhood, *J Am Coll Cardiol* 24(5):1358, 1994.

Moynihan J et al: Caring for patients with lesions increasing pulmonary blood flow, *Crit Care Nurs Clin North Am* 1(2):195, 1989.

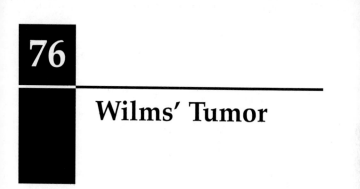

Wilms' Tumor

PATHOPHYSIOLOGY

Wilms' tumor is usually a single tumor that arises from the renal parenchyma. It is separated from the kidney by a membranous capsule. The tumor originates from renoblast cells located in the kidney's parenchyma. A larger tumor will extend across the midline. The tumor may extend to surrounding structures, causing obstruction of the inferior vena cava (from ascites or edema) and/or the intestines (obstruction or constipation). It is associated with congenital anomalies such as hypospadias, cryptorchidism, and aniridia, and with hemihypertrophy, cardiac malformations, and neurofibromatosis.

This tumor grows rapidly. Tissue type varies according to "favorable" and "unfavorable" pathologic conditions. Favorable histology includes multiocular cysts, nephroblastomatosis, and congenital mesoblastic nephromas. Unfavorable histology includes clear cell sarcoma, anaplasia, and rhabdoid tumor. Metastasis occurs through the bloodstream to the lungs and liver. The tumor may spread through the lymphatics to the retroperitoneal lymph nodes. The most common site for metastasis is in the lungs, followed by the liver, contralateral kidney, and bone (rare). The tumor should not be palpated because this can cause seeding of the tumor elsewhere or can cause a pulmonary embolization.

INCIDENCE

1. Wilms' tumor accounts for 6% of childhood cancers.
2. Age range of peak incidence is 3 to 4 years.
3. Prognosis varies according to the stage of the disease at time of diagnosis and the type of cell histology.
4. Overall survival rate of children with favorable histology and nonmetastatic disease is 90%

CLINICAL MANIFESTATIONS

The first three symptoms are the predominant clinical manifestations.

1. Flank mass
2. Pain
3. Hematuria
4. Hypertension
5. Fever
6. Malaise

COMPLICATIONS

1. Metastasis to lungs, bone marrow (anemia), contralateral kidney, and liver
2. Adverse reactions to chemotherapy and/or radiation therapy

LABORATORY AND DIAGNOSTIC TESTS

1. Intravenous pyelogram (IVP), and abdominal x-ray studies, computed tomography (CT), ultrasound, and/or magnetic resonance imaging (MRI)—to detect mass, tumor thrombus in renal veins, enlarged lymph nodes, and tumor relationship to adjoining structures
2. Serum glutamic-oxaloacetic transaminase (SGOT), serum glutamic-pyruvic transaminase (SGPT), and lactic dehydrogenase (LDH)—elevated with liver involvement
3. Complete blood count (CBC)—to assess for anemia and potential bleeding problems
4. Urinalysis—to assess for hematuria
5. Urinary catecholamines—to rule out neuroblastoma
6. Blood urea nitrogen (BUN) and creatinine—to assess renal function
7. Chest CT scan—to assess for metastasis

8. Erythropoietin levels in urine and serum—increased in presence of metastatic disease
9. Bone marrow aspiration and biopsy—to assess marrow involvement (rare)

MEDICAL MANAGEMENT

Surgery is very important in the treatment of Wilms' tumor. A nephrectomy or removal of the affected kidney is performed. In addition to removing the tumor, the surgery also serves to provide tissue for diagnosis and staging, and it provides opportunity to explore lymph nodes and abdominal organs for involvement. Staging is the exact determination of the extent of the disease at the time of diagnosis. The National Wilms' Tumor Study Group staging system consists of five stages that reflect the extent of disease. Postoperatively, radiation therapy and/or chemotherapy are initiated.

Wilms' tumor is radiosensitive. The decision to use radiation therapy or not is based on the histology and stage of the tumor. The chemotherapy drugs and dosage chosen are highly individualized. The following drugs may be given: vincristine, actinomycin-D, doxorubicin, cyclophosphamide, cisplatin, etoposide, and ifosfamide.

NURSING ASSESSMENT

1. See the section on genitourinary assessment in Appendix A.
2. Assess for enlarged abdomen in flank areas (preoperatively).
3. Assess for bowel sounds and abdominal distention postoperatively.
4. Assess for preoperative and postoperative pain.
5. Assess wound for drainage and signs of infection.
6. Assess child's and family's response to illness and surgery.
7. Assess child's developmental level.

NURSING DIAGNOSES

- Impaired tissue integrity
- High risk for injury
- Impaired gas exchange
- High risk for infection
- Anxiety

- Pain
- High risk for ineffective individual coping
- High risk for altered family processes
- High risk for ineffective management of therapeutic regimen
- High risk for altered growth and development

NURSING INTERVENTIONS
Preoperative Care

1. Avoid palpation of abdomen to prevent seeding of tumor.
2. Monitor child's clinical status; observe for signs and symptoms of complications.
   a. Vital signs
   b. Signs and symptoms of vena caval obstruction (facial plethora and venous engorgement)
   c. Signs and symptoms of renal failure
   d. Bone pain
   e. Anemia and bleeding tendencies
   f. Hypertension
3. Provide age-appropriate preprocedural and presurgical explanations to child to alleviate anxiety (see Appendix J, section on preparation for procedure/surgery).
4. Encourage child and parents to express concerns and fears about diagnosis (see Appendix J, section on supportive care).

Postoperative Care

1. Monitor child's clinical status.
   a. Vital signs (monitored as often as every 2 hours after surgery)
   b. Intake and output
   c. Hypertension (caused by removal of kidney)
2. Monitor child's abdominal functioning.
   a. Patency of nasogastric (NG) tube
   b. Bowel sounds
   c. Signs and symptoms of obstruction from vincristine-induced ileus
   d. Postoperative adhesion formation
3. Promote fluid and electrolyte balance.
   a. Monitor infusion of intravenous (IV) solutions.
   b. Monitor for electrolyte imbalances.

    c. Monitor for metabolic alkalosis (results from NG drainage).

4. Maintain and support respiratory status.
    a. Perform pulmonary toilet.
    b. Have child turn, cough, and deep breathe.
    c. Use suction as needed.
    d. Change child's position every 2 hours.

5. Monitor incisional site for intactness and healing.
    a. Observe for signs and symptoms of drainage.
    b. Monitor for intactness.
    c. Monitor for signs and symptoms of infection (redness, warmth, inflammation).
    d. Change dressing as needed.

6. Provide for child's hygienic needs.
    a. Oral and rectal care (especially important because child is immunosuppressed)
    b. Skin care—dry between folds of skin and lubricate

7. Protect child from infection resulting from immunosuppression.
    a. Maintain reverse isolation if white blood count (WBC) decreases (refer to institutional policy).
    b. Limit contacts with public.
    c. Dress child appropriately for weather changes.

8. Monitor side effects of radiotherapy; tumor is remarkably sensitive to radiation.

9. Monitor side effects of chemotherapy.
    a. Dactinomycin
    b. Vincristine

10. Monitor and alleviate child's pain (see Appendix I).

11. Provide developmentally appropriate stimulation and/or activities for child (see Appendix A).

♠ Discharge Planning and Home Care

1. Instruct parents about the various aspects of medical management.
    a. Therapeutic response to medications
    b. Untoward reactions to medications
    c. Adherence with clinic visits

2. Provide information to parents about available resources.
   a. Community (i.e., school) resources
   b. Financial resources
3. Provide emotional support and referral to support groups for parents, siblings, and affected child (see Appendix J, section on supportive care).

CLIENT OUTCOMES

1. Child will be free of complications.
2. Child's level of anxiety prior to procedures and surgery will be minimized.
3. Child and family will adhere to the long-term treatment regimen.

REFERENCES

Foley GV, Fochtman D, Mooney KH: *Nursing care of the child with cancer,* Philadelphia, 1993, WB Saunders.

Joy S et al: Wilms' tumor: diagnosis, surgical management, *AORN J* 53:437, 1991.

PART TWO

Pediatric Diagnostic Tests and Procedures

General Nursing Action

These nursing actions are applicable to all the procedures discussed in this section.

NURSING ASSESSMENT

Assess the following:
1. Developmental level of cognitive capacity as it relates to ability to understand procedure
2. Previous experience with procedure
3. Acuity level
4. Coping abilities
5. Available parental support
6. Parental understanding of procedure
7. Allergies
8. Reaction to medications taken previously

NURSING INTERVENTIONS
Preprocedural Care

1. Explain the procedure, including sensory information, in age-appropriate language; the younger child may want to practice selected aspects of the procedure (e.g., lying on abdomen).
2. Prepare child for preparatory procedural assessment (e.g., complete blood count [CBC] or urinalysis).
3. Obtain information about usual reaction and sensitivity.

4. Reinforce information given to parents about child's or infant's condition; explain purpose and anticipated outcome of procedure.

Postprocedural Care

1. Provide opportunities for the child to discuss procedure and for clarification of misconceptions.
2. Monitor child's clinical status.
   a. Vital signs
   b. Level of consciousness (LOC)
3. Provide foods and fluids when tolerated.
   a. Discontinue intravenous fluids when child is awake.
   b. Initially offer small amounts of clear fluids; assess tolerance before progressing to full liquids and solids.

77

Cardiac Catheterization

Cardiac catheterization is an invasive procedure that measures the intracardiac pressure of the heart chambers and great vessels, as well as oxygen saturation. In addition, angiography is performed when contrast dye is injected to outline the anatomic details of the cardiac malformation. A radiopaque catheter is inserted percutaneously through a large-bore needle into the right femoral artery and vein. Measurements of chamber pressures, oxygen saturation, cardiac output, and shunt flow, as well as pulmonary vascular resistance, are obtained and recorded (see the box on p. 514). Cardiac catheterization in children is used primarily to accurately diagnose complex cardiac defects. Neonates and infants with congestive heart failure (CHF) who appear pale, cyanotic, tachypneic, diaphoretic, fretful, or fatigued will be studied earlier than a stable child where the timing of further repair of a defect remains in question.

Cardiac catheterization is also performed in an interventional manner, using balloon catheters or coiled stents for such purposes as dilating stenotic valves or vessels, and coils or umbrella catheters for closing defects. This can delay or negate the need for surgery. Cardiac catheterization is also performed for electrophysiology studies, for studies of the heart's electric system, and for those infants and children with dysrhythmias refractory to medication.

NURSING ASSESSMENT

1. Assess cardiopulmonary status.
   a. Respiratory rate and quality of lung sounds
   b. Color
   c. Heart rate and cardiac sounds
   d. Pedal pulse quality
   e. Skin temperature and color
   f. Complete blood count (CBC) to obtain values necessary for hemodynamic calculations in the catheterization lab, bleeding time, and type and cross match
2. Assess whether nothing-by-mouth orders were carried out.
3. Assess child's and caregivers' knowledge of procedure and level of anxiety.

NURSING INTERVENTIONS
Preprocedural Care

1. Prepare child and caregivers for the procedure and describe the cardiac catheterization room.
2. Administer sedation and monitor child's response according to institutional guidelines.
3. Mark dorsalis pedis (pedal) pulse and posterior tibial pulse.
4. Record baseline oxygen saturation in the infant with a cyanotic heart defect.
5. Ensure safe transport to catheterization laboratory.
   a. Monitor heart rate and oxygen saturation.
   b. Provide equipment for airway management, including oxygen, suction, ventilation bag, and mask; further airway equipment (for intubation) is needed for the unstable infant or child.

Postprocedural Care

1. Assess physiologic status.
   a. Monitor vital signs every 15 minutes during first hour; every 30 minutes during second hour; then every hour for 4 hours; then every 4 hours.
   b. Assess pulses below the catheterization site for quality and symmetry.
   c. Assess color and temperature of the affected extremity.

Normal Heart Chamber and Great Vessel Pressures and Oxygen Saturations

The pressures in the systemic circuit or on the left side of the heart are normally higher than those in the pulmonary circuit or on the right side of the heart.

- Superior vena cava mean pressure: 3 to 5 mm Hg
- Right atrium mean pressure: 3 to 5 mm Hg
- Right ventricle systolic/diastolic pressure: 25/3 mm Hg
- Pulmonary artery systolic/diastolic pressure: 25/10 mm Hg
- Left atrium mean pressure: 8 mm Hg
- Left ventricle systolic/diastolic pressure: 100/6 mm Hg
- Aorta systolic/diastolic pressure: 100/60 mm Hg

It is normal for oxygen in the blood to be extracted from the tissues and return to the right side of the heart in an amount reduced by about 30% from when it entered the left atrium from the lungs. Blood entering the left atrium is less than 97% to 100% saturated in that there is mixing with blood passing through pulmonary arteriovenous and other small shunts.

- Right atrium: saturation: 65% to 75%
- Right ventricle: saturation: 65% to 75%
- Left atrium: saturation: 95%
- Left ventricle: saturation: 95%

2. Assess patency of insertion site.
   a. Intactness of dressing
   b. Signs of bleeding
   c. Formation of hematoma
3. Maintain bed rest for 6 to 12 hours after catheterization if arterial catheterization was performed, and for 4 to 6 hours if venous catheterization was performed (or per order of physician).
4. Begin administration of clear liquids and advance diet as tolerated.
5. Assess for other complications or adverse effects such as pain, cold stress (infants), dysrhythmias, dye reactions, or nausea and vomiting.
6. Provide opportunities for distraction, relaxation, and play.

REFERENCES

Betz CL, Hunsberger MM, Wright S: *Family-centered nursing care of children,* ed 2, Philadelphia, 1994, WB Saunders.

Hazinski MF: *Nursing care of the critically ill child,* ed 2, St Louis, 1992, Mosby.

Lock JE, Keane JF, Fellows KE: *Diagnostic and interventional catheterization in congenital heart disease,* Boston, 1987, Martinus Nijhoff Publishing.

Roberts PJ: Caring for patients undergoing therapeutic cardiac catheterization, *Crit Care Nurs Clinics North Am* 1(2):275, 1989.

78

Computed Tomography

Computed tomography (CT) is an invasive (with use of contrast dye) or noninvasive roentgenographic procedure that is performed to detect differences in tissue radiodensity. It is used for the entire body; for example, it provides a 360-degree view of the brain in one-degree angles, giving a view of the intracranial structures and precise location of abnormalities. It is a diagnostic tool used in the assessment of various pathologic conditions. Serial evaluations can be performed because the amount of radiation is minimal.

NURSING ASSESSMENT

1. Assess infant's or child's ability to remain still for 5 to 45 minutes.
2. Assess for allergies.
3. Assess the child's previous experience with and reaction to similar procedures and need for sedation.

NURSING INTERVENTIONS

1. Provide age-appropriate explanation of procedure as it is performed (include anticipation of sensations).
2. Monitor infant's or child's reaction to sedation.
   a. Record pulse, respiration, and pulse oximetry readings (and blood pressure, if special equipment is available) every 5 minutes.

   b. Monitor untoward allergic reactions.

   c. Secure infant or child safely on scanning table.

3. Monitor infant's or child's pretest reaction to contrast medium; report any signs or symptoms of allergic reaction.

4. If procedure is performed on an outpatient basis, instruct parents about monitoring sedated child after procedure.

   a. Child should rest or sleep until sedation has worn off.

   b. Ensure parents' understanding of the importance of maintaining an open airway when child is sleeping from sedation (especially in car seat).

REFERENCES

American Academy of Pediatrics, Committee on Drugs: Guideline for monitoring and management of pediatric patients during and after sedation for diagnostic and therapeutic procedures, *Pediatrics* 89(6):1110, 1992.

Cote C: Sedation of children for technical procedures: current standards of practice, *Pediatr Clin North Am* 41(1):31, 1994.

79

Electrocardiography

Electrocardiography is a noninvasive procedure that measures the electric activity of the heart and records it on graph paper. It provides a written account of each myocardial contraction and the electric activity generated by it. Electrocardiograms (ECG or EKG) can be used diagnostically to indicate myocardial infarction and ischemia, hypertrophy of the heart chambers, electrolyte and acid base imbalances, and effects of various drugs. The ECG is used to detect cardiac arrhythmias and conduction defects, and it can reveal a cardiac rhythm that is typically diagnostic of a specific cardiac disorder or congenital heart defect. The ECG sinus pattern changes with age. The greatest change occurs during the first year of life, reflecting the alterations in circulation.

NURSING ASSESSMENT

1. Assess the child's previous experience with procedures.
2. Assess developmental and cognitive level.
3. Assess the child's and parents' understanding of the procedure.

NURSING INTERVENTIONS

1. Explain procedure to child before it is performed.
2. Encourage child to ask questions.
3. Reassure child and encourage him or her to lie quietly during the procedure.

4. Assist in gently holding infant or child (to limit motion during procedure).
5. Remove conduction gel after procedure is completed.

REFERENCES

Ehrat K: *The art of adult and pediatric EKG interpretation,* ed 3, Dubuque, Iowa, 1990, Kendall/Hunt Publishing.

Levin D, Morriss F: *Essentials of pediatric intensive care,* St Louis, 1990, Quality Medical Publishing.

Pillitteri A: *Maternal and child health nursing,* Philadelphia, 1992, JB Lippincott.

Shively M, Fitzsimmons L, Verderber A: Research connections: nursing practice and ECG monitoring, *J Cardiovisc Nurs* 7(3): 81, 1993.

Wong D: *Whaley & Wong's essentials of pediatric nursing,* ed 4, St Louis, 1993, Mosby.

80

Endoscopy

Fiber-optic endoscopy of the upper and lower intestine is used for the diagnosis and treatment of a variety of intestinal diseases. Endoscopy provides visualization of the mucosa of the gastrointestinal tract, the ability to obtain tissue samples, and the ability to perform therapeutic procedures. The upper intestinal tract endoscopy allows the physical direct visualization of the esophagus, stomach, and duodenum. Indications for an upper intestinal tract endoscopy include bleeding, vomiting, failure to thrive, recurrent abdominal pain, foreign body and caustic ingestion, and strictures. The lower intestinal tract endoscopy allows the physician direct visualization of the mucosa of the colon. Indications for the colonoscopy include bleeding, chronic inflammatory bowel disease, and chronic diarrhea. There are few contraindications to endoscopy, and it is most often performed in an outpatient setting. Conscious sedation is used not only to sedate but to minimize discomfort during the procedure.

NURSING ASSESSMENT

1. Assess child's compliance with preprocedural preparation such as nothing-by-mouth (NPO) orders and bowel preparations as ordered.
2. Assess the child's and caregivers' understanding of the procedure.

NURSING INTERVENTIONS

1. Explain procedure to child and caregivers before it is performed.
2. Monitor vital signs including oxygen saturation during and after procedure.
3. Ensure proper positioning of the child.
4. Assist with airway maintenance.
5. Observe for evidence of bleeding or excessive abdominal pain and/or distension.

REFERENCES

Walker W et al: *Pediatric gastrointestinal disease,* vol 2, Philadelphia, 1991, BC Decker.

Wyllie R, Hay M: Gastrointestinal endoscopy in infants and children, *Pediatr Rev* 14(9):352, 1993.

81

Intracranial Pressure Monitoring

Intracranial pressure (ICP) monitoring detects intracranial hypertension. It is indicated for the following conditions: intracranial hypertension, tumors, hemorrhage, contusions, edema, and brain injury. It is used for children when there is a diagnosis of Reye's syndrome, lead poisoning, hydrocephalus, metabolic disorders and/or head trauma after neurosurgery. It is an invasive procedure, requiring the drilling of burr holes into the subarachnoid space for the placement of the pressure monitor into the epidural space. One of several techniques may be used. These include ventriculostomy, ventricular taps, shunts, subdural recordings, intraparenchymal recordings, and subarachnoid bolt. Deep sedation is induced for monitoring the child.

NURSING ASSESSMENT

Assess the child's neurologic status.

NURSING INTERVENTIONS

1. Maintain the functioning of the ICP monitoring equipment.
   a. Report variations greater than the norm.
      (1) ICP greater than 15 mm Hg

      (2) Cerebral perfusion pressure (CPP)—greater than 50 mm Hg (CPP equals mean arterial pressure [MAP] minus ICP)

  b. Note the association between elevations and sleeping and feeding respiratory rate and apical pulse.

2. Monitor for signs and symptoms of complications.
   a. Hemorrhage
   b. Infection
   c. Leakage of cerebrospinal fluid (CSF)
3. Provide explanations to parents about monitoring procedures to alleviate anxiety.
4. Monitor child's response to barbiturate coma.
   a. Monitor apical pulse, respiratory rate, blood pressure, and arterial pressure every 15 minutes during acute phase, then hourly during maintenance phase.
   b. Monitor urinary output hourly during acute phase, then every 2 to 4 hours during maintenance phase.
   c. Monitor serum level of drug.

REFERENCES

Feldman Z, Reichenthal E: Intracranial pressure monitoring, *J Neurosurg* 81(2):329, 1994.

Gambardella G, et al: Intracranial pressure monitoring in children: comparison of external ventricular device with the fiberoptic system, *Childs Nerv Syst* 9(8):470, 1993.

Levin D, Morriss F: *Essentials of pediatric intensive care,* St Louis, 1990, Quality Medical Publishing.

Raju T, Vidyasagar D, Papazafiratou C: Intracranial pressure monitoring in the neonatal ICU, *Crit Care Med* 8(10):575, 1980.

82

Intravenous Pyelogram

The intravenous pyelogram (IVP) makes it possible to identify the presence or absence and determine the size and configuration of the kidneys, ureters, and bladder through direct intravenous injection of a radiopaque dye at the time of the procedure. Distortions, strictures, scarring, and distention from obstruction can be detected. In addition, masses may be identified by their displacement of the kidneys, ureters, or bladder. Renal function is assessed by timing the clearance of the contrast medium through the kidneys. IVP is being replaced by sonogram and radionuclide scanning for diagnostic evaluation in infants and young children.

The procedure is performed by injecting IV contrast medium and assessing the passage through the kidney, ureters, and bladder through a sequence of x-ray films. Injection of the dye may cause flushing and a warm sensation. Because the dyes contain iodine, there is the potential for mild to severe allergic reactions. Antihistamine, epinephrine, steroids, oxygen, isotonic IV fluids, and resuscitation equipment must be available in case they are needed for treating an anaphylactic response.

NURSING ASSESSMENT

1. Obtain a careful history, assessing for contraindications for IVP; these include allergy or sensitivity to iodine, combined renal and hepatic disease, cardiac failure, oliguria (severe renal failure), blood urea nitrogen (BUN)

greater than 40 mg/dl, multiple myeloma, children being treated for asthma, children unable to tolerate dehydration procedures, and shock.

2. Assess the child's developmental level to plan preparation (see Appendix J, section on preparation for procedure/surgery).
3. Assess the child's previous experience with and reaction to similar procedures.

NURSING INTERVENTIONS
Preprocedural Care

1. Observe for sensitivity to skin test if test is indicated.
2. Administer cathartic or enema the evening before procedure (infants and children under 7 years of age should be excluded).
3. Provide nothing by mouth (NPO) for 4 to 6 hours before the procedure (policies vary) in infants and young children, and for 12 hours before the procedure in older children (slight dehydration is needed to concentrate the contrast medium in the urinary tract); if procedure is performed on an outpatient basis, parents should be given NPO instructions.

Postprocedural Care

1. Observe for reactions to the dye (mild reactions include nausea, vomiting, and occasional wheals); notify the physician if these reactions occur, and give antihistamines if symptoms persist.
2. Give food and fluids to replenish and to avoid dehydration.
3. Observe for signs of extravasation at the IV insertion site (elevate extremity and apply warm soaks as needed).
4. Observe for signs of post-IVP renal shutdown; support the child with hydration.

REFERENCES

Fischbach F: *A manual of laboratory diagnostic tests*, ed 3, Philadelphia, 1988, JB Lippincott.

Pagana K, Pagana T: *Diagnostic testing and nursing implications: a case study approach*, ed 4, St Louis, 1994, Mosby.

Swischuk L: *Imaging of the newborn, infant and young child*, ed 3, Baltimore, 1988, Williams & Wilkins.

83

Magnetic Resonance Imaging

Magnetic resonance imaging (MRI) is an imaging study that provides a clear anatomic display of the body. This display provides excellent tissue discrimination, and the study may be done in any plane without the use of radiation. The MRI scan is found to be superior to the computed tomography (CT) scan because MRI uses no radiation and it depicts subtle contrasts between body tissues. Magnetic resonance images are created by sending radio waves to the child who is lying in an external magnetic field. The image is created from interaction of the body tissue with the radio waves in the magnetic field. To prevent artifacts caused by movement, children under the age of eight are frequently sedated with either chloral hydrate or pentobarbital (Nembutal).

Patient and environmental safety issues are paramount in the MRI room because the magnet is always on. The resulting magnetic field will attract any ferrous object (e.g., beepers, watches, infusion pumps, and oxygen tanks) into the scanner. Patients are screened before entry for internal and external objects that may retain heat from the radio waves and cause burns.

NURSING ASSESSMENT

1. Assess for intravenous (IV) access.
2. Screen child for pregnancy or metal implanted devices before the scan (metal devices may include, but are not limited to, metal pins or screws in bones, joints, or soft tissues; Harrington rod; pacemaker; or artificial heart valve).
3. Assess for adequate oxygenation during procedure.
4. Assess child's and caregivers' understanding of the procedure.

NURSING INTERVENTIONS

1. Do not allow anyone to enter the scan room with prohibited items.
   a. Hearing aid
   b. Cochlear or lens implant
   c. Jewelry, watch, tiepin or tie tac
   d. Cardiac pacemaker
   e. Coins, magnetic-strip credit cards, money clip
   f. Keys, safety pins, bobby pins or hairpins or barrettes
   g. Beeper, metal stethoscope
2. Explain procedure to parent and child before entering the scan room.
3. Monitor child's reaction to sedation.
   a. Record pulse oximetry every 5 minutes until awake.
   b. Monitor untoward allergic reactions.

REFERENCES

Milligan D: Personal communication, December 27, 1994.
Westbrook C, Kaut, C: *MRI in practice*, Cambridge, Mass, 1993, Blackwell Science.

84

Peritoneal Dialysis

Peritoneal dialysis is the passing of solutes from the blood through the peritoneum (a semipermeable membrane) into the dialysate through osmosis and diffusion. Osmosis is the movement of a solute from an area of higher concentration to an area of lower concentration. Diffusion is the random movement of particles to form a uniform concentration. The purpose of peritoneal dialysis is to remove toxic substances, body wastes, and excess fluids. The procedure is initiated when a catheter is inserted through a stab incision into the peritoneal cavity. Gravity pulls the dialysis solution into the abdominal cavity. After equilibration between plasma and dialysis fluid has taken place (dwell time), the dialysate flows out again. The process is repeated until amelioration of the symptoms is achieved or the condition resolves. Indications for peritoneal dialysis are the following:

1. Complications of acute renal failure not controlled with medical management
2. Hypervolemia with deteriorating clinical condition (e.g., hypertension, volume overload, deterioration of neurologic status, congestive heart failure, and hypertensive encephalopathy)
3. Bleeding unresponsive to blood component therapy
4. Toxic ingestion of salicylates, phenytoin, heavy metals, or barbiturates

5. Abnormal laboratory values not responsive to medical management
   a. Blood urea nitrogen (BUN) of 125 to 150 mg/dl
   b. Metabolic acidosis
   c. Metabolic alkalosis
   d. Serum uric acid greater than 20 mg/dl
   e. Serum sodium (Na^+) greater than 160 mEq/L
   f. Serum calcium (Ca^+) greater than 12 mg/dl
   g. Serum potassium (K^+) equal to or greater than 6.5 mEq/L

NURSING ASSESSMENT

1. Assess the child's underlying condition.
2. Assess the child's ability to tolerate the procedure and therapy.
3. Assess the child's response to therapy.

NURSING INTERVENTIONS

1. Prepare the child for catheter placement.
   a. Monitor the child's reaction to sedation and pain medication (see Appendix I).
   b. Use sterile technique with procedure (i.e., use mask and sterile gloves).
   c. If possible, have child empty bladder, and weigh him or her before the procedure.
2. Monitor the child's condition during the therapy and intervene as needed.
   a. Monitor for respiratory distress (from abdominal distention, fluid overload, hydrothorax).
   b. Monitor vital signs (hypotension, tachycardia, dehydration).
   c. Monitor temperature (cold dialysate, hypothermia).
   d. Maintain patency and sterility of dialysis catheter.
      (1) Assess for flow problems.
      (2) Position without kinks.
      (3) Maintain intact system while avoiding entering the line.
      (4) Keep clamps in appropriate position.
      (5) Administer anticoagulants and antibiotics as ordered.

    e. Control pain (back pain, cramping, and incision site pain).

    f. Monitor BUN, creatinine, and blood chemistry.

    g. Assess for bowel sounds, and promote adequate nutritional intake and protein replacement.

    h. Prepare child and family for home peritoneal dialysis (as appropriate) through teaching and arranging home care support and equipment (see Appendix K).

3. Monitor the child's therapeutic and untoward responses to medications.

4. Observe for and report signs of complications.

    a. Perforation

    b. Bleeding

    c. Peritonitis

    d. Occluded catheter

    e. Dehydration

    f. Respiratory distress

    g. Cardiac compromise

    h. Electrolyte imbalance

    i. Hyperglycemia

    j. Catheter site leakage

    k. Abdominal wall hernia

    l. Protein loss

REFERENCES

Blatz S, Paes B, Steele B: Peritoneal dialysis in the neonate, *Neonatal Network* 8(6):42, 1990.

Elixson E, Clancy G: Neonatal peritoneal dialysis in acute renal failure, *Crit Care Nurs Q* 14(4):56, 1992.

McFarland K: Pediatric peritoneal dialysis, *Pediatr Nurs* 14:426, 1988.

Pagana K, Pagana T: *Diagnostic testing and nursing implications: a case study approach*, ed 4, St Louis, 1994, Mosby.

Rose A: Dialysis in the pediatric intensive care unit: a case study, *Crit Care Nurs Q* 14(4):66, 1992.

Skale N: *A manual of pediatric nursing procedures*, Philadelphia, 1992, JB Lippincott.

Appendixes

Nursing Assessments

MEASUREMENTS

1. Temperature
2. Pulse
3. Respirations
4. Blood pressure
5. Height
6. Weight
7. Head circumference (under 2 years of age)

CARDIOVASCULAR ASSESSMENT

1. Pulses
   a. Apical pulse—rate, rhythm, and quality
   b. Peripheral pulses—presence or absence; if present, rate, rhythm, quality, and symmetry; major differences between extremities
   c. Blood pressure—all extremities
2. Chest examination and auscultation results
   a. Chest circumference
   b. Presence of chest deformity
   c. Heart sounds—murmur
   d. Point of maximum impulse
3. General appearance
   a. Activity level
   b. Height, weight
   c. Apprehensive or agitated behavior
   d. Clubbing of fingers and/or toes

4. Skin
   a. Pallor
   b. Cyanosis—mucous membranes, extremities, nail beds
   c. Diaphoresis
   d. Temperature
5. Edema
   a. Periorbital
   b. Of extremities

RESPIRATORY ASSESSMENT

1. Breathing
   a. Respiratory rate, depth, and symmetry
   b. Pattern of breathing—apnea, tachypnea
   c. Retractions—suprasternal, intercostal, subcostal, and supraclavicular
   d. Nasal flaring
   e. Position of comfort
2. Chest auscultation results
   a. Equal breath sounds
   b. Abnormal chest sounds—rales, rhonchi, and wheezing
   c. Prolonged inspiratory and expiratory phases
   d. Hoarseness, cough, and stridor
3. Chest examination results
   a. Chest circumference
   b. Shape of chest
4. General appearance
   a. Color—pinkness, paleness, cyanosis, acrocyanosis
   b. Activity level
   c. Behavior—apathetic, inactive, restless, and/or apprehensive
   d. Height and weight

NEUROLOGIC ASSESSMENT

1. Vital signs
   a. Temperature
   b. Respirations
   c. Heart rate
   d. Blood pressure
   e. Pulse pressure

2. Head examination results
   a. Fontanels—bulging, flat, sunken
   b. Head circumference—under 2 years of age
   c. General shape
3. Pupillary reaction
   a. Size
   b. Reaction to light
   c. Equality of responses
4. Level of consciousness (see Glasgow coma scale in the box on p. 535)
   a. Alertness—response to name and command
   b. Irritability
   c. Lethargy and drowsiness
   d. Orientation to self, others, and environment
5. Affect
   a. Mood
   b. Lability
6. Seizure activity
   a. Type
   b. Length
7. Sensory function
   a. Reaction to pain
   b. Reaction to temperature
8. Reflexes
   a. Superficial and deep tendon reflexes (see Table B-1 in Appendix B for infant reflexes)
   b. Presence of pathologic reflexes (e.g., Babinski)
9. Intellectual abilities (dependent on developmental level)
   a. Ability to write or draw
   b. Ability to read

GASTROINTESTINAL ASSESSMENT

1. Hydration
   a. Skin turgor
   b. Mucous membranes
   c. Intake and output
2. Abdomen
   a. Pain
   b. Rigidity
   c. Bowel sounds
   d. Vomiting—amount, frequency, and characteristics

Glasgow Coma Scale

		Score
Eyes open	Spontaneously	4
	To speech	3
	To pain	2
	Not at all	1
Best verbal response	Oriented to time, place, and person	5
	Verbal response indicating confusion and disorientation	4
	Inappropriate words making little sense	3
	Incomprehensible sounds	2
	None	1
Best motor response	Obeying commands to move body part	5
	Purposefully attempting to stop painful stimuli	4
	Decorticate pain response (arm flexion)	3
	Decerebrate pain response (arm extension and internal rotation)	2
	None	1

  e. Stooling—amount, frequency, and characteristics
  f. Cramping
  g. Tenesmus

RENAL ASSESSMENT

1. Vital signs
   a. Pulse
   b. Respirations
   c. Blood pressure

2. Kidney function
   a. Flank or suprapubic tenderness
   b. Dysuria
   c. Voiding pattern—steady or dribbling
   d. Frequency or incontinence
   e. Urgency
   f. Presence of ascites
   g. Presence of edema—scrotal, periorbital, of lower extremities
3. Character of urine and urination
   a. Clear or cloudy appearance of urine
   b. Color—amber, pink, red, or reddish brown
   c. Odor—ammonia, acetone, maple syrup
   d. Specific gravity
   e. Crying upon urination
4. Hydration
5. Genitalia
   a. Irritation
   b. Discharge

MUSCULOSKELETAL ASSESSMENT

1. Gross motor function
   a. Muscle size—presence of atrophy or hypertrophy of muscles; symmetry in muscle mass
   b. Muscle tone—spasticity, flaccidity, limited range of motion
   c. Strength
   d. Abnormal movements—tremors, dystonia, athetosis
2. Fine motor function
   a. Manipulation of toys
   b. Drawing
3. Gait—arm and leg swing, heel-to-toe gait
4. Posture control
   a. Maintenance of upright position
   b. Presence of ataxia
   c. Presence of swaying
5. Joints
   a. Range of motion
   b. Contractures
   c. Redness, edema, pain
   d. Abnormal prominences

6. Spine
   a. Spinal curvature—scoliosis, kyphosis
   b. Presence of piloconidal dimple
7. Hips
   a. Abduction
   b. Internal rotation

HEMATOLOGIC ASSESSMENT

1. Vital signs
   a. Pulse
   b. Respirations
2. General appearance
   a. Signs of congestive heart failure
   b. Restlessness
3. Skin
   a. Color—pallor, jaundice
   b. Petechiae
   c. Bruises
   d. Bleeding from mucous membranes or from injection or venipuncture sites
   e. Hematomas
4. Abdomen
   a. Enlarged liver
   b. Enlarged spleen

ENDOCRINE ASSESSMENT

1. Vital signs
   a. Pulse
   b. Respirations—Kussmaul respirations
   c. Blood pressure
2. Hydration status
   a. Polyuria
   b. Polyphagia
   c. Dry skin
   d. Excessive thirst
3. General appearance
   a. Height and weight
   b. Mood
   c. Irritability
   d. Hunger
   e. Headache
   f. Shakiness

Growth and Development

INFANT (0 TO 1 YEAR)
Physical Characteristics

Age 0 to 6 months

1. Weight
   a. Birth weight doubles by 6 months.
   b. Infant gains approximately 1½ lb per month.
2. Height
   a. Average height at 6 months is 26 inches.
   b. Height increases at the rate of 1 inch per month.
3. Head circumference
   a. Head circumference reaches 17 inches at 6 months.
   b. Circumference increases by ½ inch per month.

Age 6 to 12 months

1. Weight
   a. Birth weight triples by the end of 1 year.
   b. Approximate weight at 1 year is 22 lb.
   c. Infant gains 1 lb per month.
2. Height
   a. Most extensive growth occurs in trunk.
   b. Infant grows ½ inch per month.
   c. Total height increases by 50% by 1 year.
3. Head circumference
   a. Head circumference increases by ¼ inch per month.
   b. Circumference at 1 year is 20 inches.

Gross Motor Development

Age 1 to 4 months

1. Raises head when prone
2. Can sit for short periods with firm support
3. Can sit with head erect
4. Bounces on lap when held in standing position
5. Attains complete head control
6. Lifts head while lying in supine position
7. Rolls from back to side
8. Arms and legs assume less flexed posture
9. Makes precrawling attempts

Age 4 to 8 months

1. Holds head erect continuously
2. Bounces forward and backward
3. Rolls from back to abdomen
4. Can sit with support for short intervals

Age 8 to 12 months

1. Sits from standing position without help
2. Can stand erect with support
3. Cruises
4. Stands erect alone momentarily
5. Pulls self to crawling position
6. Crawls
7. Walks with help

Fine Motor Development

Age 1 to 4 months

1. Makes purposeful attempts to grab objects
2. Follows objects from side to side
3. Attempts to grasp objects but misses
4. Brings objects to mouth
5. Watches hands and feet
6. Grasps objects with both hands
7. Holds objects momentarily in hands

Age 4 to 8 months

1. Uses thumb and fingers for grasping
2. Explores grasped objects

3. Uses shoulder and hand as single unit
4. Picks up objects with cupped hands
5. Is able to hold objects in both hands simultaneously
6. Transfers objects from hand to hand

Age 8 to 12 months

1. Releases objects with uncurled fingers
2. Uses pincer grasp
3. Waves with wrist
4. Can locate hands for play
5. Can put objects in containers
6. Feeds crackers to self
7. Drinks from cup with help
8. Uses spoon with help
9. Eats with fingers
10. Holds crayons and makes marks on paper

Sensory Development

Age 0 to 1 month

1. Distinguishes sweet and sour taste
2. Withdraws from painful stimuli
3. Distinguishes odors—able to detect mother's scent
4. Turns head away from aversive odors
5. Discriminates sounds of different pitch, frequency, and duration
6. Responds to changes in brightness
7. Begins to track objects but easily loses location
8. Prefers human face as compared to other objects in visual field
9. Has visual acuity of 20/400—able to focus on objects up to 8 inches away
10. Quiets at sound of voices

Age 1 to 4 months

1. Discriminates mother's face and voice from those of female stranger
2. Evidences accurate visual tracking
3. Discriminates between visual patterns
4. Distinguishes familiar and unfamiliar faces

Age 4 to 8 months

1. Responds to changes in color

2. Follows object from midline to side
3. Follows objects in any direction
4. Tries to locate sounds
5. Attempts hand-eye coordination
6. Has highly developed sense of smell
7. Reaches adult limits of visual acuity
8. Responds to unseen voice
9. Demonstrates taste preference

Age 8 to 12 Months

1. Has increased depth perception
2. Knows own name

Cognitive Development (Sensorimotor Stage)

Child learns through physical activities and sensory modalities.

Age 0 to 1 month

1. Involuntary behavior
2. Primarily reflexive
3. Autistic orientation
4. No concept of self or others

Age 1 to 4 months

1. Reflexive behavior is gradually replaced by voluntary movement
2. Activity is centered around body
3. Makes initial attempts to repeat and duplicate actions
4. Engages in much trial-and-error behavior
5. Attempts to modify behavior in response to varied stimuli (sucking breast vs. bottle)
6. Demonstrates symbiotic orientation
7. Is unable to differentiate self from others
8. Engages in activity because it is pleasurable

Age 4 to 8 months

1. Demonstrates purposeful repetition of actions
2. Demonstrates emergence of goal-directed behavior
3. Discriminates differences in intensity (sounds and sights)
4. Imitates simple actions

Table B-1. Infant's Reflexes

Reflex	Description	Appearance	Disappearance
Babinski	Fanning of toes with upward extension when sole of foot is stroked	Birth	9 months
Galant	Arching of trunk toward stimulated side when infant is stroked along spine	Birth	Neonatal period
Moro (startle)	Sudden outward extension of arms with midline return when infant is startled by loud noise or rapid change in position	Birth	4 months
Palmar (grasp)	Grasping of object with fingers when palm is touched	Birth	4 months
Parachute	Extension forward of arms and legs in protective manner when infant is held in horizontal prone and moving-downward position	8 months	Indefinite

Placing	Attempting to raise and place foot on edge of surface when touched on top	Birth	12 months
Plantar	Inward flexion of toes when balls of feet are stroked	Birth	12 months
Righting	Attempting to maintain head in upright position	Birth	24 months
Rooting	Turning head toward stimulated side of cheek when touched	Birth	6 months
Sucking	Initiation of sucking when object is placed in mouth	Birth	Indefinite
Swimming	Mimicking swimming movement when held horizontally in water	Birth	4 months
Walking	Making stepping movements when held upright with feet touching a surface	First weeks; reappears at 4 to 5 months	12 months

5. Demonstrates beginnings of object permanence
6. Anticipates future events (feedings)
7. Demonstrates awareness that self is separate from others

Age 8 to 12 months

1. Anticipates event as pleasant or unpleasant
2. Demonstrates emergence of intentional behavior
3. Demonstrates goal-directed behavior
4. Evidences object permanence
5. Looks for lost objects
6. Can imitate larger number of actions
7. Understands meaning of simple words and commands
8. Associates gestures and behaviors with symbols
9. Becomes more independent of mothering figure

Language Development

Age 1 month

1. Coos
2. Makes vowel-like sounds
3. Makes whimpering sounds when upset
4. Makes gurgling sounds when content
5. Smiles in response to adult speech

Age 1 to 4 months

1. Makes sounds and smiles
2. Can make vowel sounds
3. Vocalizes
4. Babbles

Age 4 to 8 months

1. Uses increasing number of vocalizations
2. Uses two-syllable words ("boo-boo")
3. Is able to form two-vowel sounds together ("baba")

Age 8 to 12 months

1. Speaks first word
2. Uses sounds to identify objects, persons, and activities
3. Imitates wide range of word sounds
4. Can say series of syllables

5. Understands meaning of prohibitions such as "no"
6. Responds to own name and those of immediate family members
7. Evidences discernible inflection of words
8. Uses three-word vocabulary
9. Uses one-word sentences

Psychosexual Development (Oral Stage)

1. Body focus—mouth
2. Developmental task—gratification of basic needs (food, warmth, and comfort) as supplied by primary caretakers
3. Developmental crisis—weaning; infant is forced to give up pleasures derived from breast or bottle feedings
4. Common coping skills—sucking, crying, cooing, babbling, thrashing, and other forms of behavior in response to irritants
5. Sexual needs—pleasurable body sensations are generalized, although focused on the oral needs; infant derives physical pleasure from being held, cuddling, rocking, and sucking
6. Play—tactile stimulation provided through caretaking activities

Psychosocial Development (Trust vs. Mistrust)

1. Developmental task—development of sense of trust with primary caretaker
2. Developmental crisis—weaning from breast or bottle
3. Play—interactions with caretakers form the basis for development of relationships later in life
4. Role of parents—infant formulates basic attitudes toward life based on experiences with parents; parents can be perceived as reliable, consistent, available, and caring (sense of trust) or as the negative counterpart (sense of mistrust)

Socialization Behavior

Age 0 to 1 month

The infant smiles indiscriminately.

Age 1 to 4 months

1. Smiles at human face
2. Is awake greater portion of day
3. Establishes sleep-awake cycle
4. Crying becomes differentiated
5. Distinguishes familiar and unfamiliar faces
6. Prefers gazing at familiar face
7. "Freezes" in presence of strangers

Age 4 to 8 months

1. Is constrained in presence of strangers
2. Begins to play with toys
3. Fear of strangers emerges
4. Is easily frustrated
5. Flails arms and legs when upset

Age 8 to 12 months

1. Plays simple games (peekaboo)
2. Cries when scolded
3. Makes simple requests with gestures
4. Demonstrates intense anxiety with separation
5. Prefers caretaker figures to other adults
6. Recognizes family members

Moral Development

Moral development does not begin until the toddler years, when initial cognition is evident.

Faith Development (Undifferentiated Stage)

Feelings of trust and interactions with caretakers form the basis for subsequent faith development.

TODDLER (1 TO 3 YEARS)
Physical Characteristics

1. Weight
   a. Toddler gains approximately 5 lb per year.
   b. Weight gain decelerates considerably.

2. Height
   a. Height increases by approximately 3 inches per year.
   b. Body proportions change; arms and legs grow at faster rate than head and trunk.
   c. Lumbar lordosis of spine is less evidenced.
   d. Toddler is achieving a less pudgy appearance.
   e. Legs have a "bowing" appearance (tibial torsion).
3. Head circumference
   a. Anterior fontanel closes by 15 months.
   b. Head circumference increases by 1 inch per year.
4. Teeth—first and second molars and canines erupt

Gross Motor Development

Age 15 months

1. Walks alone with wide-base gait
2. Creeps up stairs
3. Can throw objects

Age 18 months

1. Begins to run; seldom falls
2. Climbs up and down stairs
3. Climbs onto furniture
4. Plays with pull toys
5. Can push light furniture around room
6. Seats self on chair

Age 24 months

1. Walks with a steady gait
2. Runs in more controlled manner
3. Walks up and down stairs using both feet on each step
4. Jumps crudely
5. Assists in undressing self
6. Kicks ball without losing balance

Age 30 months

1. Can balance momentarily on one foot
2. Uses both feet for jumping
3. Jumps down from furniture
4. Pedals tricycle

Fine Motor Development

Age 15 months

1. Builds tower of two blocks
2. Opens boxes
3. Pokes fingers in holes
4. Uses spoon but spills contents
5. Turns pages of book

Age 18 months

1. Builds tower of three blocks
2. Scribbles in random fashion
3. Drinks from cup

Age 24 months

1. Drinks from cup held in one hand
2. Uses spoon without spilling
3. Builds tower of four blocks
4. Empties contents of jar
5. Draws vertical line and circular shape

Age 30 months

1. Holds crayons with fingers
2. Draws cross figure crudely
3. Builds tower of six blocks

Psychosexual Development (Anal Stage)

1. Body focus—anal area
2. Developmental task—learning to regulate elimination of bowel and bladder
3. Developmental crisis—toilet training
4. Common coping skills—temper tantrums, negativism, playing with stool and urine, regressive behaviors such as thumb sucking, curling hair into knot, crying, irritability, and pouting
5. Sexual needs—sensations of pleasure are associated with excretory functions; child actively explores body
6. Play—child enjoys playing with excreta as evidenced by fecal smearing
7. Role of parents—to help child achieve continence without overly strict control or overpermissiveness

Psychosocial Development (Autonomy vs. Shame and Doubt)

1. Developmental task—learning to assert self in the expression of needs, desires, and wants
2. Developmental crisis—toilet training; child experiences, for the first time, social constraints on behavior by parents
3. Common coping skills—temper tantrums, crying, physical activity, negativism, breath holding, affection seeking, play, and regression
4. Play—child initiates and seeks play opportunities and activities; seeks attention from caretakers; explores body; enjoys sensations from gross and fine motor movements; plays actively with objects; learns to interact in socially approved ways
5. Role of parents—to serve as socializing agents for basic rules of conduct; impose restrictions for first time on child's behavior; direct focus from primary and immediate gratification of child's needs

Moral Development (Preconventional Stage)

1. Toddler's concept of right and wrong is limited.
2. Parents have significant influence on the toddler's conscious development.

Faith Development (Intuitive-Projective Stage)

1. Faith beliefs are learned from parents.
2. Child imitates family's religious practices and gestures.

PRESCHOOLER (3 TO 6 YEARS)
Physical Characteristics

1. Weight
   a. Preschooler gains less than 2 kg (5 lb) per year.
   b. Mean weight is 18 kg (40 lb).
2. Height
   a. He or she grows 5 to 7 cm (2 to 2½ inches) per year.
   b. Mean height is 108 cm (42 inches).

3. Posture—lordosis is no longer present
4. Teeth—preschooler is losing temporary teeth

Gross Motor Development
Age 36 months
1. Dresses and undresses self
2. Walks backward
3. Walks up and down stairs, alternating feet
4. Balances momentarily on one foot

Age 4 years
1. Hops on one foot
2. Climbs and jumps
3. Throws ball overhand with increased proficiency

Age 5 years
1. Jumps rope
2. Runs with no difficulty
3. Skips well
4. Plays catch

Age 6 years
1. Runs skillfully
2. Runs and plays games simultaneously
3. Begins to ride bicycle
4. Draws a person with a body, arms, and legs
5. Includes features such as mouth, eyes, nose, and hair in drawing

Fine Motor Development
Age 36 Months
1. Strings large beads
2. Copies cross and circle
3. Unbuttons front and side buttons
4. Builds and balances 10-block tower

Age 4 years
1. Uses scissors
2. Cuts out simple pictures
3. Copies square

Age 5 years

1. Hits nail on head with hammer
2. Ties laces on shoes
3. Can copy some letters of alphabet
4. Can print name

Age 6 years

1. Is able to use a fork
2. Begins to use a knife with suspension

Sensory Development

Age 4 years

1. Has a very limited space perception
2. Can identify names of one or two colors

Age 5 years

1. Can identify at least four colors
2. Can make distinctions between objects according to weight
3. Imitates parents and other adult role models

Cognitive Development (Preoperational Stage)

Child progresses from sensorimotor behavior as a means of learning and interacting with the environment to the formation of symbolic thought.

1. Develops ability to form mental representations for objects and persons
2. Develops concept of time
3. Has egocentric perspective; supplies own meaning for reality

The following are characteristics of thoughts:

1. Animism: belief that objects have feelings, consciousness, and thoughts as humans do
2. Artificialism: belief that a powerful agent (natural or supernatural) causes the occurrence of events
3. Centration: ability to focus on only one aspect of a situation
4. Participation: belief that events occur to meet the needs and desires of the child

5. Syncretism: use of a specific explanation for an event as an answer to describe situations that are different in nature from the original one
6. Juxtaposition: rudimentary form of association and reasoning; connects two events but does not imply a causal relationship
7. Transduction: rudimentary form of association and reasoning; associates nonsignificant facts in a causal relationship
8. Irreversibility: inability to reverse the process of thinking; inability to backtrack through the content of thoughts from conclusion to beginning

Language Development

Age 2 years

1. Uses two- and three-word sentences
2. Uses holophrases
3. More than half of speech is understandable

Age 3 years

1. Constantly asks questions
2. Talks whether audience present or not
3. Uses telegraphic speech (without prepositions, adjectives, adverbs, etc.)
4. Enunciates the following consonants: *d, b, t, k,* and *y*
5. Omits *w* from speech
6. Has vocabulary of 900 words
7. Uses three-word sentences (subject-verb-object)
8. States own name
9. Makes specific sound errors (*s, sh, ch, z, th, r,* and *l*)
10. Pluralizes words
11. Repeats phrases and words aimlessly

Age 4 years

1. Has vocabulary of 1500 words
2. Counts to three
3. Narrates lengthy story
4. Understands simple questions
5. Understands basic cause-effect relationships of feelings
6. Conversation is egocentric
7. Makes specific sound errors (*s, sh, ch, z, th, r,* and *l*)
8. Uses four-word sentences

Age 5 years

1. Has 2100-word vocabulary
2. Uses five-word sentences
3. Uses prepositions and conjunctions
4. Uses complete sentences
5. Understands questions related to time and quantity (how much and when)
6. Continues specific sound errors
7. Learns to participate in social conversations
8. Can name days of week

Age 6 years

1. Speech sound errors disappear
2. Understands cause-effect relationships of physical events
3. Uses language as medium of verbal exchange
4. Speech resembles adult form in terms of structure
5. Expands vocabulary according to environmental stimulation

Psychosexual Development (Phallic Stage)

1. Body focus—genitals
2. Developmental task—increased awareness of sex organs and interest in sexuality
3. Developmental crises—Oedipal and Electra complexes; castration fears; fear of intrusion to body; development of prerequisites for masculine or feminine identity; identification with parent of same sex (in families with only one parent, resolution of crisis during this stage may be more difficult)
4. Common coping skills—reaction formation; transition of negative feelings toward parent of opposite sex to positive feelings; masturbation during periods of stress and isolation
5. Temperament—amount of jealousy and behaviors vary according to child's past experiences and family environment
6. Play—dramatic play in which children enact parent roles and same-sex roles

The following are age-specific characteristics:

1. Age 5 years—decreased sex play; child is modest and evidences less exposure; interested in where babies come from; aware of adult sex organs

2. Age 6 years—mild sex play, with increased exhibitionism; mutual investigation of sexes

Psychosocial Development (Initiative vs. Guilt)

1. Developmental task—development of conscience; increased awareness of self and ability to function in the world
2. Developmental crisis—modeling appropriate sex roles; learning right and wrong
3. Common coping skills
   a. Beginning problem-solving skills
   b. Denial
   c. Reaction formation
   d. Somatization (usually in gastrointestinal system)
   e. Regression
   f. Displacement
   g. Projection
   h. Fantasy
4. Play—child has an active fantasy life; evidences experimentation with new skills in play; increases play activities in which child has control and uses self
5. Role of parents—supervision and direction are accepted by 5-year-olds; 6-year-olds respond more slowly and negatively to parental requests and directions; parents are role models for the preschooler, and their attitudes have a great influence on the child's behavior and attitudes
6. Plan—to provide appropriate play activities and self-care opportunities

Socialization Behavior

1. Sees parents as most important figures
2. Is possessive; wants things own way
3. Is able to share with peers and adults
4. Imitates parents and other adult role models

Moral Development (Preconventional Stage)

1. Preschooler sees rules as rigid and inflexible.
2. Negative consequences are seen as punishment for misdeeds.

3. Parents are seen as the ultimate authorities for determining right and wrong.
4. Child begins process of internalizing sense of right and wrong.

Faith Development (Intuitive-Projective Stage)

1. Religious practices, trinkets, and symbols begin to have practical meaning for the preschooler.
2. God is viewed in human terms.
3. God is understood as being part of nature, such as in the trees, flowers, and rivers.
4. Evil can be imagined in frightening terms such as monsters or the devil.

SCHOOL-AGE CHILD
Physical Characteristics

A growth spurt begins. Great variation may be normal. Developmental charts are for reference only. Girls may begin to develop secondary sex characteristics and begin menstruation during this stage. Age of onset of menstruation has decreased in the past decade.

1. Weight—child gains 2 to 4 kg (4 to 7 lb) per year
2. Height—at 8 years of age arms grow longer in proportion to body; height increases at age 9
3. Teeth—begins to lose baby teeth; has 10 to 11 permanent teeth by 8 years of age and approximately 26 permanent teeth by age 12

Gross Motor Development

1. Age 7 to 10 years—gross motor activities under control of both cognitive skills and consciousness; gradual increase in rhythm, smoothness, and gracefulness of muscular movements; increased interest in perfection of physical skills; strength and endurance also increase
2. Age 10 to 12 years—high energy level and increased direction and control of physical abilities

Fine Motor Development

1. Shows increased improvement of fine motor skills because of increased myelinization of central nervous system

2. Demonstrates improved balance and eye-hand coordination
3. Is able to write rather than print words by age 8
4. Demonstrates increased ability to express individuality and special interests such as sewing, building models, and playing musical instruments
5. Exhibits fine motor skills equal to those of adults by 10 to 12 years of age

Cognitive Development (Concrete Operations—Age 7 to 11 years)

1. Child's thinking becomes increasingly abstract and symbolic in character; ability to form mental representations is aided by reliance on perceptual senses
2. Weighs a variety of alternatives in finding best solutions
3. Can reverse operations; can trace the sequence of events backward to beginning
4. Understands concept of past, present, and future
5. Can tell time
6. Can classify objects according to classes and subclasses
7. Understands the concept of height, weight, and volume
8. Is able to focus on more than one aspect of a situation

Language Development

1. Uses language as medium for verbal exchange
2. Comprehension of speech may lag behind understanding it
3. Is less egocentric in orientation; able to consider another perspective
4. Understands most abstract vocabulary
5. Uses all parts of speech, including adjectives, adverbs, conjunctions, and prepositions
6. Incorporates use of compound and complex sentences
7. Vocabulary reaches 50,000 words at end of this period

Psychosexual Development (Latency Stage)

1. Body focus—sexual concerns become less conscious
2. Developmental task—gradual integration of previous sexual experiences and reactions (in recent years there

has been increased documentation that latency is not a neutral period in the development of sexuality)
3. Developmental crisis—increased reference to preadolescent sexual concerns, beginning at approximately 10 years of age
4. Common coping skills—nail biting, dependence, increased problem-solving skills, denial, humor, fantasy, and identification
5. Role of parents—major role in educating child about rules and norms governing sexual behavior and sexuality and in influencing gender-specific behavior

The following are age-specific characteristics:
1. Age 7 years—decreased interest in sex and less exploration; increased interest in opposite sex, with beginning of girl-boy "love" feelings
2. Age 8 years—high sexual interest; increase in activities such as peeping, telling dirty jokes, and wanting more sexual information about birth and sexual lovemaking; girls—increased interest in menstruation
3. Age 9 years—increased discussion with peers about sexual topics; division of sexes in play activities; relating of self to process of reproduction; self-consciousness about sexual exposure; interest in dating and relationships with opposite sex in some children
4. Age 10 years—increasing interest in own body and appearance; many children begin to "date" and relate to the opposite sex in group and couple activities
5. Age 11 to 13 years—concerns about appearance; social pressures to look thin and attractive are a source of stress; misconceptions about intercourse and pregnancy are evident in many children

Psychosocial Development (Industry vs. Initiative)

1. Developmental task—learning to develop a sense of adequacy about abilities and competencies as opportunities for social interactions and learning increase; child strives to achieve in school
2. Developmental crisis—child is in danger of developing a sense of inferiority if he or she does not feel competent in the achievement of tasks

3. Play—child enjoys playing loosely structured activities with peers (e.g., baseball or foursquare); play tends to be sex segregated; rough-and-tumble play is characteristic of outdoor unstructured play; personal interests, activities, and hobbies develop at this age
4. Role of family and parents—parents are becoming less significant figures in terms of being agents for socialization; association with peers tends to diminish the predominant effect parents have had previously; parents are still perceived and responded to as the primary adult authorities; expectations of teachers, coaches, and religious figures have significant impact on the child's behavior

Moral Development (Conventional Stage)

1. Child's sense of morality is determined by external rules and regulations.
2. Child's social relationships and contact with authority figures influence his or her sense of right and wrong.
3. Child's sense of right and wrong is strict and rigid.

Faith Development (Mythical-Literal Stage)

1. Child's beliefs are heavily influenced by authority figures.
2. Child is learning to distinguish what is natural vs. supernatural.
3. Child begins to develop personal sense of God.

ADOLESCENT
Physical Characteristics

Adolescence is characterized by rapid growth and initial awkwardness in gross motor activity and by heightened emotionality because of hormonal changes.

1. Somatic changes—girls mature an average of 2 years earlier than boys because of rapid maturation of central nervous system
2. Height and weight—greater averages occur in boys because of greater velocity of growth spurt and 2-year delay in puberty

Table B-2. Changes during Puberty

Male	Female	Both Sexes
Thickening and strengthening of pelvic bone structure	Increased diameter of internal pelvis	Increased broadening of body frame
Increased size of scrotum and testicles	Enlargement of breasts, ovaries, and uterus	Darkening and coarsening of pubic hair
Increased sensitivity of genital area	Increased growth of labia	Increased axillary hair
Increased size of penis	Increased size of vagina	Changes in vocal pitch

3. Dentition
   a. Definition is completed during late adolescence.
   b. Eighty percent of adolescents need to have one or more wisdom teeth removed.
4. Puberty
   a. Average age of onset is 12½ years in female individuals and 15½ years in male individuals (Table B-2).
   b. Nocturnal emissions are commonly reported at 14½ years (age range is 11½ to 17½ years).
   c. Menarche is identification criterion for postpubertal female individual; average age is 12½ to 13 years.

Gross Motor Development and Fine Motor Development

Gradual increases in gross motor and fine motor control are evidenced throughout this period. Both neurologic development and increased practice of skills account for the changes.

Common difficulties associated with physical changes during adolescence are as follows:

1. Skin problems and/or disorders
   a. Eczema
   b. Acne vulgaris
2. Poor posture
   a. Lordosis
   b. Scoliosis
3. Dentition problems
   a. Removal of wisdom teeth
   b. Malocclusion
4. Headaches
5. Weight problems and/or disorders
   a. Juvenile obesity
   b. Anorexia nervosa
   c. Bulimia

Cognitive Development (Formal Operations)

The ability to think approaches a level comparable to adult competencies. The adolescent acquires the capacity to reason symbolically about more global and altruistic issues and uses a more systematic approach to problems. Characteristics of thinking include the following:

1. Takes another perspective into account when processing information
2. Thinking is not limited by actual circumstances; can apply theoretic concepts to hypothesized or imagined circumstances
3. Develops an altruistic orientation (fairness and justice)
4. Develops own value system
5. Can form deductive and inductive conclusions

Language Development

1. Uses language as a medium to convey ideas, opinions, and values

2. Incorporates complex structural and grammatical forms
3. Makes evident use of slang and peer-accepted terminology

Psychosocial Development (Identity vs. Role Diffusion)

1. Developmental task—development of a sure sense about own unique individuality, based on the needs, desires, preferences, values, and belief system that have evolved continuously throughout childhood
2. Developmental crisis—adolescent feels a sense of role diffusion; cannot identify accurately what factors are necessary for optimal self-growth; is heavily influenced by the opinions and judgments of peers
3. Play—strenuous and structured physical activities (e.g., football and soccer) tend to be sex segregated. Heterosexual relationships evolve, laying the foundation for intimate long-term relationships. Strong, intimate friendships develop. Cliques appear, providing strong social and emotional support for teenagers. The adolescents begin to assume adult activities (e.g., voting, drinking, and working). They use fantasy to imagine sexual encounters and relationships, and they enhance sexuality by focusing on male and female stereotypic activities such as driving fast cars, wearing "sexy" clothing, and lifting weights. Romance novels have become popular with adolescent girls. Activities such as shopping and spending time in clothing and department stores increase.
4. Coping skills—problem solving; use of defenses (e.g., reaction formation, displacement, identification, suppression, rationalization, intellectualization, denial, conversion, reaction); use of humor; increased socialization
5. Role of parents and family—conflicts with parents may arise, primarily out of adolescent's need to be independent; parents are influential, subconsciously and unconsciously, in the adaptation and use of values and beliefs in making decisions
6. Plan—facilitate and support the social development

Moral Development (Postconventional Stage)

1. This stage is not universally attained by adolescents.
2. Adolescent may apply ideals to moral predicaments (justice, charity).

Faith Development (Individuating-Reflexive Stage)

1. Adolescent may become very religious or reject religious beliefs entirely.
2. Adolescent may regress to earlier stages of development for comfort.
3. Beliefs may be influenced by peer group in terms of acceptance and rejection.

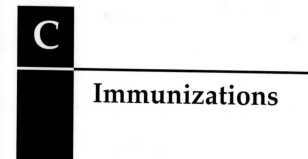

Immunizations

A major role of the nurse caring for infants and children is educating parents about immunizations and reviewing the immunization status of each child. Continuing active immunization efforts is necessary to ensure that infectious disease continues to be a rare occurrence in the United States.

Some terms must be understood. *Immunity* is the resistance to or protection against a specific disease or infectious agent. There are basically three types of immunity: active, artificial, and passive. *Active immunity* is a long-lasting immunity that results when the body is stimulated to produce its own antibodies. *Artificial immunity* is a type of active immunity wherein antibody production is caused by the introduction of antigens in the form of toxoids and vaccines rather than by a specific disease entity. A *toxoid* is a bacterial toxin that has been chemically treated or heat treated to reduce its virulence without destroying its ability to stimulate the production of antibodies (e.g., the diphtheria and tetanus toxoids). A suspension of the actual microorganisms in weakened or killed form is a *vaccine*. Typhoid, pertussis, measles, mumps, and rubella are examples of diseases for which there are vaccines. Last, *passive immunity* is a form of immediate but transient protection against infectious disease. This type of immunity can be obtained through the administration of preparations of convalescent serum or adult blood products that contain antibodies previously formed against an infectious agent. Passive immunity provides only limited protection against infectious disease.

Table C-1 gives a recommended schedule for the immunization of normal or well children. Because there are frequent changes to the immunization schedule, the reader should double-check information with the American Academy of Pediatrics Committee on Infectious Diseases.

Table C-1. Recommended Ages for Immunizations and Screenings*

Age	Immunizations and Screenings
2 months	DTP, OPV, HBC, HBV
4 months	DTP, OPV, HBC, HBV
6 months	DTP, HBC, HBV
12 months	Tuberculin test (depending on the risk of exposure, it may be administered yearly or every other year after this age), varicella vaccine
15 months	MMR, HBC
15 to 18 months	DTP, OPV, HBC
4 to 6 years	DTP, OPV
10 to 14 years	MMR
14 to 16 years	Adult tetanus toxoid (repeated every 10 years for lifetime)

*DTP: diphtheria and tetanus toxoids with pertussis vaccine; OPV: oral, attenuated, or weakened poliovirus vaccine; HBC: *Haemophilus influenzae* type B conjugate vaccine; HBV: hepatitis B vaccine; MMR: live measles, mumps, and rubella viruses combined in a vaccine.

VARIOUS VACCINES AND TOXOIDS
Diphtheria, Tetanus, and Pertussis

A mixture of all three antigens (diphtheria and tetanus toxoids and pertussis vaccine) and a mineral substance that prolongs and enhances the antigenic properties by delaying absorption make up the diphtheria, tetanus, and pertussis (DTP) vaccine. Although the diphtheria toxoid does not produce absolute immunity, when it is given as recommended by the schedule, protective levels of antitoxin continue for 10 years or more. There are three forms of the tetanus toxoid: tetanus toxoid, tetanus immune globulin (human), and tetanus antitoxin (usually horse serum).

Poliomyelitis

The Sabin vaccine, or oral (trivalent) poliovirus (OPV) vaccine, is very successful in providing immunity to all three types of poliovirus that cause paralytic poliomyelitis.

Measles, Mumps, and Rubella

Live viruses for measles, mumps, and rubella (MMR) are usually combined into one vaccine. That one vaccine may provide lifelong immunity to each disease. The rubella portion is extremely important in controlling congenital rubella syndrome.

Haemophilus Influenzae Type B   *Hib*

The *Haemophilus influenzae* type B vaccine is a polysaccharide inactive vaccine. There are three types of this vaccine currently available, all of which appear to be equally effective: HBOC, PRP-OMP, or PRP-D (refer to American Academy of Pediatrics guidelines for recommendations for vaccine regimen). This vaccine provides protection against the *H. influenzae* bacteria, which can cause meningitis, epiglottitis, septic arthritis, sepsis, and bacterial pneumonia.

Hepatitis B

Hepatitis B is a potentially fatal viral infection that can cause cirrhosis or liver cancer. The hepatitis B virus (HBV) vaccine can be administered at different sites simultaneously with the DTP, MMR, and *H. influenzae B* conjugate (HBC) vaccines. Pain and soreness at the injection site is the most common side effect. Hepatitis B vaccine is considered appropriate for all children, adolescents who are sexually active with multiple partners, persons with developmental disabilities, and health professionals. Protection is estimated to last a lifetime.

Varicella

Children targeted for vaccination against varicella are infants between 12 and 18 months of age and older school-age children who have not had chicken pox and who have not been previously immunized. Children over the age of 12 should receive two doses of the vaccine, 6 to 12 weeks apart. Side effects include a maculopapular rash with up to five lesions at the injection site or elsewhere and pain or redness at the injection site. This vaccine can be given with diphtheria, tetanus, DTP, polio, hepatitis B, and *H. influenzae* type B vaccines. Duration of immunity is not known.

TUBERCULIN SKIN TEST

The tuberculin skin test is not an immunization but is a screening device for tuberculosis. The purified protein derivative (PPD) of tuberculin is most widely used in testing for tuberculosis. There are two types of PPD tests: (1) the Mantoux test, which consists of one intradermal injection, and (2) a multiple-puncture test such as the tine test. A positive reaction indicates that the person has been infected by and has developed a sensitivity to the protein of the tuberculin bacillus. Once a positive test result is obtained, the individual will continue to react positively and should be monitored through chest x-ray examinations.

POSSIBLE REACTIONS

It is not unusual to have slight reactions to the DTP vaccine. Local reactions (redness and edema) at the infection site are common. Mild to moderate temperature elevations and irritability may occur, but they usually resolve within a few hours. Seizures or neurologic damage rarely occur after the administration of the DTP vaccine. If severe reactions occur, the pertussis portion of the vaccine may be eliminated in future vaccinations. Very rarely, vaccine-induced disease occurs; however, this occurrence is usually in immunosuppressed children. Fever and rash have occurred after the administration of the MMR vaccine.

CONTRAINDICATIONS

Any time an acute febrile illness is present, immunizations should be postponed. Administration of live virus vaccines is contraindicated, and a physician's consent must be obtained before administering other immunizations, in individuals with leukemia, lymphoma, malignancies, or immunodeficiency diseases; children with marked sensitivity to eggs, chicken, or neomycin; children on immunosuppressive therapy; children who have recently received immune serum globulin plasma or blood products; or pregnant female individuals. The pertussis vaccine is contraindicated in those children with a history of previous reaction to the DTP vaccine.

REFERENCES

ACIP: Measles prevention: recommendation of the immunization practices advisory committee, *MMWR* 38(9):1, 1989.

American Academy of Pediatrics: *AAP News* 6(11), 1990.

American Academy of Pediatrics: *Report of the committee on infectious diseases*, ed 22, Elk Grove Village, Ill, 1991, The Academy.

Centers for Disease Control: Measles: United States, *MMWR* 39(13):211, 1990.

Edelman CL, Mandle CL: *Health promotion throughout the life span*, St Louis, 1994, Mosby.

Frank J, Loh J: SSPE: but we thought measles was gone, *J Pediatr Nurs* 6(2):87, 1991.

Frenkel LD: Routine immunizations for American children in the 1990's, *Pediatr Clin North Am* 37(3):531, 1990.

Garber RM, Mortimer EA: Immunizations: beyond the basics, *Pediatrics in Review* 13:98, 1992.

Gershon A: Immunization practices in children, *Hosp Pract* 25(9):91, 1990.

Jurgrau A: Why aren't we protecting our children? *RN* 53(11):30, 1990.

US Preventive Services Task Force: Childhood, immunization, *Am Fam Physician* 40(4):115, 1989.

D

Taking Blood Pressure and Age-Appropriate Cuff Size

1. Determine cuff size (Table D-1).
   a. Width of cuff to be not less than one half or greater than two thirds of upper arm length
   b. Length of cuff to be equal to width of cuff plus 50% of extremity length
   c. Use largest size in which rubber bladder fits comfortably and completely encircles extremity
2. Position manometer at observer's eye level.
3. Take blood pressure with patient in relaxed environment.
4. Take reading with patient in supine position.
5. Do not deflate cuff at rate less than 2 to 3 mm Hg per second.
6. Take reading on three separate occasions (Table D-2).

   Blood pressures may be taken using electronic equipment. Oscillometric devices and Doppler techniques are used extensively in pediatric hospitals. Oscillometry provides accurate systolic and diastolic pressures and mean arterial pressures and pulses. The Doppler provides reliable systolic blood pressure measurements; it is not reliable for diastolic pressures. The benefit of electronic equipment is that it provides fast and dependable readings; however, the equipment is expensive.

Table D-1. Age-Appropriate Cuff Size

Cuff Name	Width (cm)	Length (cm)
Newborn	2.5-4	5-10
Infant	6-8	12-13.5
Child	9-10	17-22.5
Adult	12-13	22-23.5
Large adult arm	15.5	30
Adult thigh	18	36

From Report on the Task Force on Blood Pressure Control in Children, *Pediatrics* 59(suppl):797, 1977. Reproduced by permission of *Pediatrics*.

Table D-2. Normal Blood Pressures

Age (Years)	Diastolic (mm Hg)	Systolic (mm Hg)
Boys		
3-5	>60	>95
6-10	>70	>100
11-18	>80	>120
Girls		
3-5	>60	>95
6-10	>70	>110
11-14	>80	>120
15-18	>80	>130

E

Laboratory Values

The following are normal laboratory values unless otherwise stated.

1. Acetone, ketone bodies (serum)
   a. Newborn to age 1 week: slightly higher than values for ages over 1 week
   b. Ages over 1 week
      (1) Acetone: 0.3 to 2.0 mg/dl; 51.6 to 344.0 μmol/L (SI units)
      (2) Ketones: 2 to 4 mg/dl
2. Albumin (serum)
   a. Newborn: 2.9 to 5.4 g/dl
   b. Infant: 4.4 to 5.4 g/dl
   c. Child: 4.0 to 5.8 g/dl
3. Albumin in meconium: negative
4. Ammonia (serum)
   a. Newborn: 64 to 107 μg/dl
   b. Child: 29 to 70 μg/dl; 29 to 70 μmol/L (SI units)
5. Amylase dehydrogenase (serum)—child: 45 to 200 dye U/dl
6. Arterial blood gases
   a. Partial pressure of oxygen (Po_2): 75 to 100 mm Hg
   b. Partial pressure of carbon dioxide (Pco_2)
      (1) Infant: 27 to 40 mm Hg
      (2) Remaining ages: 35 to 45 mm Hg
   c. pH
      (1) Premature infant (cord): 7.15 to 7.35

    (2) Premature infant (age 48 hours): 7.35 to 7.5
    (3) Newborn: 7.27 to 7.47
    (4) Infant: 7.35 to 7.45
    (5) Child: 7.35 to 7.45
7. Bilirubin
  a. Total
    (1) Newborn: 2.0 to 6.0 mg/dl
    (2) Age 48 hours: 6.0 to 7.0 mg/dl
    (3) Age 5 days: 4.0 to 12.0 mg/dl
    (4) Age 1 month to adult: 0.3 to 1.2 mg/dl
  b. Indirect (unconjugated)—age 1 month to adult: 0.3 to 1.1 mg/dl
  c. Direct (conjugated)—age 1 month to adult: 0.1 to 0.4 mg/dl
8. Bleeding time
  a. Normal time: 2 to 7 minutes
  b. Borderline time: 7 to 11 minutes
9. Blood urea nitrogen (BUN) (serum)
  a. Newborn: 8 to 18 mg/dl
  b. Infant or child: 5 to 18 mg/dl
  c. Adolescent: 8 to 17 mg/dl
10. Calcium (serum)
  a. Premature infant: 6 to 10 mg/dl
  b. Full-term infant: 7.5 to 11 mg/dl
  c. Child: 8.8 to 10.8 mg/dl
  d. Adolescent: 8.4 to 10.2 mg/dl
11. Carotene (serum)—child: 40 to 130 μg/dl
12. Cerebrospinal fluid (CSF)
  a. Specific gravity: 1.007 to 1.009
  b. Glucose
    (1) Infant or child: 60 to 80 mg/dl
    (2) Remaining ages: 40 to 80 mg/dl
  c. Protein
    (1) Newborn: 45 to 100 mg/dl
    (2) Child: 10 to 20 mg/dl
    (3) Adolescent: 15 to 40 mg/dl
  d. pH: 7.33 to 7.42
  e. Cell count
    (1) Neonate: 0.5 polymorphonuclear; 0 to 5 mononuclear; 0 to 5 red blood cells (RBCs) per mm^3

    (2) Remaining ages: 0 polymorphonuclear; 0 to 5 mononuclear; 0 to 5 RBCs per mm^3

13. Catecholamines
   a. Values for child lower than those for adults
   b. Total
     (1) Random urine: 0 to 14 μg/dl
     (2) Twenty-four–hour urine: less than 100 g/24 hr
   c. Epinephrine: less than 10 ng/24 hr
   d. Norepinephrine: less than 100 ng/24 hr
   e. Metanephrines: less than 100 ng/24 hr

14. Cholesterol (serum)
   a. Age 1 to 4 years: less than or equal to 210 mg/dl
   b. Age 5 to 14 years: less than or equal to 220 mg/dl
   c. Age 15 to 20 years: less than or equal to 235 mg/dl

15. Copper (Cu) (serum)
   a. Newborn: 20 to 70 μg/dl
   b. Child: 30 to 190 μg/dl
   c. Adolescent: 90 to 240 μg/dl

16. C-reactive protein (CRP) (serum)—child: negative

17. Creatinine (serum)
   a. Cord: 0.6 to 1.2 mg/dl
   b. Newborn: 0.3 to 1.0 mg/dl
   c. Infant: 0.2 to 0.4 mg/dl
   d. Child: 0.3 to 0.7 mg/dl
   e. Adolescent: 0.5 to 1.0 mg/dl

18. Creatine phosphokinase (CPK)
   a. Infant: 20 to 31 U/L
   b. Infant to adolescent: 15 to 50 U/L

19. Cortisol (plasma)—child
   a. At 8 am: 15 to 25 μg/dl
   b. At 4 pm: 5 to 10 μg/dl

20. Culture results—blood, throat, sputum, wound, skin, stool, urine: negative or no growth of pathogen

21. Electrolytes (serum)
   a. Sodium (Na$^+$)
     (1) Premature infant: 132 to 140 mmol/L
     (2) Infant: 139 to 146 mmol/L
     (3) Child: 138 to 145 mmol/L
     (4) Adolescent: 136 to 146 mEq/L
   b. Potassium (K$^+$)
     (1) Infant: 4.1 to 5.3 mEq/L

      (2) Child: 3.4 to 4.7 mmol/L

      (3) Adolescent: 3.5 to 5.1 mmol/L

  c. Chlorine (Cl^-): 98 to 106 mmol/L

  d. Carbon dioxide (CO_2)

      (1) Infant: 27 to 41 mmol/L

      (2) Child

         (a) Male: 35 to 48 mmol/L

         (b) Female: 32 to 45 mmol/L

22. Erythrocyte sedimentation rate (ESR, sed rate)

  a. Newborn: 0 to 2 mm/hr

  b. Age 4 to 14 years: 0 to 10 mm/hr

23. Fasting blood glucose

  a. Newborn: 30 to 80 mg/dl

  b. Child: 60 to 100 mg/dl

24. Ferritin concentration (serum)—abnormal: less than 10 to 12 μg/L

25. Ferritin determination (serum)

  a. Newborn: 20 to 200 ng/mL

  b. 1 month: 200 to 500 ng/mL

  c. 2 to 12 months: 30 to 200 ng/mL

  d. 1 to 16 years: 8 to 140 ng/mL

26. Fibrin degradation products (FDP) (serum)

  a. Adult: 2 to 10 μg/ml

  b. Child: test not usually performed

27. Fibrinogen level (plasma)

  a. Newborn: 150 to 300 mg/dl

  b. Child: 200 to 400 mg/dl

28. Glucose (serum): 40 to 100 mg/dl

29. Glucose tolerance test (GTT) results (oral)—child 6 years or older:

Time (Hours)	Whole Blood (mg/dl)	Serum (mg/dl)
½	<150	<160
1	<160	<170
2	<115	<125
3	60-100	70-110

30. Hematocrit (Hct)

  a. Newborn: 44% to 75%

    b. Infant: 28% to 42%

    c. Age 6 to 12 years: 35% to 45%

    d. Age 12 to 18 years (male): 37% to 49%

    e. Age 12 to 18 years (female): 36% to 46%

31. Hemoglobin (Hb)

    a. Age 1 to 3 days: 14.5 to 22.5 g/dl

    b. Age 2 months: 9.0 to 14.0 g/dl

    c. Age 6 to 12 years: 11.5 to 15.5 g/dl

    d. Age 12 to 18 years (male): 13.0 to 16.0 g/dl

    e. Age 12 to 18 years (female): 12.0 to 16.0 g/dl

32. Hemoglobin electrophoresis (hemoglobin F [Hb, F])

    a. Newborn: Hb F, 50% to 80% total Hb

    b. Infant: Hb F, 8% total Hb

    c. Child: Hb F, 1% to 2% total Hb after 6 months

33. Human immunodeficiency virus type 1 (HIV-1) (serum)—child: seronegative

34. Immunoglobulin (Ig) values (serum):

(%) of Total		New-born	3 mo.	6 mo.	1 to 3 Years	4 to 6 Years	6 to 16 Years
IgG	80	650-1250	275-750	200-1100	300-1400	550-1500	700-1650
IgA	15	0-12	5-55	10-90	20-150	50-175	50-225
IgM	4	5-30	15-70	10-80	20-230	20-100	22-260
IgD	0.2	—	—	—	—	—	—
IgE	0.0002	—	—	—	<10	<25	<62

35. Iron (serum): 50 to 120 μg/dl

36. Iron concentration (serum): 30 to 70 μg/g

37. Lactic dehydrogenase (LDH) (serum)

    a. Newborn: 300 to 1500 IU/L

    b. Child: 50 to 150 IU/L; 100 to 295 U/L

38. Lead (serum)—child: normal range, 10 to 20—μg/dl

39. Lipase (serum)

    a. Infant: 9 to 105 U/L

    b. Remaining ages: 20 to 180 U/L

40. Magnesium (serum)

    a. Newborn: 1.4 to 2.9 mEq/L

    b. Child: 1.6 to 2.6 mEq/L

41. Osmolality (serum)—child: 270 to 290 mOsm/kg

42. Osmolality (urine)
    a. Newborn: 100 to 600 mOsm/kg/H_2O
    b. Child: 50 to 1200 mOsm/kg/H_2O; usual range, 300 to 900 mOsm/kg/H_2O
43. Ova and parasites (O and P) (feces)
    a. Child: negative
    b. Parasites most often found in stool—roundworms, ameba, hookworms, protozoa, tapeworms
44. Partial thromboplastin time (PTT) and activated partial thromboplastin time (APTT)
    a. Newborn to age 3 months: higher than adult times
    b. Child: higher than adult times
    c. Adult: PTT, 30 to 45 seconds; APTT, 35 to 45 seconds
45. Phosphorus (serum)
    a. Premature infant: 4.6 to 8.0 mg/dl
    b. Newborn: 5.0 to 7.8 mg/dl
46. Plasminogen (plasma)—adult: 2.5 to 5.2 U/ml; 20 mg/dl
47. Platelet count
    a. Newborn: 84,000 to 478,000/μl
    b. Remaining ages: 150,000 to 400,000/μl
48. Protein (serum)
    a. Premature infant: 4.2 to 7.6 g/dl
    b. Newborn: 4.6 to 7.4 g/dl
    c. Infant: 6.0 to 6.7 g/dl
    d. Child: 6.2 to 8.0 g/dl
49. Protein (urine)
    a. Values higher in children
    b. Random urine specimen: negative, 0 to 5 mg/dl; positive, 6 to 2000 mg/dl
    c. Twenty-four hour urine specimen: 25 to 150 mg/24 hr
50. Prothrombin time (PT, pro time)
    a. Newborn: 12 to 21 seconds
    b. Remaining ages: 11 to 15 seconds
51. Red blood cells (RBCs)
    a. Infant (1 to 18 months): 2.7 to 5.4
    b. Preschooler: 4.27
    c. School-ager: 4.31
    d. Adolescent: 4.60
52. Reticulocyte count
    a. Newborn: 3.2% ± 1.4%

  b. Neonate: 0.6% ± 0.3%

  c. Infant: 0.3% to 2.2%

  d. Remaining ages: 0.5% to 1.5%

53. Serum glutamic-pyruvic transaminase (SGPT)

  a. Age 6 to 12 months: 16 to 36 IU

  b. Age 2 to 17 years: 622 IU

54. Serum glutamic-oxaloacetic transaminase (SGOT)

  a. Age 6 to 12 months: less than or equal to 40 IU

  b. Age 2 to 17 years: 10 to 30 IU

55. Sweat test results: negative

56. Transferrin (serum): 200 to 400 mg/dl

57. Thyroid-stimulating hormone (TSH) (serum)—newborn: less than 25 uIU/ml by the third day

58. Toxoplasmosis, rubella, cytomegalovirus (CMV), and herpes simplex (TORCH) titer—infant under 2 months: negative

59. Triglycerides (serum)

  a. Infant: 5 to 40 mg/dl

  b. Child (5 to 11 years): 10 to 135 mg/dl

  c. Adolescent or young adult (12 to 29 years): 10 to 140 mg/dl

60. Uric acid (serum)

  a. Female: 2.0 to 6.0 mg/dl

  b. Male: 3.0 to 7.0 mg/dl

61. Urinalysis

  a. Specific gravity: 1.003 to 1.035

  b. pH

   (1) Infant: 5.0 to 7.0

   (2) Remaining ages: 4.8 to 7.8

  c. Protein: negative

  d. Blood: negative

  e. Sugar: negative

  f. Ketones: negative

62. White blood count (WBC)

  a. Infant: 6000 to 17,500

  b. Preschooler: 5500 to 15,500

  c. School-ager: 4500 to 13,500

  d. Adolescent: 4500 to 11,000

63. White blood cell differential:

Cell Type	Percentage (%) of Total	Values (μl/mm^3)
Neutrophils	61 (newborn)	—
Total	32 (1 yr)	—
Segments	50-70 (>1 yr)	2500-7000
	50-65 (>1 yr)	2500-6500
Bands	0-5 (>1 yr)	0-500
Eosinophils	1-3	100-300
Basophils	0.4-1.0	40-100
Monocytes	4-9 (1-12 yr)	—
	4-6 (>12 yr)	200-600
Lymphocytes	34 (newborn)	—
	60 (1 yr)	—
	42 (6 yr)	—
	38 (12 yr)	—
	25-35 (>12 yr)	1700-3500

REFERENCES

Kee JL: *Laboratory and diagnostic tests with nursing implications,* ed 4, East Norwalk, Conn, 1995, Appleton & Lange.

Watson J, Jaffe M: *Nurse's manual of laboratory and diagnostic tests,* Philadelphia, 1995, FA Davis.

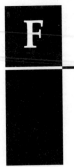

Abbreviations

<	Less than
>	Greater than
AAP	American Academy of Pediatrics
ABC	Airway, breathing, and circulation
ABG	Arterial blood gas
ABVD	Adriamycin, bleomycin, vinblastine, and dacarbazine
ACE	Angiotensin-converting enzyme
ADA	American Diabetic Association
ADH	Antidiuretic hormone
ADHD	Attention-deficit/hyperactivity disorder
AGN	Acute glomerulonephritis
AIDS	Acquired immunodeficiency syndrome
ALA	δ-Aminolevulinic acid
ALG	Antilymphocyte globulin
ALL	Acute lymphoid, or lymphocytic, leukemia
ALT	Alanine aminotransferase
ALTE	Apparent life-threatening event
AMA	American Medical Association
AML	Acute myelogenous leukemia
ANA	Antinuclear antibody
ANLL	Acute nonlymphoid leukemia
AOM	Acute otitis media
A/P	Anteroposterior
AP	Apical pulse
APTT	Activated partial thromboplastin time
ARF	Acute renal failure
AROM	Active range of motion

ASO	Antistreptolysin O
AST	Aspartate aminotransferase
ATG	Antithymocyte globulin
AV	Atrioventricular
Ax	Axillary
BAL	Dimercaprol
bid	Twice a day
BMA	Bone marrow aspiration
BMT	Bone marrow transplant
BPD	Bronchopulmonary dysplasia
BUN	Blood urea nitrogen
C and S	Culture and sensitivity
Ca^+	Calcium
CaEDTA	Calcium disodium edetate
Cal	Calories
CAT	Computerized axial tomography
CBC	Complete blood count
cc	Cubic centimeter
CCK	Cholecystokinin
CDC	Centers for Disease Control
CF	Cystic fibrosis
CHF	Congestive heart failure
CID	Cytomegalic inclusion disease
Cl	Chloride
cm	Centimeter
CMV	Cytomegalovirus
CNS	Central nervous system
CO_2	Carbon dioxide
COM	Chronic otitis media
COMP	Cyclophosphamide, Oncovin, methotrexate, prednisone
CPAP	Continuous positive airway pressure
CPK	Creatine phosphokinase
CPP	Cerebral perfusion pressure
CPR	Cardiopulmonary resuscitation
CRF	Chronic renal failure
CRP	C-reactive protein
CSF	Cerebrospinal fluid
CT	Computed tomography
CUG	Cystourethrogram
CVA	Cerebrovascular accident
CVP	Central venous pressure
d	Day

D5W	5% dextrose in water
DC	Discontinue
DIC	Disseminated intravascular coagulation
DKA	Diabetic ketoacidosis
dl	Deciliter (100 ml)
DMARD	Disease-modifying antirheumatic drug
DNA	Deoxyribonucleic acid
DSM IV	*Diagnostic and Statistical Manual of Mental Disorders,* 4th edition
DTP	Diphtheria, tetanus, and pertussis
EAT	Eating Attitudes Test
EBV	Epstein-Barr virus
ECG	Electrocardiogram
ECHO	Echocardiogram
ECMO	Extracorporeal membrane oxygenation
EDI	Eating Disorders Inventory
EEG	Electroencephalogram
EIA	Enzyme immune assay
ELISA	Enzyme-linked immunosorbent assay
EMG	Electromyogram
EN	Enteral nutrition
EP	Erythrocyte protoporphyrin
ESR	Erythrocyte sedimentation rate
ET	Endotracheal tube
EUG	Excretory urogram
FB	Foreign body
5-FC	5-fluorocytosine
FDP	Fibrin degradation product
Fe	Iron
FEP	Free erythrocyte porphyrin
FET	Force-expiration technique
FFP	Fresh frozen plasma
FTT	Failure to thrive
g	Gram
GER	Gastroesophageal reflux
GI	Gastrointestinal
gr	Grain
GTT	Glucose tolerance test
HAV	Hepatitis A virus
Hb	Hemoglobin
HBC	*Haemophilus influenzae* type B conjugate
HBV	Hepatitis B virus
Hct	Hematocrit

HCV	Hepatitis C virus
HDV	Hepatitis D virus
HEV	Hepatitis E virus
HIDA	Dimethyacetanilide iminodiacetic acid
HIV	Human immunodeficiency virus
HLA	Human lymphocyte antigens
H_2O	Water
HOB	Head of bed
hr	Hour
HSV	Herpes simplex virus
I and O	Intake and output
ICP	Intracranial pressure
ICV	Ileocecal valve
IDDM	Insulin-dependent diabetes mellitus
IDM	Infant of diabetic mother
I/E	Inspiratory/expiratory
IEP	Individualized education plan
Ig	Immunoglobulin
IG	Immune globulin
IM	Intramuscular
IPPB	Intermittent positive pressure breathing
IPV	Inactivated poliovirus
IQ	Intelligence quotient
ITP	Idiopathic thrombocytopenic purpura
IU	International unit
IV	Intravenous
IVFD	Intravenous fast drip
IVGG	Intravenous gamma globulin
IVH	Intraventricular hemorrhage
IVIG	Intravenous immune globulin
IVP	Intravenous pyelogram
JRA	Juvenile rheumatoid arthritis
K^+	Potassium
kg	Kilogram
L	Liter
LAG	Lymphangiogram
lb	Pound
LDH	Lactic dehydrogenase
LFT	Liver function test
LIP/PLH	Lymphoid interstitial pneumonia or pulmonary lymphoid hyperplasia
LOC	Level of consciousness
LP	Lumbar puncture

m	Meter
m^2	Square meter
MAO	Monoamine oxidase
MAP	Mean arterial pressure
mcg	Microgram
MCH	Mean corpuscular hemoglobin
MCHC	Mean corpuscular hemoglobin concentration
MCNS	Minimal change nephrotic syndrome
MCV	Mean corpuscle volume
mEq	Milliequivalent
mg	Milligram
Mg	Magnesium
MIBG	Metaiodobenzylguanidine
min	Minute
ml	Milliliter
mm	Millimeter
mm^3	Cubic millimeter
mM	Millimolar
MMR	Measles, mumps, and rubella
MOPP	Mechlorethamine, Oncovin, procarbazine, and prednisone
mOsm	Milliosmole
MRI	Magnetic resonance imaging
MTX	Methotrexate
Na$^+$	Sodium
NA	Non–hepatitis A
NADase	Nicotinamide adenine dinucleotidase
NaHCO$_3$	Sodium bicarbonate
NAS	No added salt
NB	Non–hepatitis B
NEC	Necrotizing enterocolitis
ng	Nanogram
NG	Nasogastric
NGT	Nasogastric tube
NHL	Non-Hodgkin's lymphoma
NICU	Neonatal intensive care unit
NPO	Nothing by mouth
NS	Normal saline
NSAID	Nonsteroidal antiinflammatory drug
NSE	Neuron-specific enolase
NWTS	National Wilms' tumor study group
O and P	Ova and parasites

OOB	Out of bed
OPV	Oral poliovirus
P	Phosphate
PBI	Protein-bound iodine
PCA	Patient-controlled analgesia
PCO$_2$	Partial pressure of carbon dioxide
PCP	*Pneumocystis* carinii pneumonia
PCR	Polymerase chain reaction
PDA	Patent ductus arteriosus
PE tubes	Pressure equalizer tubes
PEEP	Positive end-expiratory pressure
PERL	Pupils equal, react to light
PERLA	Pupils equal, react to light, accommodate
PET	Positron emission tomography
pHct	Platelet count
PHN	Public health nurse
PN	Parenteral nutrition
po	Oral; by mouth
PO$_2$	Partial pressure of oxygen
PPD	Purified protein derivative
pr	By rectum
PRBC	Packed red blood cell
prn	As needed
PROM	Passive range of motion
PT	Prothrombin time
PTT	Partial thromboplastin time
q	Every
qd	Daily
qid	Four times a day
qod	Every other day
RBC	Red blood cell; red blood count
RDS	Respiratory distress syndrome
RNA	Ribonucleic acid
ROM	Range of motion
ROP	Retinopathy of prematurity
RSV	Respiratory syncytial virus
SAARD	Slower-acting antirheumatic drug
SBS	Short bowel syndrome
SES	Socioeconomic status
SGOT	Serum glutamic-oxaloacetic transaminase
SGPT	Serum glutamic-pyruvic transaminase
SI	International System of Units (Système Internationale)

SIDS	Sudden infant death syndrome
SLE	Systemic lupus erythematosus
SOB	Shortness of breath
SOM	Serous otitis media
SQ	Subcutaneous
SSRI	Selective serotinin reuptake inhibitors
TB	Tuberculosis
TCDB	Turn, cough, and deep breathe
TCM	Transcutaneous monitoring
TENS	Transcutaneous electric nerve stimulation
tid	Three times a day
TLSO	Thoracic-lumbar-sacral orthotics
TORCH	Toxoplasmosis, rubella, cytomegalovirus, and herpes simplex
TPN	Total parenteral nutrition
TSH	Thyroid-stimulating hormone
tx	Treat or treatment
U	Unit
UA	Urinalysis
UGI	Upper gastrointestinal
URI	Upper respiratory tract infection
UTI	Urinary tract infection
VCUG	Voiding cystourethrogram
VLBW	Very low birth weight
VNA	Visiting Nurses' Association
VS	Vital signs
VSD	Ventricular septal defect
WBC	White blood cell; white blood count
WISC III	Wechsler Intelligence Scale for Children, 3rd edition
WNL	Within normal limits

West Nomogram

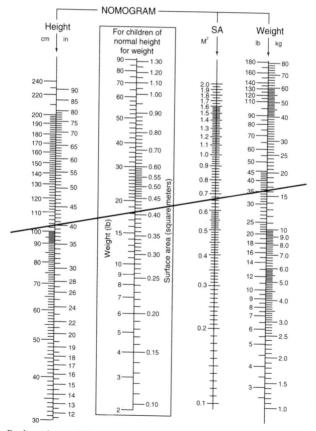

NOMOGRAM

Height		For children of normal height for weight	SA	Weight	
cm	in		M²	lb	kg

For legend see p. 586.

For estimation of surface area: surface area is given by the point at which a straight line connecting height and weight intersects surface area (SA) column, or if patient is roughly of normal proportion, is given by weight alone (enclosed area). Line shows SA determination (0.68 m^2) for child 41 inches tall who weighs 35 lb.

Nomogram modified from data of E Boyd by CD West. From Behrman RE, Vaughan VC, editors: *Nelson textbook of pediatrics*, ed 12, Philadelphia, 1983, WB Saunders.

Height and Weight Growth Curves

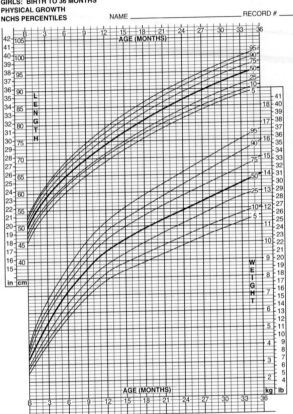

Girls: birth to 36 months. Length and weight. These charts were constructed with data from the National Center for Health Statistics, United States Public Health Service. The data on these charts are considered representative of the general United States population. Reproduced with permission from Ross Laboratories.

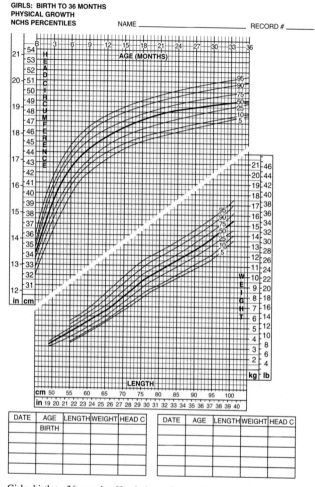

Girls: birth to 36 months. Head circumference, length, and weight.

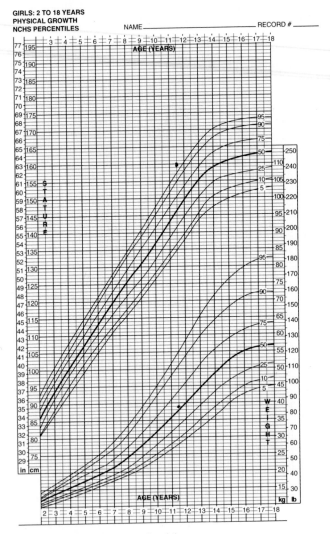

Girls: 2 to 18 years. Stature and weight.

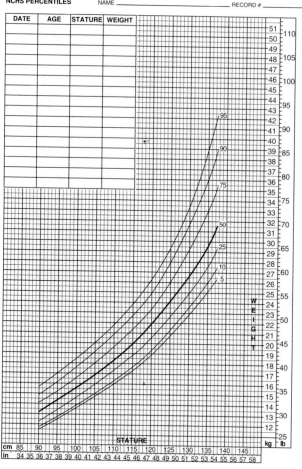

Girls: prepubescent. Physical growth.

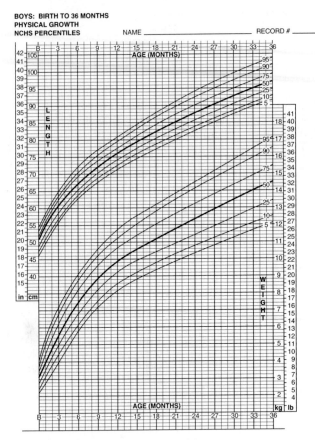

Boys: birth to 36 months. Length and weight.

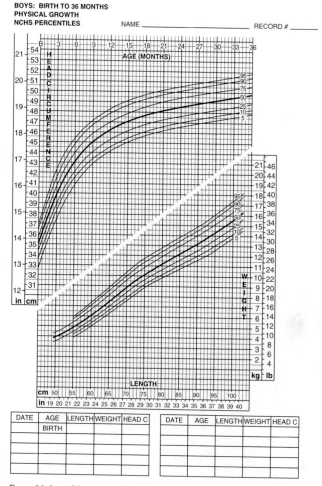

BOYS: BIRTH TO 36 MONTHS
PHYSICAL GROWTH
NCHS PERCENTILES

NAME _____   RECORD # _____

Boys: birth to 36 months. Head circumference, length, and weight.

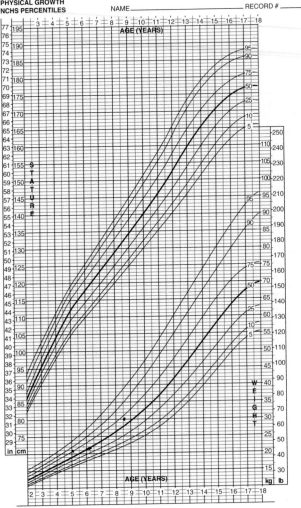

Boys: 2 to 18 years. Stature and weight.

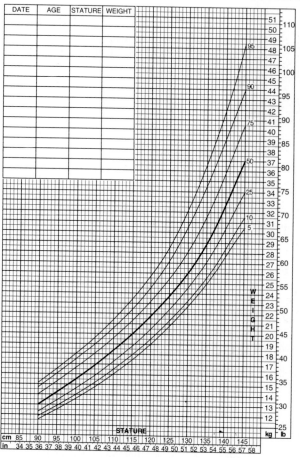

Boys: prepubescent. Physical growth.

Pain in Children

DEFINITIONS

The International Association for the Study of Pain (1979) defines pain as "an unpleasant sensory and emotional experience associated with actual or potential tissue damage, or described in terms of such damage." McCaffrey and Beebe (1989) state that "pain is whatever the person experiencing it says it is, existing whenever the experiencing person says it does." This definition does not necessarily imply that the child must verbalize pain. Pain may also be expressed through crying, vocalizations, or behavioral cues.

PHYSIOLOGY

Pain is a complex physiologic process that can be divided into three neurochemical events: transduction, transmission, and modulation (Figure 2).

Transduction occurs at the site of initiation of pain. Pain receptors (nociceptors) in the periphery are stimulated by a mechanical, thermal, or chemical event. This stimulus results in the release of pain-producing substances.

Transmission of the impulse continues as it travels into the dorsal horn of the spinal cord via large thinly myelinated A-delta fibers and small unmyelinated C fibers. From here the impulse is carried via the anterolateral pathway on to the thalamus and then the cortex. It is in the cortex that the impulse is perceived as pain. Many factors, including culture, past experience, the meaning of the pain, and

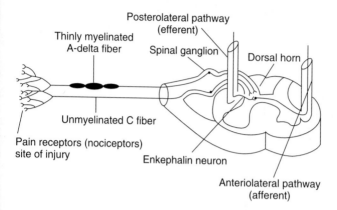

Figure 2. Transduction, transmission, and modulation of pain.

emotional state, all contribute to the individual's perception of pain. Both transduction and transmission occur at afferent pathways.

Modulation of pain occurs in the brain at the level of the periaqueductal gray matter and medulla oblongata, as well as in the dorsal horn of the spinal cord, as endogenous opioids (enkephalins) are released in the posterolateral pathway, an efferent pathway.

Figure 2 demonstrates transduction, transmission, and modulation of pain in the dorsal horn.

THE NATURE OF PAIN

Table I-1 provides a brief overview of the types of pain with descriptions and examples of each.

ASSESSMENT

Self-report is the most accurate means of obtaining information regarding the location and intensity of the child's pain. Input from the family is very important and may be necessary if the child is unwilling or unable to report for himself or herself. Obtaining a pain history is helpful in developing a plan of care for the child. Ask questions regarding the child's previous experience with painful events, how the child responds to pain, and what methods of pain management have been successful in the past. Also

Table I-1. Nature of Pain

Type	Description	Examples
Acute	Brief; associated with tissue damage or inflammation; with intensity steadily diminishing over days to weeks	Surgical pain, burns, fractures
Chronic persistent	Persistent or near-persistent pain over a period of 3 months or more	Arthritis, sickle cell crisis
Recurrent	Repetitive painful episode alternating with pain-free intervals	Headache; abdominal, chest, or limb pain
Neuropathic	Persistent pain related to persistent or abnormal excitability in the peripheral or central nervous system with no ongoing tissue injury; often described as "burning," "strange," or "pins and needles"	Amputation pain syndromes, plexus injuries, reflex sympathetic dystrophy
Psychogenic	Persistent pain that is a manifestation of a psychiatric disease	Somatization disorder, somatoform pain disorder, conversion disorder

learn what word the child uses to describe pain (boo-boo, owie). The pain assessment should be tailored to the child's developmental level.

Physiologic signs are neither specific nor sensitive indicators of pain but may be used as adjunct to behavioral assessment and self-report in all age groups. Assess behavioral manifestations with caution, because many children will play, watch television, or sleep as a means of coping with pain. If the child is receiving sedatives in addition to analgesics, behavioral response to pain may be blunted.

Neonates and Infants (Birth to 1 Year)

Use of behavioral indexes is the best method of assessing pain in neonates. Facial grimaces, alterations in tone and activity, and crying are the most often used indicators of pain in this age group. Premature and critically ill neonates may not respond as vigorously to pain as healthy, full-term neonates. This lack of response does not indicate a lack of perception.

Behavioral indexes are also the most useful indicators of pain for infants beyond the neonatal period. In addition to facial grimaces, alterations in tone and activity, and crying, these infants demonstrate deliberate withdrawal from the painful stimulus and a wide variety of vocalizations.

Toddlers (1 to 3 Years)

Behavioral responses also continue to be the standard for pain assessment in toddlers. However, their behavior repertoire is expanded to include rubbing the site of pain and aggressive behavior (biting, hitting, and kicking). Some toddlers are capable of verbalizing where something hurts, but they cannot describe the intensity of the pain.

Preschoolers (3 to 5 Years)

By age 3 to 4 years, most children can begin to use self-report tools such as the Oucher Scale (Figure 3). These tools provide the most accurate measure of a child's pain. Preschoolers are better able to describe the intensity of their pain. This age group may also display aggressive behavior in response to pain.

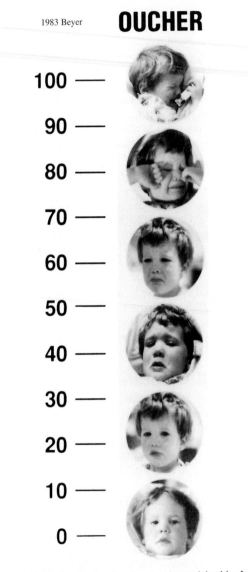

Figure 3. The Caucasian Oucher, developed and copyrighted by Judith E. Beyer, RN, PhD, 1983. This tool is also available in Hispanic and African American versions.

School-Agers (5 to 13 Years)

The Oucher Scale is also useful for school-agers. Children in this age group may use either the faces shown on the scale or the numeric scale. By age 7 or 8 many children can use a numeric scale. These children should have an understanding of the concept of order and number. Children in this age group can describe the intensity and location of their pain in greater detail. They may tend to act brave, demonstrating less overt behavior patterns, such as clenching their fists and teeth or remaining very still or rigid.

Adolescents (13 to 19 Years)

Any of the tools described here are useful for the adolescent. They can also respond to being asked, "On a scale of 0 to 10, with 0 being no pain and 10 being the worst pain you have ever had, where is your pain now?" Adolescents are capable of describing the intensity, location, and duration of their pain. They also display a variety of behavioral responses including mood swings and regression to an earlier developmental stage. Adolescents tend to dismiss their pain and refuse intervention in the presence of their peers.

MANAGEMENT

Pain management, ideally, is a multidisciplinary effort. The pain management "team" may include any or all of the following professionals: nurse, physician, child life specialist, respiratory therapist, occupational and physical therapist, and chaplain, along with the child and the family.

Strategies for pain management should include both pharmacologic and nonpharmocologic approaches. The following sections describe both types of management strategies.

Pharmacologic Management

Acute pain is managed with opioid and nonopioid analgesics. Table I-2 provides a selected list of medications used for the management of acute pain in the pediatric population. Patient-controlled analgesia and epidural analgesia are described in the following sections.

Table I-2. Selected Medications Used for Acute Pain in Pediatrics

Drug	Dose (mg/kg)*	Route	Frequency	Comments
Opioids				
Morphine	0.3	po	Every 3-4 hr	The standard for opioid therapy; most commonly used opioid in neonates
	0.1	IV	Every 3-4 hr	
Codeine	1	po	Every 3-4 hr	Not recommended for parenteral use; decreased incremental analgesic effect with doses greater than 65 mg
Hydromorphone (Dilaudid)	0.06	po	Every 3-4 hr	—
	0.015	IV	Every 3-4 hr	
Hydrocodone	0.2	po	Every 3-4 hr	Doses of aspirin and acetaminophen in combination products must be adjusted as appropriate for body weight

Drug	Dose	Route	Interval	Comments
Meperidine (Demerol)	0.75	IV	Every 3-4 hr	Reserve for very brief courses of opioid use in patients who have demonstrated allergy to morphine or hydromorphone; accumulation of the metabolite normerperidine may result in seizures
Methadone	0.2 / 0.1	po / IV	Every 6-8 hr / Every 6-8 hr	—
Oxycodone	0.2	po	Every 3-4 hr	Doses of aspirin and acetaminophen in combination products must be adjusted as appropriate for body weight
Nonopioids				
Acetaminophen	10-15	po or pr	Every 4 hr	No antiinflammatory activity
Nonsteroidal antiinflammatory drugs (NSAIDs)				
Aspirin	10-15	po	Every 4 hr	Inhibits platelet aggregation; may cause postoperative bleeding; do not administer salicylate to children with suspected or confirmed viral infection (i.e., chicken pox)

Continued

Table I-2. Selected Medications Used for Acute Pain in Pediatrics—cont'd

Drug	Dose (mg/kg)*	Route	Frequency	Comments
Choline magnesium salicylate	25	po	Twice a day	May have minimal antiplatelet activity; oral liquid available; do not administer salicylate to children with suspected or confirmed viral infection (i.e., chicken pox)
Ibuprofen	10	po	Every 6-8 hr	Oral suspension available
Naproxen	5	po	Every 12 hr	Oral liquid available
Ketoralac	0.5	IV	Every 6-8 hr	Ketoralac, the only parenteral NSAID, has not been approved for use in the pediatric population; there are presently ongoing clinical trials regarding the use of the intra-muscular preparation as an IV preparation in the pediatric and adult population

po, by mouth; IV, intravenous; pr, by rectum.
*Recommended dose for children less than 50 kg.

Because intramuscular injections are painful and frightening for children, this route of administration should be reserved for exceptional circumstances.

Patient-controlled analgesia

Patient-controlled analgesia (PCA) is a method of intravenous administration of small boluses of opiates used in the treatment of postoperative pain. The child uses a hand-operated device to signal the PCA pump to deliver a bolus dose of the medication. The pump will deliver the medication directly into the child's intravenous (IV) line, provided that a set period of time ("lockout interval") has passed since the previous dose. In addition to the boluses, many PCA pumps have the capability to deliver a background or continuous infusion of the opiate. Delivery of a continuous infusion helps maintain a steady therapeutic drug level even when the child is sleeping.

The child must have the cognitive ability to understand the principles of PCA. By the age of 7 most children can use PCA without difficulty. Each individual child's developmental level must be assessed prior to initiation of this method of drug administration. Teaching the child about PCA preoperatively is helpful.

Benefits of PCA include elimination of delay in analgesic administration, high levels of patient satisfaction, usefulness for all types of acute pain, potential reduction in total medication requirement, and reduction in nursing staff work load.

Complications are the same as those for other methods of opiate administration—respiratory depression, urinary retention, pruritus, nausea, and vomiting.

Epidural analgesia

Epidural analgesia may be used on children who have undergone any of a variety of surgical procedures, including thoracic, abdominal, and genitourinary tract procedures. The epidural catheter is placed by an anesthesiologist and provides access for continuous opiate infusion or boluses of opiates and/or local anesthetics.

Compared to traditional intravenous or PCA administration of opiates, smaller doses of opiate given via an epidural catheter provide adequate pain control with less sedation. Because of increased comfort level, the child is better able to participate in postoperative care. Additional benefits include earlier ambulation and increased ability to deep breathe. Potential side effects of epidural analgesia include respiratory depression, urinary retention, pruritus, infection, spinal headache, nausea, and vomiting.

Nonpharmacologic Management

Behavioral and other nonpharmacologic techniques may be used in conjunction with pharmacologic management of acute pain. Table I-3 lists selected nonpharmacologic pain management strategies. These techniques often allow for a reduction in the amount of analgesic required. It is important to assess the child's individual response to any strategy. Involving families in these strategies often enhances their success.

PROCEDURAL PAIN

Invasive procedures are essential in diagnosis and treatment for many hospitalized children. These procedures include venipunctures, intravenous catheter insertions, circumcisions, cardiac catheterizations, chest tube insertions, central line insertions, bone marrow aspirations, and biopsies. Some dressing changes may also cause significant pain and stress in children.

The child and the family should be adequately prepared for the procedure. The type of preparation should be based on the child's developmental level. Be aware of the environment in which the procedure is to be performed. Minimize noise, provide adequate lighting, and ensure privacy. The child's room and bed are considered safe places. Procedures should not be performed in the room or the bed unless absolutely necessary.

Allow a family member (ideally, mother and/or father, if present) to be with the child before, during, and after the procedure. The family member should be prepared for his or her role, which usually involves assisting in nonpharmacologic pain relief measures.

If anxiolytics are used to reduce anxiety associated with procedures, it is important to remember that these medications will blunt the child's response to pain but will not provide pain relief.

A key principle in the management of procedural pain is the provision of maximal treatment for the pain and anxiety of a first procedure, particularly if the child must undergo repeated procedures. This helps to reduce the development of anticipatory anxiety prior to subsequent procedures.

REFERENCES

Acute Pain Management Guideline Panel: *Acute pain management in infants, children, and adolescents: operative and medical procedures—quick reference guide for clinicians,* AHCPR Pub No 92-0020, Rockville, Md, 1992, Agency for Health Care Policy Research, Public Health Service, US Department of Health and Human Services.

International Association for the Study of Pain Subcommittee on Taxonomy: Pain terms: a list with definitions and notes usage, *Pain* 6:249, 1979.

Jeans ME, Melzack R: Conceptual basis for nursing practice: theoretical foundations of pain. In Watt-Watson JH, Donovan MI, editors: *Pain management: nursing perspective,* St Louis, 1992, Mosby.

Kachoyeanos, MK, Friedhoff M: Cognitive and behavioral strategies to reduce children's pain, *MCN,* 18:14, 1993.

Lincoln LM: Children's response to acute pain: a developmental approach, *Journal of the American Academy of Nurse Practitioners,* 4:139, 1992.

McCaffrey, M, Beebe A: *Pain: clinical manual for nursing practice,* St Louis, 1989, Mosby.

Schechter NL, Berde CB, Yaster, M: *Pain in infants, children and adolescents,* Baltimore, 1993, Williams & Wilkins.

Table I-3. Nonpharmacologic Pain Management Techniques

Age Group	Techniques
Neonates	<ul><li>Pacifiers</li><li>Music (fetal heart sounds)</li><li>Swaddling, blanket nests, or boundaries</li><li>Speaking in soft quiet tones</li><li>Minimizing noxious stimuli: frequent handling, noise, bright lights (premature neonates may be overwhelmed by increased sensory stimuli)</li></ul>
Infants	<ul><li>Visual stimuli</li><li>Speaking in quiet tones</li><li>Pacifiers</li><li>Rocking</li><li>Swaddling (for younger infants)</li><li>Music</li><li>Cutaneous stimulation: transcutaneous electric nerve stimulation (TENS), heat, cold, massage</li></ul>
Toddlers	<ul><li>Magic wands</li><li>Kaleidoscopes</li><li>Pop-up books</li><li>Music</li><li>Controlled breathing—blowing bubbles</li><li>Cutaneous stimulation</li></ul>
Preschoolers	<ul><li>Magic wands</li><li>Kaleidoscopes</li><li>Pop-up books</li></ul>

Table I-3. Nonpharmacologic Pain Management Techniques

- Finding hidden picture (*Where's Waldo?*)
- Listening to music or a story through a headset
- Watching videos
- Emotive imagery—using a child's favorite superhero to "fight" the pain
- Controlled breathing
- Behavior rehearsal—becoming familiar with a procedure through play
- Cutaneous stimulation

School-agers
- Imagery
- Listening to music or a story through a headset
- Watching videos
- Controlled breathing
- Behavior rehearsal
- Cutaneous stimulation
- Modeling—observing another child during a procedure; the child models or demonstrates behavior that assists in mastering the procedure (can be live or with videotape)

Adoles-cents
- Imagery
- Music
- Controlled breathing
- Watching videos
- Cutaneous stimulation
- Modeling

Psychosocial Interventions

PREPARATION FOR PROCEDURES OR SURGERY

1. Prepare child and parents for procedure or surgery.
   a. Provide age-appropriate explanations.
      (1) For younger children, the use of sensory materials such as graphics (e.g., pictures) or props (e.g., bandages, surgical mask) enhances the child's comprehension.
      (2) For older children, use of illustrations such as film or pictures (e.g., anatomic figures) is helpful to supplement explanation.
   b. Explain the procedure or surgery and preoperative routine in terms of the sequence of events to occur, including sensory information (e.g., mouth will feel dry, child will feel sleepy).
   c. For younger children, encourage preprocedural play such as using medical equipment, doll, or stuffed animal as a means of explaining the procedure or surgery.
   d. Use age-appropriate means for explaining body changes following the procedure or surgery and for eliciting concerns from child.
   e. Provide and reinforce information for parents about child's condition and treatment to answer their child's questions or relieve their own anxiety.
   f. Assure the child that the procedure is not being done because the child is "bad."

610

2. Prepare child and parents emotionally for surgery.
   a. Provide understandable explanations in lay terms.
   b. Use active listening to elicit concerns.
   c. Encourage ventilation of feelings (e.g., guilt, anger, anxiety, feeling of being overwhelmed).
   d. Encourage ventilation of fears concerning child's well-being.
   e. Provide anticipatory information about emotional responses to surgery.
   f. Encourage parents to room in and participate in child's care as means of promoting security and decreasing anxiety.
   g. Encourage parental participation during selected procedures; some procedures such as bone marrow aspiration can be very traumatic for the parent and convey the erroneous message to the younger child that the parent cannot "protect" the child from harm.
   h. Encourage parental participation during the induction of anesthesia and during recovery (if applicable).
   i. Provide for physical comforts (e.g., sleeping and hygiene).
   j. Encourage use of preexisting support systems such as family members, close friends, and clergy.
   k. Encourage incorporation of some home routines—such as child's blanket, use of prayers, and storytelling—into hospital routine.
   l. Assist parents in providing support and information to siblings while child is hospitalized.
   m. If needed, provide information to parents about sibling needs such as disclosing information about child's clinical status, maintenance of household routines, and communicating with school personnel.
3. Assist and support child during preoperative laboratory and diagnostic tests.
   a. Prepare or provide information about upcoming procedures (e.g., complete blood count [CBC], urinalysis, laboratory and diagnostic tests).
   b. Assist in the collection of preoperative laboratory and diagnostic data.
   c. Prepare child for surgery by obtaining nursing assessment data such as nursing assessment of body systems and nursing history.

d. Monitor child's reactions to presurgical or preprocedural preparations.
4. Monitor child's baseline status prior to surgery or procedure.
    a. Vital signs
    b. System assessment

SUPPORTIVE CARE

1. Alleviate anxiety caused by various aspects of the hospital experience, including invasive procedures for diagnostic tests, pain, a threatening and confusing hospital environment, unfamiliar hospital personnel, knowledge deficit pertaining to the hospital routines and treatments, and age-related fears.
    a. Provide therapeutic play during all phases of illness and for each new procedure based on the child's developmental level (see the previous section, on preparation for procedures or surgery, for additional information).
    b. Explain each procedure or hospital routine at child's and parents' cognitive levels; allow enough time for child and parents to ask questions and express anxieties.
    c. Suggest ways for parents to support their child during hospitalization and procedures (e.g., holding the child after the procedure).
    d. Consult parents and child about preferences among "quiet" toys and activities during acute phase of illness; encourage parents and volunteers to play with child, allowing for rest periods and then passive participation (see Appendix B, Growth and Development).
    e. Encourage and promote socialization with peers as a means to cope adaptively with impact of disease.
2. Provide emotional support to parents.
    a. Provide and reinforce explanations about the hospital experience.
    b. Encourage use of preexisting support systems (e.g., relatives, friends, clergy).
    c. Encourage ventilation of feelings through active listening techniques.

    d. Provide for physical comforts (e.g., sleeping arrangements, bathing).

    e. Refer to social service if appropriate.

    f. Refer to in-hospital parent support group; encourage parents to network with other parents in hospital for support.

3. Provide comfort measures to ease the anxiety and discomfort of the child during hospitalization.

    a. Teach parents how to hold and comfort the child who has intravenous (IV) support and other medical equipment.

    b. Encourage parents to participate in aspects of child's care such as bathing and feeding; however, if parents are uncomfortable or otherwise unable to provide care, they should not feel pressured to do so.

    c. Keep stimulation to a minimum; arrange procedures or treatments so as to keep interruptions to a minimum, especially at night.

    d. Teach parents nonpharmacologic pain relief measures to use with child (see Appendix I, Pain in Children).

4. Provide developmentally appropriate visual, auditory, and tactile stimulation (see Appendix B, Growth and Development).

5. Provide consistent nursing care to promote trust and to alleviate anxiety.

6. Encourage use of recreational and diversional activities (see Appendix B, Growth and Development).

K

Home Care

1. Instruct parents verbally and with detailed written information about the following aspects of medical management to enhance adherence:
   a. Disease process—signs, symptoms, complications, and treatment regimen
   b. Administration of medications—therapeutic response to medications, untoward reactions to medications
   c. Treatment procedures—steps of the procedures and schedule
   d. Activity restrictions
   e. Equipment needs—care and maintenance, phone number of vendor
   f. Name and phone number of appropriate follow-up contact (e.g., private medical doctor, clinic, health maintenance organization, clinical nurse specialist, nurse practitioner, case manager)
2. Instruct parents about identifying symptoms that indicate worsening of conditions and need to report to physician.
3. Provide child and family with information about community support systems for long-term adaptation.
   a. School reintegration program—refer to appropriate school personnel such as school nurse, teacher, or specialist
   b. Parent groups for ongoing support, information, and advocacy

   c. Children's groups for ongoing support

   d. Siblings groups for ongoing support

   e. Financial resources and information about third-party providers

   f. Community specialists and programs for ongoing therapy and/or services

   g. Community organizations for ongoing support and information (e.g., American Cancer Society, United Cerebral Palsy)

4. Instruct parents about parenting issues.

   a. Need to maintain usual expectations for behavior and misbehavior

   b. Continuing with disciplinary measures, e.g., use of "time out" discipline (note that parents may need additional training for this)

   c. Strategies to assist child in living normally and dealing with concerns

   d. Use of child-rearing practices that avoid labeling child's behavior as deviant, a practice that may have a self-fulfilling result

   e. Use of strategies that encourage interactions with peers

5. Facilitate adherence to long-term management during follow-up visits by reinforcing information pertaining to procedures and community resources to prevent complications; ask questions that explore adherence potential.

   a. Means of transportation

   b. Resources for child care

   c. Finances

   d. Level of motivation

   e. Understanding of need for long-term follow-up

6. Monitor disruptions in family functioning.

   a. Ensure that all interventions are based on the family's cultural, religious, educational, and socioeconomic background.

   b. Involve siblings as much as possible because they have many concerns and feelings about the changes in the child and the family's functioning.

   c. Consider the possibility that siblings feel self-blame and guilt.

   d. Encourage parents to ventilate feelings of insecurity and concerns about caring for child at home, as well as about long-term management and prognosis.

e. Refer parents to support groups and/or counseling because parental relationships may be strained as a result of the intense pressures and care expectations of the ill child.

Index

A

Abbreviations, 578-584

Abuse, child; *see* Child abuse

ABVD drug regimens, for Hodgkin's disease, 207

ACE-inhibitors
for hypertension, 234
for nephrotic syndrome, 337

Acetaminophen, for cellulitis, 64

Acquired immunodeficiency syndrome; *see* AIDS/HIV

Actinomycin-D, for Wilms' tumor, 505

ADHD; *see* Attention-deficit/ hyperactivity disorder (ADHD)

Adolescents
growth/development in, 558-562

Adolescents—cont'd
growth/development in—cont'd
cognitive, 560
faith, 562
gross/fine motor, 559-560
language, 560-561
moral, 562
physical, 558-559
psychosocial, 561-562
puberty changes, 560*t*
incidence in
of anorexia nervosa, 4
of appendicitis, 20
of bulimia, 47
of diabetes mellitus, 116-117
of drowning, 131
of hypertension, 232-233
of inflammatory bowel disease, 255
of iron deficiency anemia, 266

Adolescents—cont'd
  incidence in—cont'd
    of nonaccidental
      trauma, 347
    of osteogenic
      sarcoma, 358
    of scoliosis, 437
  pain management and,
    601, 609*t*
Adriamycin, for Hodgkin's
  disease, 208
African Americans
  facial expression pain
    scale and, *600*
  incidence in
    of cleft palate, 73
    of cystic fibrosis, 104
    of HIV/AIDS, 213
    of hypertension,
      232-233
    of hypertrophic
      pyloric stenosis,
      236
    of leukemia, 300
    of nonaccidental
      trauma, 347
    of sickle cell anemia,
      461
    of SIDS, 476
AIDS/HIV, 212-224
  classification of,
    215-217, 219*t*, 220*t*
  diagnosis of, 213-214,
    217-218, 221
  discharge/home care of,
    224
  incidence of, 213
  interventions for,
    221-223
  management of, 218,
    219*t*, 220, 220*t*

AIDS/HIV—cont'd
  nursing assessments of,
    220-221
  pathophysiology of,
    212-213
Air pollution, croup and, 99
Albuterol
  for asthma, 27
  for cystic fibrosis, 106
Alcoholism, bulimia
  nervosa and, 47
ALG; *see* Antilymphocyte
  globulin (ALG)
Alkylating agents, for
  nephrotic syndrome,
  337
ALL; *see* Leukemia
Allopurinol, for leukemia,
  302, 306
ALTE; *see* Apparent
  life-threatening event
  (ALTE)
Amenorrhea, anorexia
  nervosa and, 6
Amoxicillin, for otis
  media, 372
Amphetamine sulfate
  (Benzedrine), for
  ADHD, 34
Amputation, osteogenic
  sarcoma and,
  359-360, 361-363
Analgesia, epidural, 605-606
Anemia, aplastic; *see*
  Aplastic anemia
Anemia, iron deficiency,
  265-268
  diagnosis of, 266-267
  discharge/home care of,
    268
  incidence of, 266

Anemia, iron
    deficiency—cont'd
    interventions for,
        267-268
    management of, 266,
        267
    nursing assessments of,
        267
    pathophysiology of, 265
ANLL; see Leukemia
Anorexia nervosa
    diagnosis of, 3, 4-5, 5-7
    discharge/home care of,
        7
    incidence of, 4
    interventions for, 7
    management of, 6
    nursing assessments of,
        6
Antiacids, for
    gastroesophageal
    reflux, 165
Antibiotics
    for acute rheumatic
        fever, 433
    for aplastic anemia, 11
    for cellulitis, 64
    for cystic fibrosis, 106
    for epiglottitis, 139
    for foreign body
        aspiration, 145
    for glomerulonephritis,
        170
    for meningitis, 320
    for osteomyelitis, 366
    for otis media, 372
    for postsurgical hernia,
        195
    for RDS, 417
    for renal failure, 397
    for renal transplant, 411

Antibiotics—cont'd
    for sickle cell anemia,
        463
    for spina bifida, 469
    for tetralogy of fallot,
        483
    for urinary tract
        infections, 494
Anticholinergics, for spina
    bifida, 470
Anticoagulants
    for hemolytic-uremic
        syndrome, 176
    for Reye's syndrome, 427
Anticonvulsants, 447-448
Antidepressants
    for anorexia nervosa, 6
    for bulimia nervosa, 50
Antidiarrheal agents, for
    inflammatory bowel
    disease, 257
Antiepileptic drug
    therapy, 447-448
Antihypertensives, for
    coarctation of the
    aorta, 83
Antiinflammatory agents
    for inflammatory bowel
        disease, 257
    for juvenile rheumatoid
        arthritis, 275, 276t,
        277
Antilymphocyte globulin
    (ALG), for aplastic
    anemia, 11
Antiplatelet agents, for
    hemolytic-uremic
    syndrome, 176
Antithymocyte globulin
    (ATG), for aplastic
    anemia, 11

Anxiety, anorexia nervosa
and, 6
Aplastic anemia, 9-13
diagnosis of, 10, 12
discharge/home care of, 13
incidence of, 9-10
interventions for, 12-13
management of, 11
nursing assessments of,
11-12
pathophysiology of, 9
Apnea
ALTE and, 15
bronchiolitis and, 37
Apparent life-threatening
event (ALTE), 15-18
diagnosis of, 16-17
discharge/home care of,
18
incidence of, 15-16
interventions for, 17-18
management of, 16-17
pathophysiology of, 15
Appendectomy, 20-24
Appendicitis, 20-24
diagnosis of, 20-22
discharge/home care of,
24
incidence of, 20
interventions for, 22-23
management of, 21-22
nursing assessment of, 22
pathophysiology of, 20
surgery for, 23
Arteriolar dilators, for
CHF, 95
Artificial airways, for
croup, 100
Asians, incidence in
of cleft palate, 73
of cystic fibrosis, 104

Asians, incidence
in—cont'd
of hypertrophic pyloric
stenosis, 236
of Kawasaki disease,
281-282
of SIDS, 476
Asparaginase, for
leukemia, 302, 303-304
Aspirin, for Kawasaki
disease, 284
Asthma, 25-28
diagnosis of, 26-27
discharge/home care of,
28
incidence of, 25
interventions for, 27-28
management of, 27
nursing assessment of,
27
pathophysiology of, 25
ATG; see Antithymocyte
globulin (ATG)
Attention-deficit/
hyperactivity
disorder
(ADHD), 29-35
diagnosis of, 30-35
discharge/home care of,
35
incidence of, 33
interventions for, 34-35
management of, 33, 34
nursing assessment of,
34
pathophysiology of, 29-33
Azathioprine, for renal
transplant, 411
Azidothymidine
(zidovudine), for
HIV/AIDS, 218

B

Barlow's maneuver, 89

Beck Depression
    Inventory, anorexia
    nervosa and, 6

Behavior modification, for
    ADHD, 34

Beta-agonists
    for asthma, 27
    for cystic fibrosis, 106

Beta-blockers, for
    hypertension, 234

Bisexual males,
    HIV/AIDS in, 213

Bleomycin, for Hodgkin's
    disease, 208

Blindness, in meningitis,
    319

β-blockers, for
    hypertension, 234

Blood pressure testing,
    568-569, 569t

Blood products
    for acute renal failure,
        397
    for aplastic anemia, 11
    for chronic renal failure,
        405
    for disseminated
        intravascular
        coagulation, 127
    for hemophilia, 182
    for RDS, 417

Bone marrow transplants
    (BMT)
    for aplastic anemia, 11
    for leukemia, 300
    for neuroblastoma, 343

BPD; see
    Bronchopulmonary
    dysplasia

Bronchiolitis, 36-39
    apnea and, 37
    diagnosis of, 37-38
    discharge/home care of,
        39
    incidence of, 36
    interventions for, 38-39
    management of, 37-38
    nursing assessment of, 38
    pathophysiology of, 36

Bronchodilators
    for asthma, 27
    for bronchopulmonary
        dysplasia, 43
    for croup, 100
    for cystic fibrosis, 106
    for foreign body
        aspiration, 145
    for RDS, 417

Bronchopulmonary
    dysplasia, 41-46
    diagnosis of, 42-43
    discharge/home care of,
        45
    incidence of, 41-42
    interventions for, 43-45
    management of, 42-43
    nursing assessments of,
        43
    pathophysiology of, 41

Bronchoscopy, for foreign
    body aspiration, 145

Bulimia nervosa, 47-51
    diagnosis of, 47-50
    discharge/home care of,
        50
    incidence of, 47
    interventions for, 50
    management of, 49-50
    nursing assessments of, 50
    pathophysiology of, 47

Burns, 52-60
  classification of, 53
  diagnosis of, 53, *54, 55,*
    56-57
  discharge/home care of,
    60
  incidence of, 53
  interventions for, 57-60
  management of, 56-57
  nursing assessments of,
    57
  pathophysiology of,
    52-53

C
Calcium, chronic renal
    failure and, 405
Calcium antagonists, for
    hypertension, 234
California, HIV/AIDS in,
    213
Captopril (Capoten), for
    coarctation of the
    aorta, 83
Carbamazepine, for
    seizure disorders, 448
Cardiac catheterization,
    512-515
  interventions and, 513,
    515
  normal pressures and,
    514
  nursing assessments
    and, 513
Cardiac disorders,
    anorexia nervosa and,
    7
Casting, for fractures, 151
Caucasians
  facial expression pain
    scale of, *600*

Caucasians—cont'd
  incidence in
    of anorexia nervosa, 4
    of cystic fibrosis, 104
    of HIV/AIDS, 213
    of inflammatory
      bowel disease, 255
    of ITP, 241-242
    of nonaccidental
      trauma, 347
    of SIDS, 476
Cellulitis, 62-65
  diagnosis of, 63-65
  discharge/home care of,
    65
  incidence of, 62
  interventions for, 65
  management of, 64
  nursing assessments of, 64
  pathophysiology of,
    62-63
Central nervous system,
    near drowning and,
    134
Cerebral edema, in
    meningitis, 320
CF; *see* Cystic fibrosis (CF)
Charcoal, activated, for
    poisoning, 391
Chelation therapy, for
    lead poisoning, 292
Chemotherapy
  for cytomegaloviral
    infection, 112
  for leukemia, 302
  for neuroblastoma, 343
  for non-Hodgkin's
    lymphoma, 353
  for Wilms' tumor, 505
CHF; *see* Congestive heart
    failure (CHF)

Child abuse, 67-72
  diagnosis of, 69-71
  discharge/home care
    and, 72
  incidence of, 67-68
  interventions for, 71-72
  management of, 68
  nursing assessments of,
    71
  pathophysiology of, 67
Chinese; see also Asians
  hypertrophic pyloric
    stenosis and, 236
Cimetidine, for
  gastroesophageal
  reflux, 165
Cisapride, for
  gastroesophageal
  reflux, 165
Cisplatin, for Wilms'
  tumor, 505
Cleft lip/palate, 73-78
  diagnosis of, 74-75
  discharge/home care of,
    78
  incidence of, 73
  interventions for, 75-78
  management of, 74-75,
    76-78
  nursing assessments of,
    75
  otis media and, 371
  pathophysiology of, 73
  surgery for, 74-75,
    76-78
Clonazepam (Klonopin),
  for seizure disorders,
  448
CMV-immune globulin,
  for cytomegaloviral
  infection, 112

Coarctation of the aorta,
  80-86
  diagnosis of, 81-82, 84
  discharge/home care of,
    86
  incidence of, 80
  interventions for,
    84-86
  management of, 82-83
  nursing assessments of,
    83
  pathophysiology of, 80
  surgery and, 82-83,
    84-86
Coma scale, Glasgow, 535
COMP drug regimen, for
  non-Hodgkin's
  lymphoma, 353
Compresses, for cellulitis,
  64
Computed tomography
  (CT), 516-517
  nursing assessments
    and, 516
  nursing interventions
    and, 516-517
Congenital hip
  dislocation; see Hip
  dislocation,
  congenital
Congestive heart failure
  (CHF), 93-97
  diagnosis of, 94-95
  discharge/home care of,
    96-97
  incidence of, 94
  interventions for,
    95-96
  management of, 95
  nursing assessments of,
    95

Congestive heart
  failure (CHF)—cont'd
 pathophysiology of,
    93-94
Corticosteroids
 for acute rheumatic
    fever, 433
 for bronchopulmonary
    dysplasia, 43
 for foreign body
    aspiration, 145
 for hemolytic-uremic
    syndrome, 176
 for Hodgkin's disease,
    208
 for inflammatory bowel
    disease, 257
 for ITP, 243
 for RDS, 417
 for renal transplants,
    411
Crohn's disease, 256-258
Croup, 98-102
 diagnosis of, 99, 100
 discharge/home care of,
    101
 incidence of, 98-99
 interventions for, 100-101
 management of, 100
 nursing assessments of,
    100
 pathophysiology of, 98
Cryoprecipitate, for
    hemophilia, 182
CT; *see* Computed
    tomography (CT)
Cyclophosphamide
 for ITP, 243
 for neuroblastoma, 343
 for non-Hodgkin's
    lymphoma, 353

Cyclophosphamide—cont'd
 for Wilms' tumor, 505
Cyclophosphamide
    (Cytoxan), for
    leukemia, 302, 306
Cyclosporin A, for
    aplastic anemia, 11
Cyclosporine, for renal
    transplants, 411
Cystic fibrosis (CF),
    103-109
 diagnosis of, 104-105, 107
 discharge/home care of,
    108
 incidence of, 104
 interventions for,
    107-108
 management of,
    105-107
 nursing assessments of,
    107
 pathophysiology of,
    103-104
Cytarabine (Cytosar,
    Cytosine,
    Arabinoside), for
    leukemia, 302, 305
Cytomegaloviral infection,
    110-114
 diagnosis of, 111-112,
    113
 discharge/home care of,
    113-114
 incidence of, 111
 interventions for, 113
 management of,
    112-113
 nursing assessments of,
    113
 pathophysiology of,
    110-111

Cytotoxic agents, for juvenile rheumatoid arthritis, 275, 277

D

Dacarbazine, for Hodgkin's disease, 208

Daunorubicin (Daunomycin), for leukemia, 302

Deafness, in meningitis, 319

Debridement, for burns, 56

Depression, anorexia nervosa and, 6

Desferol, for sickle cell anemia, 463

Desipramine, for anorexia nervosa, 6

Desmopressin, for hemophilia, 182

Developing countries, hepatitis in, 188

Dextroamphetamine sulfate (Dexedrine), for ADHD, 34

Diabetes mellitus insulin-dependent type I, 115-124
  diagnosis of, 117, 118-120
  discharge/home care of, 122
  incidence of, 116-117
  interventions for, 120-121
  management of, 117-118, 120
  nursing assessments of, 120

Diabetes mellitus—cont'd insulin-dependent type I—cont'd
  pathophysiology of, 115-116
  RDS in preterm infants and, 415

Dialysis
  for acute renal failure, 396
  for chronic renal failure, 405

DIC; see Disseminated intravascular coagulation (DIC)

Diet
  for anorexia nervosa, 6
  for burns, 57
  for CHF, 95
  for cystic fibrosis, 106
  for diabetes mellitus, 120, 123-124
  for gastroenteritis, 161
  for gastroesophageal reflux, 165
  for hepatitis, 190
  for hypertension, 234
  for hypertrophic pyloric stenosis, 236
  for inflammatory bowel disease, 257
  for nephrotic syndrome, 337
  for renal failure, 397, 405
  for rheumatic fever, acute, 433
  for short bowel syndrome, 454, 455-456
  for tetralogy of fallot, 483

Digitalis, for tetralogy of fallot, 483

Dilators, for CHF, 95

Dimercaprol, for lead poisoning, 292

Diphtheria, tetanus, pertussis (DTP) immunization, 565
contraindications and, 567
reactions and, 566-567

Dislocations
in child abuse, 70
congenital hip, 87-92

Disseminated intravascular coagulation (DIC), 125-129
diagnosis of, 126-127
discharge/home care of, 129
incidence of, 125-126
interventions for, 128-129
management of, 126, 127
nursing assessments of, 127
pathophysiology of, 125

Dopamine (Intropin), for ventricular septal defect, 498

Down syndrome
leukemia and, 300
ventricular septal defect and, 497

Doxorubicin
for neuroblastoma, 343
for non-Hodgkin's lymphoma, 353
for Wilms' tumor, 505

Drainage, for cellulitis, 64

Drowning/near drowning, 130-137
diagnosis of, 132-134
discharge/home care of, 135
incidence of, 131-132
interventions for, 134-135
management of, 132-133, 134
nursing assessments of, 134
pathophysiology of, 130-131

DTP; see Diphtheria, tetanus, pertussis (DTP) immunization

Duchenne muscular dystrophy; see Muscular dystrophy

E

Eat-26, for anorexia nervosa, 6

Eating Attitudes Test (EAT), for anorexia nervosa, 6

Eating Disorders Inventory (EDI), for anorexia nervosa, 6

ECG; see Electrocardiography (ECG)

Edetate disodium calcium, for lead poisoning, 292

Electrocardiography (ECG), 518-519
interventions and, 518-519

Electrocardiography (ECG)—cont'd
nursing assessments and, 518
Emergency care
for burns, 57
for foreign body aspiration, 145
for near drowning, 134
Emetic agents, for poisoning, 391
Endocrine systems, nursing assessments in, 537
Endoscopy, 520-521
interventions and, 521
nursing assessments and, 520
Enemas, bulimia nervosa and, 47
Epidural analgesia, 605-606
Epiglottitis, 138-141
diagnosis of, 138-140
discharge/home care of, 141
incidence of, 138
interventions for, 140-141
management of, 139-140
nursing assessments of, 140
pathophysiology of, 138
Epilepsy, 443-450
Epinephrine
for asthma, 27
for croup, 100
Epstein-Barr, aplastic anemia and, 9
Escherichia coli, urinary tract infections and, 492

Eskimos, congenital hip dislocation and, 88
Estrogen, for anorexia nervosa, 6
Ethosuximide (Zarontin), for seizure disorders, 448
Etoposide, for Wilms' tumor, 505
Exercise
for diabetes mellitus, 120
for hypertension, 234
for juvenile rheumatoid arthritis, 275

F
Facial injuries, in child abuse, 69
Fall season
croup during, 98
hemolytic-uremic syndrome during, 173-174
Falls, in child abuse, 69
Family counseling
for ADHD, 34
for bulimia nervosa, 50
for child abuse, 71
for SIDS, 478
Fanconi's anemia, 9
Fats, cystic fibrosis and, 106
Fear, child abuse and, 71
Feeding
for gastroesophageal reflux, 165
for post surgical hernia, 195
Females, incidence in
of anorexia nervosa, 4
of aplastic anemia, 10

Females, incidence
in—cont'd
of bulimia nervosa in,
47
of cleft palate in, 73
of congenital hip
dislocation, 87
of cytomegaloviral
infection, 111
of HIV/AIDS, 213
of IDDM, 116-117
of iron deficiency
anemia, 266
of juvenile rheumatoid
arthritis, 271
of leukemia, 300
of muscular dystrophy,
330
of patent ductus
arteriosus, 376
of scoliosis, 437
of sexual abuse, 67-68
of spina bifida, 468
of urinary tract
infections, 492-493
Florida, HIV/AIDS in, 213
Fluoxetine, for anorexia
nervosa, 6
Foreign body aspiration,
143-147
diagnosis of, 144-146
discharge/home care of,
146-147
incidence of, 144
interventions for, 146
management of, 144,
145
nursing assessments of,
146
pathophysiology of,
143-144

Fractures, 148-153
in child abuse, 70
diagnosis of, 149-151
discharge/home care of,
153
incidence of, 150
interventions for,
151-152
management of, 151,
152-153
nursing assessments of,
151
pathophysiology of, 148
Fundoplication, for
gastroesophageal
reflux, 165

G
Galeazzi's sign,
assessment of, 89
Ganciclovir, for
cytomegaloviral
infection, 112
Gastroenteritis, 155-163
diagnosis of, 160-162
discharge/home care of,
163
incidence of, 160
interventions for,
162-163
management of, 161
pathophysiology of,
155, 156t-159t
Gastroesophageal reflux,
164-167
diagnosis of, 164-166
discharge/home care of,
167
incidence of, 164
interventions for,
166-167

Gastroesophageal
reflux—cont'd
management of, 165-166
nursing assessments of,
166
pathophysiology of, 164
Gastrointestinal systems,
nursing assessments
in, 534-535
Gay males, HIV/AIDS in,
213
Glasgow coma scale, 535
nursing assessments
and, 535
Glomerulonephritis,
168-172
chronic renal failure
and, 402
diagnosis of, 169-171
discharge/home care of,
171
incidence of, 168-169
interventions for, 171
management of, 170
nursing assessments of,
170
pathophysiology of, 168
Glucocorticoids, for glomerulonephritis, 170
Glucocorticosteroids, for
juvenile rheumatoid
arthritis, 277
Grafting, for burns, 56
Growth/development
criteria, 538-562
adolescents, 558-562
infants, 538-546
preschoolers, 550-555
school-age children,
555-558
toddlers, 546-550

H
Haemophilus influenzae type
B, immunizations for,
565
Hair loss, child abuse
and, 69
HBIG, for hepatitis, 190
Head injuries, in child
abuse, 69
Hearing
cleft lip/palate and, 74
otis media and, 371
Heart transplants, cystic
fibrosis and, 106-107
Height/weight
anorexia nervosa and, 6
growth curves in,
588-595
females, 588-591
males, 592-595
Heimlich maneuver, for
foreign body
aspiration, 145
Hematology, nursing
assessments in, 537
Hemolytic-uremic
syndrome, 173-178
diagnosis of, 174-177
discharge/home care of,
178
incidence of, 173-174
interventions for,
177-178
management of, 176
nursing assessments of,
176
renal failure and, 395
Hemophilia, 180-184
diagnosis of, 182-183
discharge/home care of,
184

Hemophilia—cont'd
  incidence of, 181
  interventions for,
      183-184
  management of, 181,
      182
  nursing assessments of,
      183-184
  pathophysiology of, 180
Heparin, for disseminated
    intravascular
    coagulation, 127
Hepatitis, 186-192
  aplastic anemia and, 9
  diagnosis of, 188-191
  discharge/home care of,
      192
  immunizations for,
      565-566
  incidence of, 188
  interventions for,
      191-192
  management of,
      190-191
  nursing assessments of,
      191
  pathophysiology of,
      186-187
Hernia, 194-197
  diagnosis of, 195-196
  discharge/home care of,
      196-197
  incidence of, 194
  management of, 195, 196
  nursing assessments of,
      195
  pathophysiology of, 194
  surgery for, 196
Hip dislocation,
    congenital, 87-92
  diagnosis of, 88-90

Hip dislocation,
    congenital—cont'd
  discharge/home care, 91
  incidence of, 87-88
  interventions for, 90-91
  management of, 88-89
  nursing assessments of,
      89, 90
  pathophysiology of, 87
Hirschsprung's disease,
    198-204
  diagnosis of, 199-201
  discharge/home care of,
      203
  incidence of, 198
  interventions for,
      201-202
  management of, 199-200
  nursing assessments of,
      200
  pathophysiology of, 198
  surgery and, 199-203
Hispanics, facial
    expression pain scale
    for, *600*
HIV/AIDS; see AIDS/HIV
Hodgkin's disease,
    205-211
  diagnosis of, 206-207, 209
  discharge/home care of,
      210
  incidence of, 205
  interventions for,
      209-210
  management of, 207-208
  nursing assessments of,
      209
  pathophysiology of, 205
Holy-Oram syndrome,
    ventricular septal
    defect and, 497

Home care; *see also* specific disorders procedures for, 614-616

Human immunodeficiency virus; *see* AIDS/HIV

Hydrocephalus, 225-229
diagnosis of, 225-226, 227
discharge/home care of, 229
incidence of, 225
interventions for, 228-229
management of, 227-229
nursing assessments of, 227
pathophysiology of, 225
surgery and, 227-229

Hydrocortisone, for non-Hodgkin's lymphoma, 354

Hyperkalemia, burns and, 58

Hypertension, 231-235
diagnosis of, 233-234
discharge/home care of, 235
glomerulonephritis and, 170
incidence of, 232-233
interventions for, 235
management of, 234
nursing assessments of, 234
pathophysiology of, 231-232

Hypertransfusion, for sickle cell anemia, 463

Hypertrophic pyloric stenosis, 236-240
diagnosis of, 236-238

Hypertrophic pyloric stenosis—cont'd
discharge/home care of, 239-240
incidence of, 236
interventions for, 238
management of, 237
nursing assessments of, 238
pathophysiology of, 236
surgery and, 237-239

Hypocalcemia, burns and, 58

Hypoglycemia, chronic renal failure and, 405

Hyponatremia, burns and, 58

I
Ibuprofen, for juvenile rheumatoid arthritis, 275

ICP; *see* Intracranial pressure monitoring (ICP)

IDDM; *see* Diabetes mellitus, insulin-dependent type I

Idiopathic thrombocytopenic purpura (ITP), 241-245
diagnosis of, 242-244
discharge/home care of, 245
incidence of, 241-242
interventions for, 244-245
management of, 243
nursing assessments of, 244
pathophysiology of, 241

Ifosfamide, for Wilms'
tumor, 505
Ig; *see* Immune globulin (Ig)
Imipramine
for anorexia nervosa, 6
for bulimia nervosa, 50
Immune globulin (Ig)
for hepatitis, 190
for ITP, 243
Immunizations, 563-567
contraindications and,
567
diphtheria, tetanus,
pertussis, 565
Haemophilus influenzae
type B, 565
hepatitis B, 565-566
for HIV/AIDS children,
220
measles, mumps,
rubella, 565
poliomyelitis, 565
reactions to, 566-567
recommended ages/
screening for, 564*t*
varicella, 566
Immunosuppressants
glomerulonephritis and,
170
ITP and, 243
Immunotherapy
for aplastic anemia, 11
for neuroblastoma, 343
Imperforate anus,
247-252
diagnosis of, 248-250
discharge/home care of,
252
incidence of, 248
interventions for,
250-252

Imperforate anus—cont'd
nursing assessments of,
250
pathophysiology of,
247, 248*t*
surgery and, 249-252
Inactivated poliovirus
(IPV) immunizations,
for HIV/AIDS
children, 220
Indomethacin (Indocin), for
juvenile rheumatoid
arthritis, 275
Infants; *see also* Neonates;
Preterm infants
growth/development
in, 538-546
cognitive, 541-544
faith, 546
fine motor, 539-540
gross motor, 539
language, 544-545
moral, 546
physical, 538-539
psychosexual, 545
psychosocial, 545-546
reflexes, 542*t*-543*t*
sensory, 540-541
socialization, 545-546
height/weight growth
curves in, 588-589,
592-593
incidence in
of bronchiolitis, 36
of cellulitis, 62
of CHF, 94
of coarctation of the
aorta, 81
of congenital hip
dislocation, 88-89
of croup, 98

Infants—cont'd
  incidence in—cont'd
    of cystic fibrosis, 104
    of cytomegaloviral
        infection, 111
    of foreign body
        aspiration, 144
    of gastroenteritis, 161
    of hemolytic-uremic
        syndrome, 173-174
    of hernia, 194
    of HIV/AIDS, 213
    of hydrocephalus,
        225-226
    of hypertrophic
        pyloric stenosis,
        236
    of iron deficiency
        anemia, 266
    of ITP, 241-242
    of juvenile
        rheumatoid
        arthritis, 271
    of Kawasaki disease,
        281-282
    of lead poisoning, 290
    of meningitis, 318
    of mental retardation,
        325
    of neuroblastoma, 341
    of otis media, 371
    of patent ductus
        arteriosus, 376
    of pneumonia, 383
    of RDS, 414-415
    of renal failure, 393
    of respiratory
        syncytial virus,
        420-422
    of Reye's syndrome,
        424

Infants—cont'd
  incidence in—cont'd
    of spina bifida, 468
    of tetralogy of fallot,
        481
  management of
    AIDS/HIV, 212-224
    apparent
        life-threatening
        event, 15-18
    bronchopulmonary
        dysplasia, 41-46
    child abuse, 67-72
    cleft lip/palate, 73-78
    croup, 98-102
    gastroesophageal
        reflux, 164-167
    Hirschsprung's
        disease, 199
    hypertrophic pyloric
        stenosis, 236-240
    imperforate anus,
        247-250
    meningitis, 317-322
    neuroblastoma,
        341-345
    pain, 599, 608t
    respiratory syncytial
        virus, 420-422
    shaken infant
        syndrome, 70
    spina bifida, 467-473
    tetralogy of fallot,
        480-490
  SIDS and, 474-478
Inflammatory bowel
    disease, 254-264
  diagnosis of, 255-257, 259
  discharge/home care of,
        263-264
  incidence of, 255

Inflammatory bowel
disease—cont'd
interventions for, 260-263
management of, 257-259
nursing assessments of,
259
pathophysiology of,
254-255
surgery for, 258-259,
261-263
Inhalers
for asthma, 27
for foreign body
aspiration, 145
Injuries, documented
child abuse, 68
Insulin-dependent
diabetes mellitus; see
Diabetes mellitus,
insulin-dependent
type I
Intermittent positive
pressure breathing, for
cystic fibrosis, 106
Intracranial hypertension,
near drowning and,
134
Intracranial pressure
monitoring (ICP),
522-523
interventions and,
522-523
nursing assessments
and, 522
Intravenous gamma
globulin (IVGG), for
Kawasaki disease, 284
Intravenous
hyperalimentation,
for inflammatory
bowel disease, 257

Intravenous immune
globulin (IVIG), for
ITP, 243
Intravenous pyelograms
(IVP), 524-525
interventions and, 525
nursing assessments
and, 524-525
Ipecac syrup, for
poisoning, 391
Iron deficiency anemia; see
Anemia, iron
deficiency
Isoproterenol (Isuprel),
ventricular septal
defect, 498
ITP; see Idiopathic
thrombocytopenic
purpura (ITP)
IVGG; see Intravenous
gamma globulin
(IVGG)
IVP; see Intravenous
pyelograms (IVP)

J
Japanese, Kawasaki
disease and, 281-282
Juvenile rheumatoid
arthritis (JRA),
270-280
diagnosis of, 271-275,
277
discharge/home care of,
279-280
incidence of, 271
interventions for,
277-279
management of,
273-274, 275, 276t,
277

Juvenile rheumatoid arthritis (JRA)—cont'd
    nursing assessments of, 277
    pathophysiology of, 270-271

K

Kawasaki disease, 281-287
    diagnosis of, 282-284
    discharge/home care of, 287
    incidence of, 281-282
    interventions for, 284-287
    management of, 284
    nursing assessments of, 284
    pathophysiology of, 281

L

Laboratory values, 570-577
Lasix, for near drowning, 134
Latinos, SIDS in, 476
Law, compliance with; *see* Legal compliance
Laxatives, bulimia nervosa and, 47
Lead poisoning, 289-298
    diagnosis of, 290-291, 296
    discharge/home care of, 297-298
    incidence of, 290
    interventions for, 296-297
    management of, 292, 293t-295t

Lead poisoning—cont'd
    nursing assessments of, 296
    pathophysiology of, 289-290
Legal compliance, child abuse and, 68, 71
Leukemia, 299-316
    diagnosis of, 300-302, 307
    discharge/home care of, 316
    incidence of, 300
    interventions for, 314-316
    management of, 302-307, 308t-314t
    nursing assessments of, 307
    pathophysiology of, 299
Lung transplants, cystic fibrosis and, 106-107

M

Magnetic resonance imaging (MRI), 526-527
    interventions and, 527
    nursing assessments and, 527
Males, incidence in
    of acute rheumatic fever, 430
    of ADHD, 33
    of anorexia nervosa, 4
    of aplastic anemia, 10
    of appendicitis, 20
    of bulimia nervosa, 47
    of cellulitis, 62
    of cleft lip, 73
    of croup, 98

Males, incidence
in—cont'd
of drowning, 132
of glomerulonephritis,
168-169
of hemophilia, 184
of hernia, 194
of HIV/AIDS, 213
of Hodgkin's disease, 205
of hypertension,
232-233
of IDDM, 116-117
of Kawasaki disease,
281-282
of leukemia, 300
of meningitis, 318
of mental retardation,
325
of muscular dystrophy,
330
of nephrotic syndrome,
335
of nonaccidental
trauma, 347
of non-Hodgkin's
lymphoma, 352
of osteomyelitis, 366
of RDS, 414-415
Malnutrition,
hypertrophic pyloric
stenosis and, 236
Mannitol
for near drowning, 134
for Reye's syndrome,
427
MAO inhibitors; see
Monoamine oxidase
(MAO) inhibitors
Measles, mumps, rubella
(MMR)
immunizations, 565

Measles, mumps, rubella
(MMR) immuniza-
tions—cont'd
contraindications and, 567
reactions and, 567
Measurements, nursing
assessments and,
532-533
Mechanical supports, for
muscular dystrophy,
331
Mechlorethamine, for
Hodgkin's disease, 207
Medical records, of child
abuse, 68, 71
Meningitis, 317-322
diagnosis of, 318-320
discharge/home care of,
322
incidence of, 318
interventions for,
321-322
management of, 320
nursing assessments of,
320
pathophysiology of,
317-318
Mental retardation, 323-327
diagnosis of, 324-326
discharge/home care of,
327
incidence of, 325
interventions for, 327
management of, 326
nursing assessments of,
326
pathophysiology of,
323, 324
Mercaptopurine, for
leukemia, 302,
304-305

Metaiodobenzylguanidine (MIBG), for neuroblastoma, 343
Methotrexate
  for juvenile rheumatoid arthritis, 275, 277
  for leukemia, 304
  for non-Hodgkin's lymphoma, 354
Methylphenidate (Ritalin), for ADHD, 34
Metoclopramide, for gastroesophageal reflux, 165
Milwaukee braces, for scoliosis, 437
MMR; see Measles, mumps, rubella (MMR) immunizations
Monoamine oxidase (MAO) inhibitors, for bulimia nervosa, 50
MOPP drug regimen, for Hodgkin's disease, 207
Morphine, for tetralogy of fallot, 483
MRI; see Magnetic resonance imaging (MRI)
Mucolytics, for cystic fibrosis, 106
Mucosal edema, asthma and, 27
Muscular dystrophy, 329-333
  diagnosis of, 330-331
  discharge/home care of, 332
  incidence of, 330

Muscular dystrophy—cont'd
  interventions for, 332
  management of, 331
  nursing assessments of, 331
  pathophysiology of, 329
Musculoskeletal systems, nursing assessments in, 536-537

N
Naproxen (Naprosyn), for juvenile rheumatoid arthritis, 275
Narcotics
  for burns, 56
  for inflammatory bowel disease, 257
Native Americans, incidence in
  of congenital hip dislocation, 88
  of SIDS, 476
Near drowning; see Drowning/Near drowning
Near-miss sudden infant death syndrome; see Apparent life-threatening event (ALTE)
Neglect, child abuse and, 71
Neonates; see also Infants; Preterm Infants
  incidence in
  of congenital hip dislocation, 89
  of Hirschsprung's disease, 199

Neonates—cont'd
management of
bronchopulmonary
dysplasia, 41
cleft lip/palate, 73-78
imperforate anus,
247-250
pain, 599, 608*t*
sickle cell anemia,
461, 463
Nephrectomy, for Wilms'
tumor, 505
Nephrotic syndrome, 334-340
diagnosis of, 336-338
discharge/home care of,
340
incidence of, 335
interventions for,
338-340
management of, 337
nursing assessments of,
338
pathophysiology of,
334-335
Neuroblastoma, 341-345
diagnosis of, 342-344
discharge/home care of,
345
incidence of, 341
interventions for, 344
management of, 343,
344-345
nursing assessments of,
344
pathophysiology of, 341
surgery and, 344
Neurology
muscular dystrophy
and, 331
nursing assessments in,
533-534

New Jersey, HIV/AIDS in,
213
New York, HIV/AIDS in,
213
Nomograms, West,
585-586
Nonaccidental trauma,
347-349
diagnosis of, 348
discharge/home care of,
349
incidence of, 347
interventions for, 349
management of, 348
nursing assessments of,
348
Non-Hodgkin's
lymphoma, 350-356
diagnosis of, 352-353
discharge/home care of,
356
incidence of, 352
interventions for, 355-356
management of,
353-354
nursing assessments of,
354
pathophysiology of,
351-352
Nonsteroidal
antiinflammatory
agents (NSAIDs), for
juvenile rheumatoid
arthritis, 275
Nursing assessments, 510,
532-537; *see also*
specific disorders
endocrine, 537
gastrointestinal, 534-535
Glasgow coma scale,
535

Nursing assessments—
  cont'd
  hematologic, 537
  measurements, 532-533
  musculoskeletal,
    536-537
  neurologic, 533-534
  renal, 535-536
  respiratory, 533
Nursing interventions,
  510-511; see also
  specific disorders
Nutrition; see Diet
Nystatin, for renal
  transplants, 411

O

Obsessive-compulsive
  behaviors, in anorexia
  nervosa, 6
Occupational therapy
  for juvenile rheumatoid
    arthritis, 275
  for muscular dystrophy,
    331
Oncovin (vincristine), for
  Hodgkin's disease,
    207
Oral injuries, in child
  abuse, 69
Oral poliovirus (OPV)
  immunizations,
  HIV/AIDS children
  and, 220
Orogastric lavage, for
  poisoning, 391
Orthopedics, muscular
  dystrophy and, 331
Orthoplast jackets, for
  scoliosis, 437
Ortolani's maneuver, 89

Osteogenic sarcoma,
  358-364
  diagnosis of, 359, 361
  discharge/home care of,
    363-364
  incidence of, 358
  interventions for, 361-363
  management of,
    359-360
  nursing assessments of,
    360-361
  pathophysiology of, 358
  surgery and, 359-360,
    361-363
Osteomyelitis, 365-369
  diagnosis of, 366-367
  discharge/home care of,
    369
  incidence of, 366
  interventions for,
    367-369
  management of, 367
  nursing assessments of,
    367
  pathophysiology of,
    365-366
Otis media, 370-374
  diagnosis of, 371-372,
    373
  discharge/home care of,
    374
  incidence of, 371
  interventions for,
    373-374
  management of, 372
  nursing assessments of,
    373
  surgery and, 374
Oxygen
  for asthma, 27
  for bronchiolitis, 37

Oxygen—cont'd
  for bronchopulmonary
      dysplasia, 43
  for burns, 56
  for croup, 100
  for near drowning, 134
  for pneumonia, 387
  for RDS, 416

P

Pain management,
    596-609
  for adolescents, 601
  assessments in, 597-599,
      598*t*
  epidural, 605-606
  facial pain scale and,
      600
  for neonates/infants,
      599
  nonpharmacologic,
      608*t*-609*t*
  patient-controlled, 605
  pharmacologic, 601,
      602*t*-604*t*, 605-606
  for preschoolers, 599
  procedural, 606-607
  for school-age children,
      601
  for toddlers, 599
Pancreatic enzymes, for
    cystic fibrosis, 106
Parent counseling
  for child abuse, 71-72
  for SIDS, 478
Parent education
  in ADHD, 34
  in bulimia nervosa, 50
  in cystic fibrosis, 106
Paroxetine, for anorexia
    nervosa, 6

Patent ductus arteriosus
    (PDA), 375-382
  diagnosis of, 376-377
  discharge/home care of,
      381-382
  incidence of, 376
  interventions for,
      379-381
  management of,
      377-379
  nursing assessments of,
      372
  pathophysiology of, 375
  surgery and, 380-381
Patient history, child
    abuse and, 68
Patient-controlled pain
    management, 605
PDA; *see* Patent ductus
    arteriosus (PDA)
Pedialyte, for
    gastroenteritis, 161
D-penicillamine, for lead
    poisoning, 292
Pentamidine, for
    HIV/AIDS
    pneumonia, 218
Perineal anoplasty,
    249-252
Peritoneal dialysis,
    528-530
  interventions and,
      529-530
  nursing assessments
      and, 529
Persantine, for Kawasaki
    disease, 284
Phenobarbital, for seizure
    disorders, 448
Phenytoin (Dilantin), for
    seizure disorders, 448

Physical examinations,
child abuse and, 68
Physical therapy
for juvenile rheumatoid
arthritis, 275
for muscular dystrophy,
331
Plasma
for disseminated
intravascular
coagulation, 127
for hemophilia, 182
Platelets, for disseminated
intravascular
coagulation, 127
Pneumonia, 383-388
diagnosis of, 384-387
discharge/home care of,
388
incidence of, 383, 385
interventions for, 387-388
management of, 387
nursing assessments of,
387
pathophysiology of,
383-388
Poisoning, 390-392
diagnosis of, 390-392
discharge/home care of,
392
incidence of, 390
interventions for, 392
lead; see Lead poisoning
management of, 391
nursing assessments of,
391
Poliovirus (OPV),
immunizations for,
565
HIV/AIDS children
and, 220

Posterior spinal fusion, for
scoliosis, 438
Prednisone
for Hodgkin's disease,
208
for leukemia, 302, 303
for nephrotic syndrome,
337
for non-Hodgkin's
lymphoma,
353-354
Preschoolers
growth/development
in, 550-555
cognitive, 551-552
faith, 555
fine motor, 551
gross motor, 550-551
language, 552-553
moral, 555
physical, 550
psychosexual,
553-554
psychosocial, 554
sensory, 551
socialization, 554
pain management in,
599, 608t-609t
Preterm infants; see also
Infants; Neonates
incidence in
of cytomegaloviral
infection, 111
of hernia, 194
of patent ductus
arteriosus, 376
of respiratory distress
syndrome, 414-415
of respiratory
syncytial virus,
420-422

Preterm infants—cont'd
management of
apparent
life-threatening
event, 15
cytomegaloviral
infection
treatment, 113
RDS, 415
Primidone, for seizure
disorders, 448
Procarbazine (Matulane),
for Hodgkin's
disease, 207
Propranolol (Inderal)
for coarctation of the
aorta, 83
for tetralogy of fallot, 483
Protein, cystic fibrosis
and, 106
Psychopharmacologic
treatment
for anorexia nervosa, 6
for bulimia nervosa, 50
Psychosocial interven-
tions, 610-613
for supportive care,
612-613
for surgical procedures,
610-612
Psychostimulants, for
ADHD, 34
Psychotherapy
for anorexia nervosa, 6
for bulimia nervosa, 50
Purging behaviors
in anorexia nervosa, 2
in bulimia nervosa, 47
Pyloromyotomy, for
hypertrophic pyloric
stenosis, 237

R
Radiation therapy
for neuroblastoma,
343
for Wilms' tumor, 505
RDS; *see* Respiratory
distress syndrome
(RDS)
Red blood cells (RBC), for
disseminated
intravascular
coagulation, 127
Renal failure
acute, 393-408
diagnosis of,
395-396
discharge/home care
of, 399
incidence of, 393
interventions for,
398-399
management of,
396-397
nursing assessments
of, 397
pathophysiology of,
393-394
chronic, 401-408
diagnosis of, 402-404,
406
discharge/home care
of, 407
incidence of, 402
interventions for,
406-407
management of,
404-405
nursing assessments
of, 405-406
pathophysiology of,
401-402

Renal systems, nursing assessments in, 535-536
Renal transplants, 409-419
 diagnosis of, 410-411
 discharge/home care of, 413
 incidence of, 409-410
 interventions for, 412
 management of, 410, 411
 nursing assessments of, 411
 pathophysiology of, 409
 surgery and, 410-412
Reserpine, for coarctation of the aorta, 83
Respiratory distress syndrome (RDS), 414-419
 diagnosis of, 415-416, 418
 discharge/home care of, 419
 incidence of, 414-415
 interventions for, 418-419
 management of, 416-417
 nursing assessments of, 417
 pathophysiology of, 414
Respiratory syncytial virus, 420-422
Respiratory systems, nursing assessments in, 533
Retardation, mental; see Mental retardation
Reye's syndrome, 423-429
 diagnosis of, 424-425, 427

Reye's syndrome—cont'd
 discharge/home care of, 429
 incidence of, 424
 interventions for, 427-429
 management of, 425-427, 426t
 nursing assessments of, 427
 pathophysiology of, 423-424
Rheumatic fever, acute, 430-435
 diagnosis of, 431-432, 433
 discharge/home care of, 434-435
 incidence of, 430-431
 interventions for, 433-434
 management of, 433
 nursing assessments of, 433
 pathophysiology of, 430
Ribavirin, for bronchiolitis, 37
Ricelyte, for gastroenteritis, 161
Ringer's solution, for gastroenteritis, 161

S
Salter-Harris fracture classification, 149
SBS; see Short bowel syndrome (SBS)
School-age children growth/development in, 555-558

School-age children—cont'd
  growth/development
      in—cont'd
    cognitive, 556
    faith, 558
    fine motor, 555
    gross motor, 555-556
    language, 556-557
    moral, 558
    physical, 555
    psychosexual, 557
    psychosocial, 557-558
  pain management in,
      601, 609t
Scoliosis, 436-441
  diagnosis of, 437, 438
  discharge/home care of,
      440
  incidence of, 436-437
  interventions for, 438-440
  management of, 437
  nursing assessments of,
      438
  pathophysiology of, 436
  surgery and, 438-440
Secondary drowning; see
      Drowning/near
      drowning
Sedatives
  for near drowning, 134
  for Reye's syndrome, 427
Seizure disorders, 443-450
  diagnosis of, 444-447, 448
  discharge/home care of,
      449-450
  incidence of, 443
  interventions for, 448-449
  management of, 447-448
  nursing assessments of,
      448
  pathophysiology of, 443

Seizures, ALTE and, 15
Sepsis, ALTE and, 15
Sertaline, for anorexia
      nervosa, 6
Serum glucose, for IDDM,
      120
Sexual abuse
  assessment of, 71-72
  defined, 70
  incidence of, 67-68
Shaken infant syndrome,
      defined, 70
Shock, gastroenteritis and,
      161
Short bowel syndrome
      (SBS), 451-459
  diagnosis of, 453-454,
      457
  discharge/home care of,
      459
  interventions for, 458-459
  management of, 454-455
  nursing assessments of,
      457
  pathophysiology of,
      451-453
  surgery for, 456-457
Sickle cell anemia,
      460-466
  diagnosis of, 461-463,
      464
  discharge/home care of,
      465-466
  incidence of, 461
  interventions for,
      464-465
  management of, 463
  nursing assessments of,
      463-464
  pathophysiology of,
      460-461

Single parents, sexual abuse and, 67-68

Skin injuries, in child abuse, 69

Smoking (passive), otis media and, 371

Social services, for child abuse, 71-72

Socioeconomic groups, incidence in
of acute rheumatic fever, 430
of bulimia, 47
of child abuse, 67-68
of cytomegaloviral infection, 111
of hypertension, 232-233
of mental retardation, 325
of nonaccidental trauma, 347

Sodium bicarbonate, for tetralogy of fallot, 483

Sodium nitroprusside (Nipride), for coarctation of the aorta, 83

Solu-Cortef, for asthma, 27

Solu-Medrol, for asthma, 27

Speech, in cleft lip/palate, 74

Spina bifida, 467-473
diagnosis of, 468-469, 470
discharge/home care of, 472
incidence of, 468
interventions for, 470-471

Spina bifida—cont'd
nursing assessments of, 470
pathophysiology of, 467-468
surgical management of, 469-470, 470-471

Spinal fusion, for scoliosis, 438

Splenectomy, for ITP, 243

Spring season
bronchiolitis during, 36
hemolytic-uremic syndrome during, 173-174
ITP during, 241-242
Kawasaki disease during, 281-282
respiratory syncytial virus during, 420-422

Stepfamilies, sexual abuse incidence in, 67-68

Steroids, for renal transplant rejection, 411

Succimer, for lead poisoning, 292

Sudden infant death syndrome (SIDS), 474-478
apparent life-threatening event and, 15
care after, 477
client outcomes with, 478
diagnosis of, 476
follow-up after, 478
incidence of, 476

Sudden infant death
   syndrome (SIDS)—
   cont'd
 interventions for,
     476-477
 near-miss; *see* Apparent
     life-threatening
     event (ALTE)
 nursing assessments of,
     476
 pathophysiology of,
     474-476
 prevention of,
     476-477
 risk factors in, 475
Surgery
 appendectomy, 20-24
 for CHF, 95
 for cleft lip/palate,
     74-75
 for coarctation of the
     aorta, 82-83
 for cystic fibrosis, 106
 fundoplication, 165
 for gastroesophageal
     reflux, 165
 for hernia, 196-197
 for Hirschsprung's
     disease, 199-200
 for hydrocephalus,
     227-229
 for hypertrophic pyloric
     stenosis, 237
 for imperforate anus,
     249-252
 for inflammatory bowel
     disease, 258-259
 for ITP, 243
 for neuroblastoma, 343
 for nonaccidental
     trauma, 348

Surgery—cont'd
 for osteogenic sarcoma,
     359-360, 361-363
 perineal anoplasty,
     249-252
 psychosocial
     interventions for,
     610-612
 for renal transplants,
     410-412
 splenectomy, 243
 for ventricular septal
     defect, 498-499,
     500-501
 for Wilms' tumor, 505

T
Terbutaline, for asthma,
     27
Tetralogy of fallot, 480-490
 diagnosis of, 481-483,
     485
 discharge/home care of,
     490
 incidence of, 481
 interventions for,
     486-490
 management of, 483
 nursing assessments of,
     485
 pathophysiology of,
     480-481
 surgery for, 483-485,
     487-490
Theophylline
 for asthma, 27
 for RDS, 417
Thermal injuries, child
     abuse and, 70
Thoracotomy, for foreign
     body aspiration, 145

Time of day, SIDS and, 476
Toddlers
  growth/development in, 546-550
    faith, 550
    fine motor, 548-549
    gross motor, 547-548
    language, 549-550
    moral, 550
    physical, 546-547
    psychosexual, 549
    psychosocial, 549-550
  incidence in
    of cellulitis, 62
    of congenital hip dislocation, 87, 88
    of croup, 98-102
    of foreign body aspiration, 144
    of hemolytic-uremic syndrome, 173-174
    of ITP, 241-242
    of juvenile rheumatoid arthritis, 271
    of Kawasaki disease, 281-282
    of lead poisoning, 290
    of leukemia, 300
    of meningitis, 318
    of pneumonia, 383
    of poisoning, 390
    of respiratory syncytial virus, 420-422
    of urinary tract infections, 492-493

Toddlers—cont'd
  incidence in—cont'd
    of Wilms' tumor, 504
  pain management in, 599, 608t
Tolmetin (Tolectin), for juvenile rheumatoid arthritis, 275
Tracheostomy, for epiglottitis, 139
Traction, for fractures, 151
Transplants
  bone marrow
    for leukemia, 300
    for neuroblastoma, 343
  heart, for cystic fibrosis, 106-107
Traumatic hair loss, in child abuse, 69
Trendelenburg test, 89
Trimethoprim-sulfamethoxazole (Septra, Bactrim), for HIV/AIDS, 218
Tropical countries, hepatitis in, 188
Tuberculin skin test, 566

U
Ulcerative colitis, 256-257
United States, HIV/AIDS in, 213
Upper airway obstruction, in ALTE, 15
Urinary tract infections (UTI), 492-495
  diagnosis of, 493-494, 494-495
  discharge/home care of, 495
  incidence of, 492-493

Urinary tract infections
(UTI)—cont'd
interventions for, 495
management of, 494
nursing assessments of,
494
pathophysiology of, 492
UTI; *see* Urinary tract
infections (UTI)

V
Varicella, immunizations
and, 566
Vasodilators
for CHF, 95
ventricular septal
defect, 497
Vecuronium
for near drowning, 134
for Reye's syndrome,
427
Ventilation, for near
drowning, 134
Ventricular septal defect
(VSD), 496-502
diagnosis of, 497-498,
499-500
discharge/home care of,
501
incidence of, 497
interventions for,
500-501
nursing assessments of,
499
pathophysiology of,
496-497
surgery for, 498-499,
500-501
Videx, for HIV/AIDS, 218
Vinblastine, for Hodgkin's
disease, 208

Vincristine
for Hodgkin's disease,
207
for ITP, 243
for leukemia, 302, 303
for non-Hodgkin's
lymphoma, 353-354
for Wilms' tumor, 505
Vitamin K
for cystic fibrosis, 106
for Reye's syndrome, 427
Vitamins, for cystic
fibrosis, 106
Vomiting, bulimia nervosa
and, 2, 47
VSD; *see* Ventricular septal
defect (VSD)

W
Weight
anorexia nervosa and, 6
control for
hypertension, 234
growth curves in,
588-595
females, 588-591
males, 592-595
West nomograms, 585-586
Wilms' tumor, 503-508
diagnosis of, 504-505,
505-506
discharge/home care of,
507-508
incidence of, 504
interventions for, 506-507
management of, 505
nursing assessments of,
505
pathophysiology of, 503
surgery for, 505,
506-507

Winter season
  bronchiolitis during, 36
  croup during, 98
  epiglottitis during, 138
  IDDM during, 116-117
  ITP during, 241-242
  Kawasaki disease
      during, 281-282
  respiratory syncytial
      virus during,
      420-422

Winter season—cont'd
  Reye's syndrome
      during, 424
  SIDS during, 476

Z
Zalcitabine, for
    HIV/AIDS, 218
Zidovudine
    (Azidothymidine), for
    HIV/AIDS, 218